Diabetes Education Goals

Stuart Brink, MD, Co-Chair
Linda Siminerio, RN, MS, CDE, Co-Chair
Deborah Hinnen-Hentzen, RN, MN, CDE
Larry C. Deeb, MD
Anne S. Daly, RD, MS, CDE
Barbara J. Anderson, PhD
Richard J. Agrin, MD

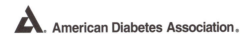

American Diabetes Association.

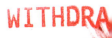

Chief Scientific and Medical Officer
Richard Kahn, PhD

Publisher
Susan H. Lau

Editorial Director
Peter Banks

Managing Editor
Christine B. Welch

Editor
Sherrye Landrum

Director of Production
Carolyn R. Segree

Diabetes Education Goals
p. cm. — (Practical approaches in diabetes care)
Includes bibliographical references
ISBN 0-945448-49-X
1. Diabetes—Study and teaching. I. American Diabetes Association
II. Series.
RC660.D4457 1995   95-10032
616.4'62'007—dc20   CIP

American Diabetes Association, Inc., 1660 Duke Street, Alexandria, VA 22314

CONTENTS

Diabetes Education Goals was first published as a manual of the American Diabetes Association in 1981 and was revised in 1986. As stated by Harold Rifkin, MD, in the second edition, "It is increasingly clear that the 'treatment of diabetes' is largely an educational process. Educational goals and objectives are critical elements in the management of diabetes and particularly in the prevention of acute and chronic complications." Treating diabetes is more than handing out a meal plan or prescribing insulin or an oral agent. Diabetes education requires a network of people following a prescribed process.

We recommend the team approach as the way to provide a comprehensive plan of care. This approach brings together diabetes health providers of all disciplines: physicians, nurses, dietitians, social workers and psychologists, exercise specialists, and other care providers as needed. The patient with his or her family, or supportive others, completes the diabetes-care team. For youngsters, teachers, camping staff, and peers also play important roles. Each member of the diabetes-care team brings expertise and provides support for the person with diabetes to improve his or her self-management skills, thereby leading to a healthy diabetes outcome.

The development of diabetes self-management skills relies heavily on the use of behavioral goals incorporated into the educational process. *Diabetes Education Goals* highlights the use of behavioral goals in an educational process that compliments the Diabetes Self-Management Standards. For this edition, we decided to group educational objectives into the three broad categories of insulin-dependent (type I) diabetes mellitus, non-insulin-dependent (type II) diabetes mellitus, and gestational diabetes. We also added sections on age-sensitive considerations for patients with type I and type II diabetes and numerous educational approaches for patients with special challenges to learning that will help make these *Diabetes Education Goals* practical.

We continue to distinguish between initial goals and continuing goals, believing that too much information provided to people with diabetes too early is just as frustrating as too little information later. All diabetes educators should be able to assess and promote patient readiness to learn and help set small, realistic goals whose achievement will strengthen further interest and success in diabetes self-management. The challenges we face include assessing initial needs and then mapping out a program to pro-

vide for these needs. After initial assessment, emphasis must be on providing an appropriate knowledge base and teaching ways to apply this
knowledge in a manner practical for the individual. This helps patients
move on to greater levels of understanding, self-care, and self-reliance.

We are convinced that educating the patient with diabetes (as well as
those around them) benefits not only the patient but also our society.
As medical care changes, more effort will be spent preventing rather than
treating a chronic illness like diabetes and its complications. *Diabetes
Education Goals* should prove valuable in enhancing professional skills
with this in mind.

Stuart Brink, MD, Co-Chair
Linda Siminerio, RN, MS, CDE, Co-Chair
Deborah Hinnen-Hentzen, RN, MN, CDE
Larry C. Deeb, MD
Anne S. Daly, RD, MS, CDE
Barbara J. Anderson, PhD
Richard J. Agrin, MD

HOW TO USE DIABETES EDUCATION GOALS

This book is designed to help diabetes educators assess and develop education goals for people with diabetes. This book emphasizes the belief that
education and counseling occur at different stages and are a continuous
process. Individual needs change as people adapt to the diagnosis of diabetes
and as they learn and refine self-management skills. As they acknowledge
the importance of making lifestyle changes and then incorporate these
changes into self-management skills, patients' needs change. Your job is to
assess and reassess these needs and to help your patients meet them. Assessing the patient's health status, knowledge, skills, attitudes, goals, and self-
care behaviors is necessary to formulate an educational plan and goals. The
educator needs to ask the following questions initially and at various times
during the educational process.

- ○ How old is the patient?
- ○ What is the patient's current state of health?
- ○ What are the patient's health goals, health beliefs, and attitudes?
- ○ How is the patient managing the diabetes, and who assists him or
  her?
- ○ How does the patient learn things most easily?
- ○ Can the patient read and process information correctly?
- ○ What are the patient's math skills? Can the patient tell time?
- ○ Is the patient able to think abstractly?
- ○ What are the patient's ongoing psychosocial restrictions, such as
  finances, concurrent medical or emotional problems, or existence
  or lack of a support system?

The educational objectives in this book are categorized by the 15
curriculum content areas recommended in the National Standards for Diabetes
Self-Management Education Programs developed by a consortium of leading
diabetes groups. You can use the 15 content areas with the initial and continuing educational objectives to design your program and develop your own
curriculum. (See National Standards for Diabetes Self-Management Education Programs and American Diabetes Association Recognition, page 51.)

INITIAL EDUCATION

Goals at diagnosis address basic needs. It is not realistic to expect the person
with diabetes and his or her family to assimilate and accept all there is to

know about diabetes immediately. The amount of new information they must process is enormous. In addition, diagnosis produces emotional turmoil, with anger, fear, guilt, depression, and frustration. For some, there is a severe metabolic disarray that must be accommodated. The crisis exists for the patient whether he or she is an inpatient or an outpatient when the diagnosis of diabetes is first made.

Initial education includes information and skills the person with diabetes needs to *begin* coping with the diagnosis of diabetes and its management. The educational objectives for this phase of training must be met before the patient and his or her significant others can move toward more in-depth, continuing education and counseling. Some people will not proceed past the initial level because of their own learning limitations or because appropriate education and counseling are not available to them. For some, initial education will be done at diagnosis, whereas, for others, initial education will be done over a period of weeks or months after diagnosis.

When diabetes has been present for some time but only some of the educational objectives have been satisfied, initial education may have to be combined with continuing education. For all patients, diabetes education must initially assess what they currently know and understand as well as their technical skills *vis-a-vis* these issues, and establish priorities for making progress in areas vital to promoting better diabetes self-management. The health-care team's open agreement with the patient about these goals helps to summarize this assessment and to establish an agenda by which the patient's progress can be measured.

ELEMENTS OF SUCCESSFUL EDUCATION

Initial Education

SETTING already shown as Goals...

GOALS

Educational objectives at the initial level provide the person and his or her family with the basic knowledge, skills, and new behaviors necessary to begin to participate in self-management of diabetes. In this book, these are given as a list of educational objectives that should be achieved by the completion of the initial education.

SETTING

At diagnosis, education begins immediately in a hospital or outpatient setting, i.e., clinic or office. Initial planning for this education requires a coordinated team effort by the physician, dietitian, nurse, and diabetes educators such as a mental health professional, i.e., social worker or psychologist, to help the patient make adjustments and accept the realities of diabetes. Although some teaching may be done in group settings at this time, most needs to be done on a one-to-one basis.

ASSESSMENT

The newly diagnosed person's awareness of diabetes and the needs of the person and his or her family must be assessed before the educator can plan what to teach and how to teach it to help the person master the self-management skills essential for survival. This assessment should include:

- ○ age(s), occupation(s)
- ○ likes, dislikes, fears
- ○ current lifestyle
- ○ evaluation of general health, attitudes about health, self-care behaviors
- ○ learning ability and style, willingness to learn,
- ○ acceptance of diabetes, current knowledge of diabetes,
- ○ skills needed, attitudes, goals,
- ○ ethnic background, language, and
- ○ home situation.

DOCUMENTATION

All information about the educational experience should be documented in the participant's permanent medical or educational record, so that different health-care professionals can share information. Documentation in the medical record includes information learned during the assessment process, a teaching plan with objectives to meet the identified needs, an evaluation of what was learned (outcomes), and a plan for follow-up education and counseling. The standards do not require a list of materials given and received, but this information may be helpful to all members of the health-care team.

Continuing Education and Counseling

The educational objectives in these sections focus on increasing the patient's knowledge, skills, and flexibility as he or she gains experience in living *well* with diabetes. These must be tailored to individual needs and learning ability. This phase begins with an in-depth assessment of current needs and leads to a formal or informal education program. This phase enriches the person's life by contributing to the flexibility, insight, and skills needed to make lifestyle changes to improve day-to-day glucose control, lipid abnormalities, and weight problems.

Patients cannot begin the in-depth process until initial educaiton has been provided. Educating patients who are ready to make the commitment to learn advanced concepts and to incorporate them into their daily life can be a major challenge. The increasing demands placed on this patient will be best supported by a team. However, some patients will not have experience being part of a team and will need to learn what each has to offer, how we interact, and how the education process functions.

Good self-management means the patient can be independent and participate safely in a wide variety of activities while maintaining diabetes control. Patients need to know what behavior changes, based on their understanding of medication, nutrition, and monitoring, can lead to increased flexibility and improvement in their metabolic control.

GOALS

Educational objectives at this level should provide patients with the skills and knowledge they need to manage their diabetes. Ultimately, the patient and his or her family will become self-sufficient in the daily management of diabetes. The educator's support helps patients make appropriate decisions and take actions to reach that goal.

SETTING

Continuing education usually takes place formally and informally over time through contact with several health-care professionals, including the physician, dietitian, nurse educator, mental health professional, exercise physiologist, pharmacist, podiatrist, and other consultants. This education, which can occur in group sessions or during one-on-one consultation, may take place in education centers, clinics, hospitals, or physicians' offices.

ASSESSMENT

Continuing education begins with an assessment of the patient's and the patient's family's current knowledge and skills. Have they acquired the knowledge and skills described in the sections on initial education? This assessment should include:

O age(s), occupation(s)
O likes, dislikes, fears
O current lifestyle
O evaluation of general health, attitudes about health, self-care behaviors
O learning ability and style, willingness to learn,
O acceptance of diabetes, current knowledge of diabetes,
O skills needed, attitudes, goals,
O ethnic background, language, and
O home situation.

To be effective the educational program content and the teaching approach must be based on this assessment. Continuing education must be individualized to both personal and family needs.

DOCUMENTATION

Documentation in the medical record includes assessment of the individual needs of the person and his or her family, a teaching plan with objectives to meet the identified needs, an evaluation or measure of what was learned (outcomes), and a plan for continued follow-up and review. The standards do not require a list of educational materials given and received, but this information may be helpful to you and other members of the health-care team.

ELEMENTS OF TEACHING AND LEARNING

Styles of Learning

Health education is defined as any combination of learning experiences designed to facilitate voluntary adaptation of behavior, or sustained behavior, conducive to health. Facilitating this adaptation of behavior involves a major process–the teaching-learning process. Teaching is a system of actions designed to bring about learning. The educator is responsible for initiating the teaching actions designed to bring about learning.

Learning is the change of behavior. Learning is an active, goal-directed process that involves transforming new knowledge, skills, and values into new behavior. To implement the teaching-learning process, health educators must recognize that people have different learning styles. In recognizing these differences, Gregorc proposed the concept of style-differentiated instruction that includes the four different learning styles below. This list is adapted from *Diabetes Youth Curriculum: A Toolbox for Educators.* (See Resources.)

Concrete sequential learners are hands-on learners and creators who prefer to work in a systematic orderly fashion. They thrive on detail and often are perfectionists. They want to be very efficient and become frustrated when goals cannot be accomplished readily. They prefer lots of preparation before trying to solve a problem and tend to make lists of things to do and create an order in which they should be done.

Abstract sequential learners are conceptual and analytical learners who prefer to work in a logical and systematic approach with ideas. They are thinkers, debaters, and intellectual critics. They are eager to learn and like to debate and challenge new concepts to help them understand these concepts. They may overintellectualize problems in an effort to control new situations and prefer to obtain several different sources of information on which their concepts can be based.

Abstract random learners are emotion-based learners and creators who prefer to focus on themes, ideas, people, and feeling through literature, media, music, and other forms of personal expression and art. They have strong emotional responses to new information and often jump from topic to topic in what appears to be random fashion. Nevertheless, they learn better in this way rather than when they are forced into a more logical, step-by-step approach. Time and deadlines are less important.

Concrete random learners are experimenters, investigators, and discovery learners who work best with minimal structure but often within certain guidelines. They are natural problem-solvers who thrive on change, diversity, and experience. They often take a leap of understanding rather than go methodically in a step-by-step fashion in creating answers and solving problems. Conventions of society are less important.

Assessing and appreciating a patient's learning style can facilitate a more productive learning experience. Using a mismatched or inappropriate teaching approach for a particular individual can frustrate the educator and the patient. As a result, much energy may be expended without the patient learning any of the material or coming any closer to attainment of a particular self-management goal.

Along with recognizing learning styles, health educators should also be familiar with educational theories and conceptual models. Conceptual models and theories are often used in health education to explain or predict an individual's learning and behavior. Diabetes educators have been encouraged to use these theoretical constructs because they serve as a framework to approach a comprehensive plan of care in behavioral outcomes, provide guidelines for teaching, and facilitate not only clinical practice but research.

Although there are many theoretical models, discussion here will be limited to the three models used frequently in diabetes education: the Health Belief Model, Locus of Control, and the Self-Efficacy model.

Health belief theorists use the Health Belief Model (HBM) as a framework for understanding patient adherence to diabetes care. HBM was developed in the 1950s to explain the widespread failure of people to participate in programs to prevent or detect disease. The HBM is based on value-expectancy theories of social psychology. It suggests that behaviors reflect a person's subjective interpretation of a situation, readiness to take action, and perception that the benefits outweigh the perceived "costs." The HBM in relation to diabetes suggests that the person's willingness to adhere to the management plan largely depends on accepting the seriousness of the condition and believing that the benefits of the health action taken outweigh the "costs."

Locus of control (LOC) is another theoretical construct of perceived control over behavior. Individuals are classified as having an internal locus of control or an external locus of control. People with an "internal" locus of control are said to believe their health is mostly determined by their own behavior. Those that believe their health is determined outside their realm of control (i.e., fate, chance, powerful others, or events) are considered to have an "external" locus of control.

Although studies report mixed findings on the relationship of diabetes-care adherence and "internal" vs. "external" locus of control, it is still helpful for diabetes educators to be cognizant of the patient's LOC orientation in planning educational strategies. For example, internally-oriented patients may need more choices and a greater emphasis on individual responsibility. Externally-oriented patients may need more emphasis on social support systems and the importance to the individual of compliance with the health providers' instruction. Because congruence between expectations and outcomes reinforces behavioral change, tailoring programs to the diabetic patient's LOC holds promise for improving control of diabetes.

Bandura's self-efficacy model has been proposed as a control concept underlying behavior and a framework for diabetes education. The Self-Efficacy Theory reports that a person's perception of his/her capabilities affects behavior, level of motivation, thought patterns, and emotional reactions in stressful situations. In other words, the more confident and capable the person feels about performing a set of behaviors, the more likely it is that the person will actually perform those behaviors.

There is evidence to suggest that self-efficacy is effective as an intervention for incorporating new behaviors into self-care regimens. Diabetes educators encourage patients to do as much for themselves as possible. The challenge is helping patients develop their own strategies for self-care. Since the effectiveness of diabetes management depends on self-care, the adoption of the self-efficacy model for diabetes care appears logical.

Theories, conceptual models, and understanding the teaching-learning process are important tools for the diabetes educator. The largest challenge, however, depends upon the educator's ability to communicate information, so that the patient can successfully self-manage his or her disease. To communicate effectively, the educator must comprehensively assess the patient's knowledge, motivation, developmental life stage, health beliefs, and attitudes. Increasingly, the responsibility for diabetes management is given back to the patients themselves. Improvements will be more likely to come from the educator's appreciation of individual needs. Using information from an assessment process will serve as a sound foundation for developing realistic individualistic goals in pursuit of healthy diabetes outcomes.

TYPE I DIABETES

Initial Education Goals

DIABETES OVERVIEW

○ Identify diabetes as a chronic metabolic disorder in which the body is unable to use food properly.

○ Describe what happens in the body when insulin is not available.

○ State that daily insulin injections, monitoring, and prescribed meal/exercise plans are necessary in the treatment of diabetes, and that pills do not work in type I diabetes.

○ State that oral diabetes medications do not contain insulin.

○ State the need to carry or wear diabetes identification.

○ Describe the difference between type I diabetes and type II diabetes.

○ State that diabetes is not contagious and the exact cause is unknown.

STRESS AND PSYCHOSOCIAL ADJUSTMENT

○ Verbalize that he or she has diabetes.

○ Verbalize and vent his or her feeling about diabetes.

○ Acknowledge peer pressure and identify family/friend resources.

○ State that there are normal feelings of denial, anger, and sadness that will become less intense as diabetes becomes more a part of everyday life.

○ Acknowledge that insulin injections, monitoring, and prescribed medication/exercise plans are necessary in the treatment of diabetes.

○ Acknowledge that discussing complications of diabetes may be scary.

○ State that stressful conditions may cause problems with blood glucose control.

○ Acknowledge that a mental health counselor may be able to help him or her prevent or cope with stress.

FAMILY INVOLVEMENT AND SOCIAL SUPPORT

○ Acknowledge diabetes to family members and close associates.

○ Involve at least one family member or support person in an educational session to learn how to give insulin, recognize and treat hypoglycemia including glucagon, and know emergency phone numbers.

NUTRITION

(See also Relationships Among Nutrition, Exercise, Medication, and Blood Glucose Levels)

○ State that dietary management is a critical component of diabetes management and control and often the most difficult to balance properly.

○ State the importance of eating meals and snacks at consistent times each day.

○ State that food is important in the control of blood glucose and lipid levels.

○ State calorie level if applicable and list the types and amounts of foods to be included in a meal plan.

○ State the importance of eating the same types and amounts of food at meals and snacks.

○ Describe how different foods affect blood glucose levels.

○ State that during periods of illness, modifications in food, (especially salty liquids) will be necessary and close contact with the health-care team will be needed.

EXERCISE AND ACTIVITY
(see also Relationships Among Nutrition, Exercise, Medication, and Blood Glucose Levels)

○ State that exercise is recommended for overall general health and for specific diabetes management.

○ State how exercise can affect blood glucose levels, i.e., usually lowers.

○ State the need for guidelines to adjust food for planned/unplanned activity.

○ State that hypoglycemia can result during or after exercise.

○ State the reason for carrying a high carbohydrate snack and list examples.

○ State the importance of keeping blood glucose records related to exercise, i.e., monitoring before, during, and after physical activity.

○ Identify situations when exercise is not appropriate, e.g., sick days or when ketonuric.

○ State the need to inform friends and/or others of the possibility of hypoglycemia related to exercise, with instructions on how to prevent, recognize, and treat it.

○ State the need to consult with the health-care team before beginning an exercise program.

MEDICATIONS
(See also Relationships Among Nutrition, Exercise, Medication, and Blood Glucose Levels)

○ State that insulin must be taken daily as prescribed, indicate at what times it must be taken, and state what to expect if insulin is omitted.

○ State what action insulin has on the blood glucose level.

○ State the type, brand, and amount of insulin to be taken.
○ State the time of onset, peak, and duration of the insulin prescribed.
○ Demonstrate how to draw up and/or mix the correct amount of insulin.
○ Demonstrate how to inject insulin correctly.
○ State where insulin is to be injected and what times.
○ Describe the type of insulin syringe he or she uses.
○ Describe the care and storage of insulin, needles, and syringes.
○ State the action of glucagon on the blood glucose level.
○ Describe the use and storage of glucagon and who has learned glucagon administration.
○ Describe the proper disposal of syringes and lancets.

MONITORING AND USE OF RESULTS
○ Describe the rationale for and methods of monitoring blood glucose levels.
○ Demonstrate how to perform blood glucose tests with appropriate testing material.
○ Demonstrate how to record the results of blood glucose tests.
○ Describe the proper disposal of lancets.
○ State the need to contact health-care providers if blood glucose tests are consistently higher or lower than the guidelines given.
○ Describe the rationale and method of monitoring urine ketones.
○ Demonstrate how to record urine ketone tests.
○ State the need to contact health-care providers if urine ketone tests are positive.

RELATIONSHIPS AMONG NUTRITION, EXERCISE, MEDICATION, AND BLOOD GLUCOSE LEVELS
○ State the relationship of food and meals to insulin, activity, and blood glucose levels.
○ Discuss timing of glucose monitoring.
○ Identify the best times to exercise.
○ State that additional food may be needed before, during, or after physical activity.
○ Describe the type and amount of food to use to prevent hypoglycemia during and after exercise.
○ Identify times for snacks.

Prevention, Detection, and Treatment of Acute Complications

- ○ List the possible causes of hypoglycemia.
- ○ State how to prevent hypoglycemia.
- ○ List the possible symptoms of hypoglycemia and define mild, moderate (need assistance), and severe (unconscious or convulsing) hypoglycemia.
- ○ State that hypoglycemia can occur without symptoms, especially nocturnal hypoglycemia.
- ○ State how to treat hypoglycemia.
- ○ State the importance of always carrying a concentrated, quickly absorbed source of carbohydrate.
- ○ State the need to wear and carry diabetes identification.
- ○ State that drinking alcohol is a risk factor for hypoglycemia.
- ○ List the possible causes of hyperglycemia.
- ○ State how to prevent hyperglycemia.
- ○ List the symptoms of hyperglycemia.
- ○ State how to treat hyperglycemia.
- ○ State when and how to contact health-care providers or emergency facilities in case of severe or persistent hypoglycemia or hyperglycemia.
- ○ State when to check for ketonuria and sick-day guidelines.
- ○ State the need for continuing insulin during illness.
- ○ State how and when to contact his or her health-care provider or emergency facility in case of illness.

Prevention, Detection, and Treatment of Chronic Complications

- ○ State that good glucose control lessens the chance of developing chronic complications.
- ○ State that attitude toward diabetes is related to long-term glucose control.
- ○ State that there may be serious chronic complications associated with diabetes and how long-term hypoglycemia, if uncorrected, increases the risk for these problems.
- ○ State that near-normal blood glucose control may prevent or delay chronic complications.
- ○ State that smoking is extremely dangerous for someone with diabetes.
- ○ State the need for an ophthalmologic examination at diagnosis and an annual dilated-pupil exam thereafter.

FOOT, SKIN, AND DENTAL CARE

○ State the need for daily foot inspection for adults or anyone with neuropathy and/or vascular insufficiency (but not kids).

○ State the need for good personal hygiene and skin care.

○ State the need for daily dental and mouth care.

BEHAVIOR-CHANGE STRATEGIES, GOAL SETTING, RISK-FACTOR REDUCTION, AND PROBLEM SOLVING

○ State that stress can affect glucose level.

○ List stress-reduction stategies.

BENEFITS, RISKS, AND MANAGEMENT OPTIONS FOR IMPROVING GLUCOSE CONTROL

○ State that following the diabetes-care plan will bring short-term and long-term benefits in terms of good health and quality of life.

○ List monitoring options needed (SMBG, glycohemoglobin, lipids, urine protein).

PRECONCEPTION CARE, PREGNANCY, AND GESTATIONAL DIABETES
(See Diabetes and Pregnancy, page 35.)

○ State the importance of preconception counseling and the use of birth control to prevent unplanned pregnancy.

○ State general guidelines for responsible sexual behavior and prevention of STDs.

○ State the blood glucose goals for pregnancy (which are lower than usual).

USE OF HEALTH-CARE SYSTEMS AND COMMUNITY RESOURCES

○ State that the responsibility for carrying out the diabetes-care plan belongs to the patient, but that resources and supports are *always* necessary.

○ State the need for a planned system of medical care, including follow-up and continuing education.

○ Name the members of the health-care team.

○ Describe when and how to obtain emergency medical care.

○ List telephone numbers to access help with daily problem-solving questions.

○ List expected schedule for follow-up medical appointments for the first year.

○ List the community resources available for diabetes care and education.

○ List the community resources available for help with other social and economic problems.

○ State how to connect with other people in the community who have diabetes.

Continuing Education and Counseling Goals

DIABETES OVERVIEW

○ List the causes of diabetes.

○ State that diabetes is a disorder of the metabolism not only of carbohydrates, but also of protein, and fat because of reduced insulin action.

○ Distinguish between the two types of diabetes (i.e., type I and type II).

○ Describe the characteristic symptoms of uncontrolled diabetes.

○ State how the diagnosis of diabetes is established.

○ State the importance of good diabetes control, and list the factors that influence it.

○ Describe the action of insulin in the body and the effects of insulin deficiency.

STRESS AND PSYCHOSOCIAL ADJUSTMENT

○ State that it is unrealistic to expect near-normal blood glucose levels all the time.

○ State the pros and cons of acknowledging diabetes to family, peers, and colleagues.

○ List the people who definitely need to be informed that one has diabetes.

○ State his or her position as the most important member of the health-care team.

○ State that diabetes requires a change in his or her lifestyle.

○ State that stress affects diabetes control in two ways: Stress affects blood glucose levels directly, and stress affects self-care patterns.

○ Describe situations that cause stress, identify your blood glucose response, and discuss several methods of stress management.

○ Acknowledge that a social worker or psychologist may help with handling stress.

FAMILY INVOLVEMENT AND SOCIAL SUPPORT

○ State that living with diabetes concerns all family members.

○ State that family members themselves may need extra support in learning to adjust to diabetes and to carry out diabetes care when needed.

○ State that family members may need extra support in adjusting to diabetes.

NUTRITION

○ Describe the role of meal planning in controlling blood glucose and lipid levels and in maintaining normal growth, weight, and general health.

14

○ Demonstrate how to plan meals to enhance flexibility in the meal plan.

○ State the importance of maintaining a reasonable body weight.

○ List types of nutrients, their effect on blood glucose and lipid levels, and their relationship to insulin.

○ Discuss antioxidants and their potential benefits for preventing or delaying complications.

○ State the calorie level and list the types and amounts of foods to be included in the meal plan.

○ Explain the importance of reducing total fat as well as saturated fat and cholesterol in the meal plan.

○ List cooking and meal-planning strategies to limit dietary fat and increase carbohydrates.

○ Explain the role of dietary fiber in treating or preventing gastrointestinal disorders.

○ List food sources of dietary fiber and strategies for adding fiber to the meal plan.

○ State the relationship of salt (sodium) to hypertension and ways to decrease sodium intake, if necessary.

○ Demonstrate correct portion sizes for the meal plan using a food scale and measuring cups and spoons.

○ Demonstrate how to select foods when eating out—e.g., restaurants, fast foods, school lunches, pizza—according to the meal plan.

○ Describe appropriate menus for special occasions—e.g., birthdays, holidays, traveling, entertaining—to suit the meal plan.

○ Demonstrate how to evaluate food products using the nutrition facts panel on the food label.

○ Define terms such as dietetic, free foods, sugar free, calorie free, low calorie, fat free, and reduced calorie, and identify examples of such products that might be appropriate for the meal plan.

○ List caloric and noncaloric sweeteners and foods that contain them, and describe how they might be used in the meal plan.

○ State the effects of alcohol on blood glucose levels and precautions to follow, if used.

○ State how to incorporate appropriate favorite recipes into the meal plan.

EXERCISE AND ACTIVITY

○ List the specific benefits and risks of exercise, especially that of delayed hypoglycemia.

○ State the need for regular aerobic exercise, and list examples.

- Distinguish between aerobic and nonaerobic exercise.
- Demonstrate how to monitor intensity of exercise, i.e., heart rate.
- State target heart rate zone during aerobic exercise for age.
- List the three stages of appropriate exercise program, i.e., warm up, aerobic, and cool down.
- State the importance of keeping blood glucose records related to exercise, i.e., monitoring before, during, and after exercise.
- List types of physical activity that the patient agrees to utilize.
- Discuss planning exercise into schedule.
- Describe proper shoes and clothing for exercise.
- State the need for ongoing evaluation of and guidance for the exercise plan.
- Describe precautions when chronic complications are present.
- State why and how to avoid dehydration.
- State the reason for carrying a high-carbohydrate source while exercising, and list examples.
- State that hypoglycemia may occur up to 12–24 hours after activity and exercise.
- State the benefit of exercising with a companion.

MEDICATIONS
- Describe the different sources of insulin, i.e., animal and human.
- Distinguish between the different types of insulin and brands available.
- Describe the rationale for the time of insulin injection.
- Describe the rationale for and method of rotation of insulin-injection sites.
- Define lipohypertrophy, and describe how to prevent this problem.
- Define lipoatrophy, and describe how to treat this problem.
- List the possible influences of other medications on insulin action.
- Discuss the reuse of disposable insulin syringes: techniques, benefits, and risks.
- Describe methods for storing and adjusting insulin during travel and how to ensure insulin that is delivered by mail is not spoiled.
- State the various methods of insulin delivery and administration, i.e., pumps and injection devices.
- Describe intensive insulin therapy, i.e., multiple daily injections and pumps.

MONITORING AND USE OF RESULTS

○ State the target blood glucose ranges determined with the diabetes-care provider.

○ Demonstrate how to use monitoring information to problem solve.

○ Describe how to use blood glucose monitoring results, including written records, to adjust the treatment plan based on approved guidelines.

○ Describe visual vs. meter methods of monitoring blood glucose.

○ State the purpose of testing for glycated hemoglobin or other glycated proteins.

○ State how glycated hemoglobin results relate to the overall management plan.

○ State the relationship between glycated hemoglobin results and daily blood glucose values.

○ Establish individual glycated hemoglobin goals.

○ Demonstrate the steps for glucose-meter quality assurance.

○ Discuss the use of computers for blood glucose data management.

RELATIONSHIPS AMONG NUTRITION, EXERCISE, MEDICATION, AND BLOOD GLUCOSE LEVELS

○ Demonstrate how to make adjustments in the insulin dosage according to guidelines provided by the health-care team.

○ State that the insulin regimen is individualized according to the planned usual food intake, activity level, and blood glucose level testing results.

○ State the relationship of exercise to insulin activity, blood glucose levels, timing of exercise, timing of meals, and insulin-injection sites.

○ State the effect of exercise on insulin absorption.

○ State how to prevent hypoglycemia by adjusting food or insulin for planned and unplanned exercise and activity.

○ State the importance of keeping blood glucose records related to exercise, i.e., before, during, and after exercise.

○ Explain and demonstrate how to alter the meal pattern according to changes in his or her physical activity and subsequent blood glucose levels.

○ Describe appropriate foods and menus to use during physical activity.

○ Describe travel-related diabetes precautions.

○ Describe how intensive insulin therapy allows for flexibility with nutrition and exercise.

Prevention, Detection, and Treatment of Acute Complications

○ List individualized symptoms and appropriate treatment of hypoglycemia.

○ Demonstrate, with family or others, how to administer glucagon.

○ State the importance of informing close friends about hypoglycemic reactions and how they can recognize and treat them.

○ State the importance of reporting hypoglycemic episodes to health-care provider.

○ State the importance of carrying a high-carbohydrate source, and list examples.

○ Describe hypoglemia unawareness.

○ Describe the "Somogyi effect" (rebound hyperglycemia) and how to prevent it.

○ Describe the "dawn phenomenon" and how to treat it.

○ Distinguish between dawn phenomenon and Somogyi effect.

○ Describe the effect of counterregulatory hormones, e.g., glucagon, growth hormones, and catecholamines, on blood glucose levels.

○ State the need for checking ketones when blood glucose is elevated.

○ List the factors, including fasting, that may cause ketone production.

○ Define the relationship between hypoglycemia and ketosis.

○ Define ketoacidosis and its causes.

○ List the signs of ketoacidosis.

○ List ways to prevent and treat ketoacidosis.

○ State the need for more frequent blood glucose and ketone monitoring during illness.

○ State how concurrent illness may affect diabetes.

○ State that fluid intake may need to be increased during illness.

○ State the general rules of care during illness.

○ State that regular insulin adjustments during illness are based on blood glucose levels.

Prevention, Detection, and Treatment of Chronic Complications

○ Describe how improved metabolic control lessens the chance of developing chronic complications.

○ Identify the organ systems particularly at risk from diabetes.

○ List ways each system will be monitored.

○ State the need for reporting any visual disturbances to health-care providers.

- ○ State that diabetes can affect the eyes without any symptoms being apparent initially.
- ○ State the need for an annual eye exam with dilated pupils by an ophthalmologist.
- ○ State that regular blood pressure monitoring is necessary because of the frequency of blood pressure problems associated with diabetes.
- ○ State the need for control of high blood pressure.
- ○ Identify the major symptoms of and factors in prevention and treatment of:
  - ○ kidney disease
  - ○ cardiovascular disease
  - ○ peripheral vascular disease
  - ○ peripheral neuropathy
  - ○ autonomic neuropathy
  - ○ periodontal disease
- ○ State that diabetes may cause adult sexual dysfunction, and identify resources for help.
- ○ State the need for children and adolescents to have height and weight plotted against standards at least quarterly.

FOOT, SKIN, AND DENTAL CARE

- ○ Demonstrate how to inspect and bathe the feet and how to trim the nails.
- ○ Identify factors that may cause injury to the feet.
- ○ Describe the basic first-aid measures for minor injuries to the feet.
- ○ State the need for well-fitting shoes and socks and that special shoes and referral for fitting are available if appropriate.
- ○ State that podiatric services are available if there are special foot-care needs.
- ○ State the value of a foot exam at follow-up visits (removal of shoes and socks during visit).
- ○ State the need for early aggressive professional treatment of any foot problems that occur.
- ○ Describe the proper care of the skin according to age and individual requirements.
- ○ State the possible effects of diabetes on dental health.
- ○ State the value of regular visits to the dentist.
- ○ State when to communicate with the dentist about dental problems and care.

Behavior-Change Strategies, Goal Setting, Risk-Factor Reduction, and Problem Solving

○ List strategies to be considered for risk reduction and improved compliance.

○ List resources available.

○ Set priorities.

○ Include smoking cessation in smokers.

Benefits, Risks, and Management Options for Improving Glucose Control

○ Summarize DCCT results.

Preconception Care, Pregnancy, and Gestational Diabetes

(See Diabetes and Pregnancy, page 35.)

○ State the importance of preconception counseling and the use of birth control to prevent unplanned pregnancy.

○ State the need for tight blood glucose control **before** conception and **during** pregnancy for the best health outcomes of mother and baby.

○ State general guidelines for responsible sexual behavior and prevention of STDs.

○ State the need for urine ketone testing every morning.

Use of Health-Care Systems and Community Resources

○ List members of the health-care team and identify their responsibilities.

○ Name and know how to contact all members of the diabetes health-care team.

○ State his or her position as the most important member of the health-care team.

○ State the need for regular follow-up visits for medical care.

○ List periodic blood/urine tests to be done by health-care provider.

○ State the importance of nutrition education and counseling on a routine basis at least annually.

○ State the need for continuing diabetes education.

○ State when support groups and counseling are appropriate and how they can help.

○ State how to access competent diabetes medical care when traveling or living away from home.

20

○ List the resources available to help with special needs and concerns, such as finances, pregnancy, visual impairment, weight management, traveling, sports, school, child care, career, marriage, and senior citizen activities and networks.

○ List the resources available for long-term psychosocial support.

○ State how to connect with other people with diabetes in the patient's community and how to connect with diabetes organizations, e.g., American Diabetes Association, Juvenile Diabetes Foundation, International Diabetes Federation, American Association of Diabetes Educators. (See Resources.)

TYPE II DIABETES

Initial Education Goals

(For patients with type II diabetes who take insulin, refer to the corresponding type I diabetes section.)

DIABETES OVERVIEW

○ Identify diabetes as a chronic metabolic disorder in which the body is unable to use food properly.

○ Describe what happens in the body when insulin is not available or does not work properly.

○ State that prescribed meal/exercise plans and monitoring are the foundation of treatment of type II diabetes and that medication may be necessary.

○ Describe the difference between type I and type II diabetes.

○ State that oral hypoglycemic agents (or "pills") are not insulin.

STRESS AND PSYCHOSOCIAL ADJUSTMENT

○ Verbalize that he or she has diabetes.

○ Verbalize and vent his or her feelings about diabetes.

○ State that there are normal feelings of denial, anger, and sadness that will become less intense as diabetes becomes more a part of everyday life.

○ Acknowledge that daily medication (if used), monitoring, and pre-scribed meal/exercise plans are necessary in the treatment of diabetes.

○ Acknowledge that discussing complications of diabetes may be scary.

○ State that stressful conditions may cause problems with blood glucose control.

○ Acknowledge that a mental health counselor may be able to help him or her prevent or cope with stress.

FAMILY INVOLVEMENT AND SOCIAL SUPPORT

○ Acknowledge diabetes to family members and close associates.

○ Involve at least one family member or support person in an education session involving giving medication (if used), recognizing and treating hypoglycemia, and knowing emergency phone numbers.

NUTRITION

○ State that medical nutrition therapy and meal planning are essential components in the control of blood glucose and lipids.

○ List the goals of medical nutrition therapy, including the importance of reaching and maintaining reasonable body weight, controling blood glucose and lipids, and achieving good nutrition.

○ State the importance of eating meals and snacks at consistent times each day.

○ List the types and amounts of foods to be included in meals as indicated in the meal plan.

○ State that even a moderate weight loss can improve blood glucose levels.

EXERCISE AND ACTIVITY

○ State that exercise is recommended for health and diabetes management.

○ State that exercise can affect blood glucose levels, i.e., usually lowers.

○ State that hypoglycemia can result from exercise if medication is used.

○ State the reason for carrying a high carbohydrate snack and list examples.

○ State that physical activity on a regular basis is recommended to control blood glucose and related risk factors, i.e., hypertension and hyperlipidemia.

○ Describe role of physical activity on a regular basis to achieve and/or maintain desirable body weight.

○ State the need to consult with the health-care team before beginning an exercise program.

MEDICATIONS

○ State what action oral medication has on blood glucose level.

○ State the name of oral medication (if used), its correct dosage, and when it is to be taken.

○ List the possible side effects of oral medication.

○ State the possible interactions of oral medication with other medications taken.

○ State that insulin may be needed temporarily, e.g., with surgery or stressful illness, or in addition to oral medications, i.e., at bedtime.

○ State that some people with type II diabetes may require insulin.

○ State that insulin must be taken daily as prescribed and indicate at what times it must be taken.

○ State what action insulin has on the blood glucose level.

○ State the type, brand, and amount of insulin to be taken.

○ State the time of onset, peak, and duration of the insulin prescribed.

○ Demonstrate how to draw up and/or mix the correct amount of insulin.

○ Demonstrate how to inject insulin correctly.

- ◯ State where insulin is to be injected and at what times.
- ◯ Describe the type of insulin syringe he or she uses.
- ◯ Describe the care and storage of insulin, needles, and syringes.
- ◯ State the action of glucagon on the blood glucose level.
- ◯ Describe the use and storage of glucagon and who has learned glucagon administration.
- ◯ Describe the proper disposal of syringes and lancets.

MONITORING AND USE OF RESULTS

- ◯ Describe the rationale for and methods of monitoring blood glucose levels.
- ◯ Demonstrate how to perform blood glucose tests with appropriate testing material.
- ◯ Demonstrate how to record the results of blood glucose tests.
- ◯ Demonstrate the proper disposal of lancets.
- ◯ State when and how to contact the health-care provider if blood glucose tests are consistently higher or lower than guidelines given.
- ◯ Demonstrate the ability to perform and record urine ketone tests with appropriate testing material if the treatment plan calls for it.
- ◯ State the need to contact his or her health-care provider if urine ketone tests are positive.

RELATIONSHIPS AMONG NUTRITION, EXERCISE, MEDICATION, AND BLOOD GLUCOSE LEVELS

- ◯ State the relationship of food and meals to blood glucose levels, medication (if used), and activity.
- ◯ State that one should monitor blood glucose levels before, during, and after physical activity, if medication is used.
- ◯ State the best times to exercise.
- ◯ Describe the type and amount of food to use to prevent hypoglycemia during and after exercise.
- ◯ Identify times for snacks.

PREVENTION, DETECTION, AND TREATMENT OF ACUTE COMPLICATIONS

- ◯ List the possible causes of hypoglycemia and how to prevent them.
- ◯ List the symptoms of hypoglycemia (if treatment includes oral medication or insulin).
- ◯ State that hypoglycemia can occur without symptoms.
- ◯ State how to treat hypoglycemia.

○ State the need to carry and wear diabetes identification, if medication is used.

○ State the importance of carrying a concentrated, quickly absorbed source of carbohydrate.

○ List the possible causes of hyperglycemia and how to prevent them.

○ List the symptoms of hyperglycemia.

○ State how to treat hyperglycemia.

○ State the need for monitoring and reporting blood and urine tests during illness.

○ State how and what medications to take during illness.

○ State when and how to contact the health-care provider or emergency facilities in case of illness.

PREVENTION, DETECTION, AND TREATMENT
OF CHRONIC COMPLICATIONS

○ Acknowledge that there may be serious chronic complications associated with diabetes.

○ State that near-normal blood glucose control may prevent or delay chronic complications.

○ State that attitude toward diabetes is related to long-term glucose control.

○ State that smoking is very risky for someone with diabetes.

○ State the need for an ophthalmologic examination on diagnosis and an annual dilated pupil exam thereafter by an ophthalmologist.

FOOT, SKIN, AND DENTAL CARE

○ State the need for daily foot inspection and well-fitting shoes.

○ Demonstrate how to trim toenails safely.

○ State the need for good personal hygiene and skin care.

○ State the need for daily dental and mouth care.

BEHAVIOR-CHANGE STRATEGIES, GOAL SETTING, RISK-FACTOR
REDUCTION, AND PROBLEM SOLVING

○ List health-related behaviors that should be changed to reduce unnecessary risks.

○ Set initial goals to begin such change.

○ Enlist the help of family and friends.

○ Include smoking cessation for smokers.

Benefits, Risks, and Management Options for Improving Glucose Control

○ State that carrying out the diabetes-care plan will bring short-term and long-term benefits in terms of good health and quality of life.

Preconception Care, Pregnancy, and Gestational Diabetes

(See Diabetes and Pregnancy, page 35.)

○ State the importance of preconception counseling and the use of birth control to prevent unplanned pregnancy.

○ State the need for tight blood glucose control before conception and during pregnancy for the best health outcomes of mother and baby.

○ Include methods to prevent STDs.

Use of Health-Care Systems and Community Resources

○ State that the responsibility for following the plans belongs to the patient but that resources and supports are *always* necessary to carry this responsibility successfully.

○ State the need for a planned system of medical care, including follow-up and continuing education.

○ Describe when and how to obtain emergency medical care.

○ List telephone numbers to access help with daily problem-solving questions.

○ List the expected schedule for follow-up medical appointments for the first year.

○ List the community resources available for diabetes care and education.

○ List the community resources available for help with other social and economic problems.

○ State how to connect with other people in the community who have diabetes.

Continuing Education and Counseling Goals

DIABETES OVERVIEW

❍ List the causes of diabetes.

❍ State that diabetes is a disorder of the metabolism of carbohydrate, protein, and fat because of reduced insulin action.

❍ State how the diagnosis of diabetes is established and the differences between type I and type II.

❍ State the importance and benefits of good diabetes control, and list the factors that influence it.

❍ Describe the actions of insulin in the body and the effects of insulin deficiency and excess.

❍ Describe insulin resistance and how it is treated with exercise, moderate weight loss, and medication.

STRESS AND PSYCHOSOCIAL ADJUSTMENT

❍ State the pros and cons of acknowledging diabetes to family, peers, and colleagues.

❍ List those people who definitely need to be informed about diabetes.

❍ State his or her position as the most important member of the health-care team.

❍ State that changes in lifestyle are required because of diabetes.

❍ Describe situations that cause stress, and discuss several methods of stress management.

❍ Acknowledge that a social worker or psychologist may be able to help the patient in preventing or coping with stress.

FAMILY INVOLVEMENT AND SOCIAL SUPPORT

❍ State that living with diabetes concerns all family members.

❍ State that at least one family member or support person must know how to give medications (if used), recognize and treat hypoglycemia, be able to carry out sick-day rules, and know emergency phone numbers.

❍ State that family members themselves may need extra support in learning to adjust to diabetes and to carry out diabetes care when needed.

NUTRITION

❍ State the need for consistent timing of food intake and medication.

❍ State the relationship of obesity to diabetes, and benefits of moderate weight loss (10–15 lb) for obese people with diabetes.

❍ Identify what reasonable body weight might be.

○ Describe how to arrange food to prevent hypoglycemia while losing weight (if an oral agent or insulin is used).

○ State how to incorporate appropriate favorite recipes into the meal plan.

○ Demonstrate correct portion sizes for the meal plan using a food scale and measuring cups and spoons.

○ Demonstrate how to plan meals to enhance flexibility in the meal plan.

○ List types of nutrients, their effect on blood glucose and lipids levels, and their relationship to insulin.

○ State the calorie level and list the types and amounts of foods to be included in the meal plan.

○ Discuss possible benefits of vitamin and mineral supplementation, e.g., antioxidants.

○ Demonstrate how to evaluate food products using the nutrition facts panel on the food label.

○ Define terms such as dietetic, free foods, sugar free, calorie free, low calorie, reduced calorie, and fat free and identify examples of such products that might be appropriate for the meal plan.

○ List caloric and noncaloric sweeteners and foods that contain them, and describe how they might be used in the meal plan.

○ Explain the importance of reducing total fat as well as saturated fat and cholesterol in the meal plan.

○ List cooking and meal-planning strategies to meet goals of individualized meal plan.

○ Explain the role of dietary fiber in treating or preventing gastrointestinal disorders.

○ List food sources of dietary fiber and strategies for adding fiber to the meal plan.

○ State the relationship of salt (sodium) to hypertension and ways to decrease sodium intake, if necessary.

○ Demonstrate how to select foods when eating out—e.g., restaurants, fast foods, others' homes—according to the meal plan.

○ Describe appropriate menus for special occasions—e.g., birthdays, holidays, entertaining, social situations—to suit the meal plan.

○ State the effects of alcohol on blood glucose levels and precautions to follow, if used.

EXERCISE AND ACTIVITY

○ List the specific benefits and risks of exercise, including weight management, glucose control, and cardiovascular health.

○ State the need for regular aerobic exercise, and list examples.

○ State the importance of keeping blood glucose records related to exercise, i.e., monitoring before, during, and after exercise.

○ State the reason for carrying a high-carbohydrate snack and list examples.

○ Demonstrate how to monitor intensity of exercise, i.e., heart rate.

○ State target heart rate zone during aerobic exercise for age.

○ List the three stages of appropriate exercise program, i.e., warm up, aerobic, and cool down.

○ List types of physical activity that patient agrees to utilize.

○ Discuss planning exercise into schedule.

○ Describe the proper shoes and clothing for exercise.

○ State the need for ongoing evaluation of and guidance for his or her exercise plan.

○ Describe precautions when chronic complications are present, especially neuropathy and existing vascular compromise.

○ State why and how to avoid dehydration.

○ If medication is used, list factors that may increase the risk of exercise-induced hypoglycemia, e.g., alcohol and b-blockers.

MEDICATIONS

○ State that in addition to diet and exercise, some individuals with type II diabetes may need either oral agents or insulin.

○ Describe the action times and maximum dose of oral hypoglycemic agents (if treatment includes oral medication).

○ List the possible influences of other medications on blood glucose.

○ List the possible interactions of other commonly used medications with oral hypoglycemic agents.

○ Describe the different sources of insulin, i.e., animal and human.

○ Distinguish between the different types of insulin and brands available.

○ Describe the rationale for the time of insulin injection.

○ Describe the rationale for and method of rotation of insulin-injection sites.

○ Define lipohypertrophy, and describe how to prevent this problem.

○ Define lipoatrophy, and describe how to treat this problem.

○ List the possible influences of other medications on insulin action.

○ Discuss the reuse of disposable insulin syringes: techniques, benefits, and risks.

○ Describe methods for storing and adjusting insulin during travel and how to ensure insulin that is delivered by mail is not spoiled.

○ State the various methods of insulin delivery and administration, i.e., pumps and injection devices.

MONITORING AND USE OF RESULTS

○ Describe visual vs. meter methods of monitoring blood glucose.

○ Demonstrate how to use monitoring information to solve problems in self-management.

○ Describe how to use blood glucose monitoring results to adjust the treatment plan based on approved guidelines.

○ State the purpose of testing for glycated hemoglobin or other glycated proteins.

○ State how glycated hemoglobin results relate to the overall management plan.

○ State the relationship between glycated hemoglobin or other glycated proteins and daily blood glucose values.

○ Establish glycated hemoglobin targets.

○ Demonstrate the steps for glucose-meter quality assurance.

○ State when to check urine ketones.

RELATIONSHIPS AMONG NUTRITION, EXERCISE, MEDICATION, AND BLOOD GLUCOSE LEVELS

(For patients with type II diabetes who take insulin, refer to the corresponding type I diabetes section.)

○ State that the oral medication level is individualized to his or her planned usual food, activity level, and blood glucose levels.

○ State the relationship of exercise to oral agent activity, timing of exercise, timing of meals, and blood glucose levels.

○ State how to prevent medication-induced hypoglycemia by adjusting food or oral medication for planned and unplanned exercise and activity.

○ State the importance of keeping blood glucose records related to exercise, i.e., before, during, and after.

PREVENTION, DETECTION, AND TREATMENT OF ACUTE COMPLICATIONS

○ State that stressful conditions may cause problems with blood glucose control.

○ List the causes of hypoglycemia and how to prevent, recognize, and treat them (if treatment includes oral medication or insulin).

○ State the importance of carrying a high-carbohydrate source, and list examples.

○ State the importance of carrying a diabetes identification card, tag, or bracelet.

○ Define ketoacidosis and hyperosmolar nonketotic coma.

○ Define hyperglycemic hyperosmolar coma.

○ List the early signs of ketoacidosis.

○ State when to report symptoms to the health-care provider.

○ State how concurrent illness may affect diabetes and may require insulin.

○ State the general rules of care during illness.

○ State that fluid intake may need to be increased during illness.

○ State the need for more frequent blood glucose and ketone monitoring during illness.

○ State that oral medication or insulin adjustments during illness are based on blood glucose levels.

PREVENTION, DETECTION, AND TREATMENT OF CHRONIC COMPLICATIONS

○ Identify the organ systems particularly at risk from diabetes.

○ Describe hyperinsulinemia and state why it may be harmful.

○ State the need to report any visual disturbances to the health-care providers.

○ State that diabetes can affect the eyes without any symptoms being initially apparent.

○ State the need to see an ophthalmologist for annual eye exams with dilated pupils.

○ State that regular blood pressure monitoring is necessary.

○ State the need for control of high blood pressure.

○ State that monitoring of cholesterol and triglycerides is necessary and the differences between HDL and LDL.

○ State why control of cholesterol and triglycerides is important.

○ Identify the symptoms of, treatment of, and major factors in prevention of:
   ○ kidney disease
   ○ cardiovascular disease
   ○ peripheral vascular disease
   ○ peripheral neuropathy
   ○ autonomic neuropathy
   ○ periodontal disease

○ Identify how the diseases listed above will be monitored (BUN, CCR, AER, EKG, etc.)

○ State that diabetes may cause sexual dysfunction and identify resources for help.

FOOT, SKIN, AND DENTAL CARE
○ Demonstrate how to inspect and bathe the feet and how to trim the nails.
○ Identify factors that may cause injury to the feet.
○ Describe the basic first-aid measures for minor injuries to the feet.
○ State the need for well-fitting shoes and socks and that special shoes and referral for fitting are available if appropriate.
○ State that podiatric services are available if there are special foot-care needs.
○ State the value of a foot exam at follow-up visits (removal of shoes and socks during visit).
○ State the need for early aggressive professional treatment of any foot problems that occur.
○ Describe the proper care of the skin according to age and individual requirements.
○ State the possible effects of diabetes on dental health.
○ State the value of regular (i.e., annual) visits to the dentist.
○ State when to communicate with the dentist about dental problems and care.

BEHAVIOR-CHANGE STRATEGIES, GOAL SETTING, RISK-FACTOR REDUCTION, AND PROBLEM SOLVING
○ Establish goals and priorities that are measurable and attainable.
○ Define strategies to handle setbacks.
○ Enlist assistance of others at work or in family.

BENEFITS, RISKS, AND MANAGEMENT OPTIONS FOR IMPROVING GLUCOSE CONTROL
○ State that carrying out the diabetes-care plan will bring short-term and long-term benefits in terms of good health and quality of life.

PRECONCEPTION CARE, PREGNANCY, AND GESTATIONAL DIABETES
(See section on Diabetes and Pregnancy, page 35.)
○ State the importance of preconception counseling and the use of birth control to prevent unplanned pregnancy.
○ State the need for tight blood glucose control before conception and during pregnancy for the best health outcomes of mother and baby. State that she can't use oral medications during pregnancy.

USE OF HEALTH-CARE SYSTEMS AND COMMUNITY RESOURCES

○ State the need for regular routine follow-up visits for medical care.

○ Name and know how to contact all members of the diabetes health-care team.

○ State his or her position as the most important member of the health-care team.

○ List periodic blood/urine tests to be done by the health-care provider.

○ State the importance of nutrition education and counseling on a routine basis.

○ State the need for continuing diabetes education.

○ State when support groups and counseling are appropriate and how they can help.

○ State how to access competent diabetes medical care when traveling or living away from home.

○ List the resources available to help with special needs and concerns, such as finances, pregnancy, visual impairment, weight management, traveling, sports, school, child care, career, marriage, and senior citizen activities/networks.

○ List the resources available for long-term psychosocial support.

○ State how to connect with other people with diabetes in the patient's community and how to connect with diabetes organizations.

Special Considerations

Educators should first examine their own beliefs concerning elderly people with type II diabetes. Do you believe that tight diabetic control is appropriate for someone over the age of 65? Recall that chronic complications of diabetes such as retinopathy and nephropathy can appear within a decade of the onset, and that life expectancy at age 65 is 17 years. Add to that the current belief that many individuals have had glucose intolerance for years before they are diagnosed. Do you believe the elderly can learn new concepts? You might read "Age-related changes in human memory: normal and abnormal" in *Geriatrics* , 1988. Do you have the energy to devote to the task of educating the elderly? Teaching the elderly can require extra time—yours, the family's, and the patient's at a rate of reimbursement that does not acknowledge this.

Your sessions with an older individual will be more productive if you give the caregiver a preprinted history form to complete ahead of time, and ask for the patient's old records to be assembled and brought to the first meeting. It is important that the patient's primary-caregiver is present at all sessions. Be prepared for the possibility of your patient having decreased vision or limited mobility with the large print materials and tools described in "Diabetes Aids and Products for People with Visual or Physical Impairment" by Ruth Ann Petzinger in *The Diabetes Educator* or the Annual Buyer's Guide in the October issue of *Diabetes Forecast* (see Resources).

You should think of your client in terms of "functional age" instead of chronological age. To do this you can assess cognitive abilities with such resources as "The Mini-Mental Health Exam" or "Assessing physical function in the elderly" (see Resources). You should ask about your client's potential difficulty with shopping, preparing food, ingrained dietary habits, change in the sense of taste, and chronic changes in bowel habits. Management of diabetes can be quite expensive. Knowing the current costs in your community for oral agents, insulin, syringes, monitors, glucose strips, and discussing these with your client is important.

Be aware that symptoms of diabetes and its complications, such as hypoglycemia, can be subtle or absent in the elderly, and that changes in behavior should prompt a check of blood glucose and a call to the doctor. Loneliness may be the root of the elderly person's exaggerated expectations from healthcare providers. Create a teaching plan with the client's and the caregiver's input. "Prioritize" teaching to include two or three concepts in short, focused, slower-paced, concrete sessions with hands-on practice. The elderly often have numerous other medical conditions and can be on several medications. Simple written instructions, charts, and "pill counters" are important aids for them.

MANAGEMENT OPTIONS FOR THE ELDERLY INCLUDE:

Diet	*Simplified Healthy Food Choices* (ADA, 1988), or *The First Step in Meal Planning* (ADA/TADA, 1995) rather than more complicated exchange plans; Meals on Wheels; "Healthy Frozen Dinners," *Tufts University Nutrition Letter* (1994)
Exercise	"Armchair Fitness" videos (see Resources), after appropriate medical evaluation for risk; Classes for seniors at the local YMCA.
Oral Agents	Short-acting drugs to reduce the risk of hypoglycemia in the elderly who often have diminished real and hepatic function.
Insulin	Premixed combinations enabling the caregiver to draw up a week's supply of syringes at one time or cartridges that give greater ease of measuring doses than syringes.

DIABETES AND PREGNANCY

This section is divided into two parts. The first part identifies behavioral objectives for the woman with type I or type II diabetes before pregnancy. It assumes that the woman has met the objectives from the initial and continuing education phases. If she has not done so, the educator will need to assess which of these objectives are also applicable. The behavioral objectives listed in each content area are specific to pregnancy.

Gestational diabetes, discussed in the second part, is defined as impaired glucose tolerance that appears during pregnancy. It is usually diagnosed during the second or third trimester of pregnancy and is associated with perinatal fetal and maternal risks. All women should be routinely screened for gestational diabetes sometime between the 24th and 28th week of pregnancy. The behavioral objectives given here are specific to gestational diabetes.

Pregnancy With Preexisting Diabetes

DIABETES OVERVIEW

○ State the importance of preconception counseling to achieve glycemic control and maintain overall health as close to normal as possible for an appropriate period before conception.
○ State that pregnancy requires major efforts by her and her health-care team to prevent complications and ensure a healthy baby.
○ State that during pregnancy she will have a greater risk of problematic glycemic control, first trimester hypoglycemia, diabetic ketoacidosis, hypertension, and fluid retention.
○ State that the risk to the fetus is largely determined by the level of maternal blood glucose and glycemic control and list potential problems (i.e., prematurity, hypoglycemia, hypocalcemia, hyperbilirubinemia, fetal malformation, etc.)
○ State that special studies and examinations of the fetus are necessary during the entire pregnancy to evaluate the health of the fetus.
○ State that glycemic control must be assessed regularly by blood glucose monitoring and urine tests for ketones and glycated proteins.
○ State that during pregnancy, target blood glucose values will be lower than when she is not pregnant.
○ State that the timing and the mode of delivery will be determined by the health status of the mother and baby.

35

○ State that situations may arise at delivery that require specialized care for the baby.

○ State that breast-feeding is encouraged in women with diabetes and may even provide some protection against diabetes developing in the baby later on.

STRESS AND PSYCHOSOCIAL ADJUSTMENT

○ State the need for a high level of patient involvement during pregnancy to achieve a successful outcome.

○ Acknowledge that pregnancy is a time of uncertainty and that those feelings are complicated by diabetes.

○ Acknowledge that there is no guarantee of a healthy baby no matter how good care is.

○ Acknowledge that working at the daily insulin injections, monitoring, and prescribed meal/exercise plans is a complex task when she is not pregnant. This task is more difficult during pregnancy and requires a team effort by her, her family and close friends, and health-care providers.

FAMILY INVOLVEMENT AND SOCIAL SUPPORT

○ Involve at least one family member (or support person) in an educational session about diabetes during pregnancy. This person should be able to treat hypoglycemia and should know emergency phone numbers.

NUTRITION

○ State the role of nutrition in achieving euglycemia before conception and during pregnancy.

○ State that nutritional needs change as a result of pregnancy, e.g., increased need for calories, carbohydrates, protein, calcium, iron, and other vitamins and minerals.

○ State the importance of monitoring the pattern of weight gain during pregnancy.

○ State that pregnancy is not a time for weight loss.

○ Identify appropriate snacks, especially for bedtime, to prevent hypoglycemia.

○ State the importance of nutritional care and education during pregnancy.

○ State the need for meal-plan review after pregnancy.

○ State that adjustments in the meal plan are necessary to meet the nutritional requirements of lactation.

○ State the risks of alcohol to the developing fetal organs and the added risk of severe hypoglycemia.

Exercise and Activity
- State that pregnancy is not the time for initiation of a vigorous exercise program.
- State that moderate exercise can assist in lowering blood glucose levels. Women with an active lifestyle are encouraged to continue a program of moderate activity.
- State that with tighter metabolic control during pregnancy, the risk of hypoglycemia is increased.
- State how to prevent and treat the hypoglycemia that can occur with increased activity.

Medications
- State insulin requirements will be different from the nonpregnant state and require careful monitoring.
- State that insulin requirements may be low during the first trimester of pregnancy.
- State that during the second and third trimesters, insulin requirements may increase because the hormones from the placenta interfere with insulin action.
- State that insulin requirements will drop abruptly during active labor and in the immediate postpartum period
- State that oral hypoglycemic agents are contraindicated during pregnancy.
- If insulin is required for the first time because of pregnancy, demonstrate the correct technique for administration (refer to the corresponding type I diabetes section).
- State benefits of intensive insulin therapy, i.e., insulin pump, multiple injections.

Monitoring and Use of Results
- State that frequent blood glucose monitoring is essential during pregnancy.
- State that glucose self-monitoring at least eight times a day (before each meal, 1–2 hours after each meal, at bedtime, and in the middle of the night) is optimum.
- State that the results of monitoring will be used to determine insulin requirements.
- State that daily morning urine ketone monitoring is necessary to avoid starvation ketosis.

Relationships Among Nutrition, Exercise, Medication, and Blood Glucose Levels

○ State that pregnancy alters nutritional needs, and careful attention is required during periods of exercise to prevent hypoglycemia.

○ State that the fetus may increase her need for calories. Monitoring for ketones may show when she needs additional calories.

Prevention, Detection, and Treatment of Acute Complications

○ State that hypoglycemia and hyperglycemia during pregnancy can best be prevented by careful blood glucose monitoring, proper insulin administration, and meal planning.

○ State that hypoglycemic reactions occur most frequently during the first trimester and during the immediate postpartum period.

○ State that pregnancy can aggravate hyperglycemia.

○ State that hyperglycemia can be harmful to the fetus.

○ State the importance of carrying a concentrated, quickly absorbed source of carbohydrate.

○ State that ketones are thought to be damaging to the fetus.

○ State that during illness, ketosis may develop more rapidly than in the nonpregnant state, and immediate contact with the health-care provider is required with any illness producing fever or ketosis of over 4 hours duration.

Prevention, Detection, and Treatment of Chronic Complications

○ State that the risk of developing or worsening retinopathy and nephropathy may be increased during pregnancy.

○ State that smoking is harmful to the mother and fetus during pregnancy.

○ State the rationale for avoiding alcoholic beverages and illicit drugs during pregnancy.

Behavior-Change Strategies, Goal Setting, Risk-Factor Reduction, and Problem Solving

○ Establish goals and priorities.

○ Define strategies to handle setbacks.

○ Enlist assistance of others at work or in family.

BENEFITS, RISKS, AND MANAGEMENT OPTIONS
FOR IMPROVING GLUCOSE CONTROL

○ State that following the diabetes-care plan will bring short-term and long-term benefits in terms of good health and quality of life to the woman as well as to the fetus.

USE OF HEALTH-CARE SYSTEMS AND COMMUNITY RESOURCES

○ State the need for frequent visits with the health-care team—obstetrician, primary-care physician, endocrinologist or diabetologist, dietitian, nurse, and diabetes educator—during pregnancy.

○ State that the responsibility for carrying out the diabetes-care plan belongs to the patient, but that resources and supports are *always* necessary.

○ Identify the follow-up plan and appointments.

○ List the resources available for help with the problems and concerns of pregnancy.

Gestational Diabetes

DIABETES OVERVIEW

○ Define gestational diabetes.

○ State the rationale for normalization of blood glucose levels during pregnancy.

○ State the importance of avoiding obesity after pregnancy to prevent or delay the onset of type II diabetes.

○ State the percentage risk (i.e., 30%) of developing diabetes after pregnancy.

STRESS AND PSYCHOSOCIAL ADJUSTMENT

○ State that there is a normal grieving and adjusting process after diagnosis. It is important to understand that strong feelings of denial, anger, and sadness are normal. It is also normal to worry about the baby. Because of the short time frame from diagnosis until delivery, the patient needs to become involved in self-management very quickly.

○ State the importance of a high level of patient involvement to achieve a normal and/or safe pregnancy and delivery.

○ Acknowledge that working with diabetes is a complex task that takes a team to master. The patient will have a team to support the management of gestational diabetes.

Family Involvement and Social Support

○ Involve at least one family member (or support person) in the educational process especially if insulin is used. This person should be able to recognize and treat hypoglycemia and should know emergency phone numbers.

Nutrition

○ State the nutritional changes that must occur during pregnancy to meet the nutritional requirements of both the mother and the fetus.

○ State the importance of monitoring food intake to normalize blood glucose levels.

○ State the relationship of food and activity to insulin.

○ State the importance of consistency in planning meals and snacks (particularly if her treatment includes insulin).

○ State the importance of monitoring her weight to assess appropriate weight gain.

○ State the types and amounts of foods to be included in her meals and snacks.

○ Demonstrate the ability to plan appropriate meals and snacks.

○ Demonstrate how to select foods in proper serving sizes.

○ State the nutritional needs for lactation.

Exercise and Activity

○ State that pregnancy is not the time for initiation of a vigorous exercise program.

○ State that moderate exercise can assist in lowering blood glucose levels. Women with an active lifestyle are encouraged to continue a program of moderate activity.

○ State how to prevent and treat the hypoglycemia that can occur with increased activity (if treatment includes insulin).

Medications

○ State that insulin will be required during pregnancy if normalization of blood glucose is not attained by diet therapy alone.

○ State that insulin will most likely be discontinued after the baby is delivered.

○ Demonstrate the correct technique for insulin administration (if treatment includes insulin).

○ State that oral hypoglycemic agents are contraindicated for gestational diabetes.

MONITORING AND USE OF RESULTS

○ State that blood glucose monitoring, urine testing for ketones, and blood testing for fructosamine and/or glycated hemoglobin are necessary during gestational diabetes.
○ Demonstrate how to monitor blood glucose levels.
○ Demonstrate how to adjust the meal plan (and insulin, if used) based on blood glucose levels.
○ Demonstrate how to test the urine for ketones.

RELATIONSHIPS AMONG NUTRITION, EXERCISE, MEDICATION, AND BLOOD GLUCOSE LEVELS

○ State that pregnancy alters her nutritional needs. Careful attention is required during and after periods of exercise to prevent hypoglycemia if insulin is used.
○ State that the baby may increase her need for calories. Monitoring for ketones may show when she needs additional calories.
○ State that breast-feeding is the healthiest choice for the baby and her.

PREVENTION, DETECTION, AND TREATMENT OF ACUTE COMPLICATIONS

○ State the causes of hypoglycemia and how to prevent it (if treatment includes insulin).
○ State the importance of carrying a concentrated, quickly absorbed source of carbohydrate.
○ State how to recognize the signs and symptoms of hypoglycemia and how to treat it (if treatment includes insulin).
○ State the importance of monitoring blood glucose levels to avoid hyperglycemia.
○ Describe the signs and symptoms of hyperglycemia.
○ State the need to notify health-care providers if hyperglycemia develops.
○ State that frequent blood glucose monitoring and urine tests for ketones are important during periods of illness.

PREVENTION, DETECTION, AND TREATMENT OF CHRONIC COMPLICATIONS

○ State that gestational diabetes places her at risk to develop diabetes later in life. State that attention to weight control may prevent or delay the development of diabetes.
○ State that smoking is harmful to the mother and fetus during pregnancy.

○ State the rationale for avoiding alcoholic beverages and other illicit drugs during pregnancy.

BEHAVIOR-CHANGE STRATEGIES, GOAL SETTING, RISK-FACTOR REDUCTION, AND PROBLEM SOLVING

○ Establish goals and priorities.
○ Define strategies to handle setbacks.
○ Enlist assistance of others at work or in family.

BENEFITS, RISKS, AND MANAGEMENT OPTIONS FOR IMPROVING GLUCOSE CONTROL

○ State that following the diabetes-care plan will bring short-term and long-term benefits in terms of good health and quality of life for the woman and the fetus.

USE OF HEALTH-CARE SYSTEMS AND COMMUNITY RESOURCES

○ State the need for frequent visits with her health-care team during pregnancy.
○ State that the responsibility for carrying out the diabetes-care plan belongs to the patient, but that resources and supports are *always* necessary.
○ Identify her follow-up plan and appointments.
○ State the reason for routine screening for diabetes after pregnancy.
○ List the resources available for help with the problems and concerns of pregnancy.

DIABETES THROUGH THE LIFE STAGES

Infants and Preschool Children

In this age group, parents are the primary-care providers, so educators need to pay attention to metabolic, psychosocial, and developmental issues as well as general parenting issues and family interactions. How parents learn has to do with their current emotional state as well as their specific learning abilities. Parents confronted with diabetes often exhibit enormous guilt, fears, and frustration because of the diagnosis or because of prior stresses in their own upbringing and family situations. It's important that responsibility for parenting a small child with diabetes be shared and not shouldered completely by the child's mother. You may need to make specific and repeated efforts at involving fathers, older siblings, and other close relatives such as grandparents in the child's care. Because young children are not capable of abstract thinking, understanding the need for injections and fingerpricks is difficult. Creative, innovative teaching tools and learning through play can serve as an acceptable educational mode for this age group. Allowing the young child to act out frustrations and fears through play activities can alleviate pressure and anxiety.

Pediatric diabetes consultation is strongly recommended, even if it requires long travel because local expertise may not be available. Pediatric nurses, dietitians, physicians, and counselors should work to identify families at acute risk and those families who need frequent and/or intensified assistance to help lessen or even prevent future disasters. Severe hypoglycemia, usually with associated convulsions, is common and strategies for prevention should be acknowledged. Hypoglycemia fears can often interfere with appropriate glucose control.

Encourage parents of very young children to meet with other parents who have similar concerns. Outpatient visits are usually needed more frequently (i.e., every 1–2 months) in this age-group. Parents will need education on what and how to tell sitters and day-care providers about caring for their child.

School Children

As children grow, they move toward more independence. Going to school forces the child with diabetes to begin assuming some self-care tasks, such as recognizing hypoglycemia and making healthy meal choices. Parents and/or health-care providers should meet with school personnel and include them on the health-care team. Understanding these processes, individual differences, and how a chronic illness like type I diabetes can hamper appropriate developmental progress calls for special pediatric diabetes training, interest, and expertise. The multidisciplinary health-care team should assist the responsible adults in the home by providing information on normal limit setting, diabetes-specific limit setting, and dealing with schools and after-school activities.

Work with parents to ensure that self-care is not promoted too early, before the child is ready technically, emotionally, and developmentally. Because peer pressures begin to surface, group learning experiences like diabetes weekend retreats, day camp, and residential camp programs can help the child develop appropriate self-care habits and a strong sense of ego and self-esteem.

Adolescents

The trials and tribulations of adolescence involve major hormonal and body changes and the psychosocial stresses and challenges that are caused by or accompany the transition from child to adult. Peer pressures increase, and teenagers naturally experiment with societal and personal issues and limits. However, some research suggests that overbearing parents and/or living with type I diabetes are associated with developmental delay in children with diabetes achieving age- and sex-appropriate independence. Assistance of the diabetes health-care team can help prevent and treat such problems. Recurrent diabetic ketoacidosis (DKA) is psychosocial in origin and caused by omitted insulin until proven otherwise. An initial solution is to have a responsible adult actually prepare and inject the insulin as prescribed.

A combination of eating disorders, dysfunctional families, and type I diabetes places tremendous demands on the adolescent and his or her family as well as health-care providers. Family counseling can be more important than therapy focusing only on the teen. Once again, teen support groups, teen-only weekends, and camp programs can promote appropriate experimentation and self-growth without compromising diabetes care. Help parents recognize alcohol, nicotine, and other drug use and abuse and start a treatment plan if needed. Sexual issues impact type I diabetes in multiple ways, and preconception and birth-control counseling may help prevent unplanned pregnancies.

Young Adults

The issue of accepting responsibility for living well with type I diabetes comes to bear as young adults move away from their families, start their own jobs, begin to purchase their own diabetes-care supplies, and engage in long-lasting relationships. Independent living, buying and preparing foods, managing finances, and dealing with insurance and health-care costs impact directly on their self-management of type I diabetes. Support their efforts to counteract prior unhealthy behaviors regarding food, nutrition, smoking, and glucose monitoring. Young adults will require medical as well as stress and psychosocial adjustment assistance in dealing with early diabetes complications and with the accompanying feelings of depression, guilt, anger, and fear. Planning for ongoing medical care and relationship with the diabetes health-care team must be proactive.

Adults

As adults, people with type I diabetes face unique challenges. Diabetes can significantly affect decisions related to marriage and relationships with friends and family. When an adult with diabetes decides to marry, the spouse needs to be educated about diabetes and the role of the spouse in diabetes care. Diabetes may affect a couple's decision about whether and when to have children. As the family develops, the impact of diabetes is felt by all family members.

The cost of diabetes care is usually an issue, especially when finances are limited. In the case of dual-career families, diabetes adds to the burden of balancing parental and career responsibilities within limited time. Divorce or significant family events can affect diabetes control.

Employment also presents additional challenges resulting from diabetes. Diabetes may affect a person's occupational choice. Although most occupations are equally desirable whether or not a person has type I diabetes, jobs that involve significant physical activity or unpredictable hours will affect diabetes control. Intensive individualized diabetes education may be required. The health-care team can help construct a diabetes-care plan to fit a job that involves odd hours. Working variable hours is generally difficult for people taking insulin, and in certain situations, e.g., pregnancy, such work shifts are contraindicated for optimum glucose control. Because of diabetes, health insurance coverage is vitally necessary and may affect a client's decision about changing jobs. The health-care team must be aware of an individual's special needs and goals, assess them regularly, and develop care plans to meet them.

The Older Person

The number of people with diabetes aged 65 and over has doubled in the past 20 years. Older people with type I diabetes face many challenges in addition to aging.

The process of aging brings changes in physiological function and sensory perception. Commonly, older people experience changes in renal and bladder function, constipation, hearing loss, changes in eyesight, and loss of teeth, taste sensitivity, and touch perception. The presence of chronic disease affects 80–86% of people aged 65 and older. Arthritis, hypertension, cardiovascular disease, and emphysema are common ailments. These conditions may add to the prescribed dietary restrictions and cause an increase in the use of both prescription and over-the-counter drugs. These drugs can affect glucose control, with either hypoglycemic or hyper-glycemic effects. Also, drug and nutrient interactions increase when a person takes multiple medications.

Many older people also face changing financial situations. Fourteen percent of people over 65 live below the poverty level; 15% live just above that poverty line. Most are on a fixed retirement income that may not adequately cover the rising costs of living in addition to adequate diabetes care.

Most older people experience psychosocial stresses, such as the loss of their spouse and friends, retirement, or having to live alone. Not only is their social network disrupted, but they may be forced to leave their familiar home environment. Independence is gradually replaced by depen-dence on others. The older person may experience loneliness, worry, frustration, and feelings of helplessness and hopelessness.

To meet the needs of the older person with type I diabetes, the diabetes educator can arrange for the educational setting to be quiet and well-lit. Frequent short education sessions focused on single topics are preferable, because the older person may have a shorter attention span. The diabetes educator should check to see whether the patient usually wears eyeglasses, and make sure they are worn for educational sessions. If hearing is a problem, the educator must speak slowly at a low pitch and use short sentences. Saying the person's name, touching him or her, and ensuring eye contact before speaking are helpful in gaining attention.

The diabetes educator should use appropriate educational tools, showing examples of possible tools, and asking the older person or family member which tools they feel would work best for them. Generally, simplified materials, possibly with large print or pictures, are preferred. Including hands-on demonstrations, return demonstrations, role-playing, and visual tools, such as food models, is helpful.

The inclusion of caregivers or family members in educational sessions may increase the patient's chances of successfully achieving their goals. Older patients may need to be told about specialized equipment, such as injection aids to help those with limited manual dexterity draw up and inject insulin, and needle guides, syringe magnifiers, and non-visual insulin measurement aids to help those who are visually impaired. (See Buyer's Guide in the Resources.)

Energy-Diverting Issues
In all instances, the presence of these issues indicates need for more specialized services.

For patients of all ages:
- ○ Mental retardation
- ○ Learning disability
- ○ Preexisting stress and psychosocial adjustment or behavioral problems
- ○ Prior history of physical or sexual abuse
- ○ Alcohol, nicotine, and/or illicit drug problem
- ○ Obesity
- ○ Eating disorder
- ○ Preexisting other chronic illness (e.g., asthma, epilepsy, or celiac disease)

For families (all the above in a spouse or parent) plus:
- ○ Insurance coverage
- ○ Economic compromise
- ○ Job change or unemployment
- ○ Housing change
- ○ Marital distress (recent/possible)
  a. Single-parent family
  b. Separation
  c. Divorce

EDUCATIONAL APPROACHES FOR SPECIAL SITUATIONS

Every person with diabetes is unique and should receive an individualized assessment and plan. A thorough assessment of needs will identify not only medical and health information, but special learning needs that should be considered when developing the teaching plan. Low literacy, cultural diversity, low income, and a host of other situations do not change our educational goals for people with diabetes, but each impacts the style and format of the delivery of diabetes education.

Each special situation may be complicated by additional emotional adjustment crises or maladaptive behavior. Care partners or supporting family members are necessary in many cases to prevent hospitalization of the person with diabetes. Establishing and maintaining support for the care partner should not be overlooked. A few considerations for teaching strategies in some of the more commonly seen special populations are addressed below.

VISUALLY IMPAIRED people with diabetes may continue to want to be very independent with self-care skills and can do so if they receive education on adaptive devices. Talking blood glucose meters, devices to help people draw up insulin doses, and insulin pens with auditory clicks are a few of the products available. It is important to identify care partners and support people. They should receive basic/survival skill instructions and demonstrate skill competency. The exercise plan for the visually impaired may be modified to ensure safety. Activities of daily living will be carried out differently from the activities of the sighted person, but many resources are available in terms of food, transport, and supplies to facilitate that process. (See Resources.)

LOW LITERACY patients will need verbal explanations and printed materials with pictorial instructions and a few simple words. They'll need to demonstrate their understanding by performing the skills taught at previous sessions. Verbal feedback can demonstrate their understanding. A straightforward, sincere question, such as "Do you have any trouble reading?" may help with your assessment. However, do not simply ask, "Do you understand?" Most often, these clients will answer yes even when they do not understand. Ask in-depth questions to determine where the lesson may have gotten sidetracked. When possible, have the patient demonstrate what was learned.

CULTURAL DIVERSITY encompasses many areas of consideration, such as foreign languages, foods, and customs. You may need a professional interpreter if family members cannot act as an interpreter. Include ethnic and cultural foods in the meal plan. In fact, flexible meal plans, together with blood glucose monitoring, encourage the patient to begin self-management.

PHYSICALLY CHALLENGED people with diabetes will need an introduction to adaptive devices. Stroke victims may have to do everything single-handed. Care partners, relatives, or friends may have to predraw syringes and should be educated about insulin preparation and care. Patients with amputations need to deal with the issue of limited mobility. People with diabetes and cerebral palsy may need to live in an assisted-care environment and will experience modified independence. People who are deaf or have some hearing loss require interpreter services just as foreign language patients do.

LOW INCOME patients with diabetes often look to diabetes educators for resources. Diabetes educators should inform patients of community resources for supplies and emergency-care information, medication, food, and housing. The cost of glucose monitoring strips may necessitate cutting the strips in half. In this instance, visual readings will need to be done, because cut strips cannot be read accurately by meters. The diabetes educator should be knowledgeable about Medicare and Medicaid reimbursement, and should refer patients to social workers for additional eligibility information.

SEVERE DEBILITATING COMPLICATIONS of diabetes may be an indication for modifying your teaching approaches. The modifications may include shorter teaching segments, adapting the exercise prescription, and special attention to medication interactions. Patients with severe neuropathy or hypertension will need modifications to their exercise plan. Assisted living may be necessary for your client's safety—hypoglycemia identification and treatment as well as help managing the activities of daily living. Safety is an overriding issue for this person. For patients on dialysis, time education sessions around dialysis sessions. Adjust instruction to focus on daily life with dialysis.

MENTAL AND EMOTIONAL DISABILITY will require the identification of an alternate caregiver for diabetes care if the disability is severe. The caregiver or family member should seek support systems for themselves as well. Constant, long-term care can be draining and stressful and the caregiver deserves a respite. The major concern for these patients is consistency of daily-care routines and adherence in taking all medications. The patient's diabetes-care needs will be met best by maintaining counseling appointments and follow-ups.

LEARNING DISABILITIES are often difficult to diagnose and may remain undiagnosed. They may affect a person's ability to learn and perform the skills for diabetes self-management. For instance, dyslexia may complicate the recording and manipulation of blood glucose readings or insulin doses. Mistakes could have devastating effects on the person with diabetes. Resources include blood glucose meters with memories and written instructions on medication doses. Contact these patients often or write down follow-up instructions for them to take home to help reinforce instructions and facilitate compliance.

AMERICAN DIABETES ASSOCIATION RECOGNITION AND NATIONAL STANDARDS FOR DIABETES SELF-MANAGEMENT EDUCATION PROGRAMS

If you are offering a diabetes self-management education program, you may want to consider applying for Recognition from the American Diabetes Association (ADA). ADA Recognition is a voluntary process that formally identifies diabetes patient education programs that meet the National Standards. Achieving Recognition requires the successful completion and submission of an application with supporting documentation plus the payment of a processing fee. Although rigorous enough to differentiate quality programs, the Standards are designed to be flexible enough to be applicable in any healthcare setting, from physician's offices and health management organizations to clinics and hospitals. Each submission must include demographic data on patients served, information about the instructors and advisory committee, the program's curriculum and education materials, and patient records and follow-up evaluations. By obtaining Recognition, education programs can demonstrate that they have met the highest standards thereby entitling them to the confidence of the community and the patients they serve.

The National Standards were originally developed and tested by a committee made up of many diabetes organizations under the auspices of the National Diabetes Advisory Board (NDAB). The Standards were revised and updated in 1994, again by a group representing many diabetes and other organizations, and are designed to promote acceptable quality education nationwide for every person with diabetes. American Diabetes Association approved the original standards in 1983 and the revised standards in 1994. In 1986, a voluntary committee of the ADA developed an application and a review process to determine whether a program met the standards. The first programs were formally recognized by the ADA in 1987 as having met the standards.

Some of the benefits of ADA Recognition include:
○ ensuring that a diabetes program meets the National Standards for Diabetes Patient Education Programs.
○ providing patients with a means of identifying quality education programs that meet nationally accepted standards.

○ increasing the likelihood of obtaining third-party reimbursement.
○ helping insurers identify quality diabetes education services for reimbursement purposes.
○ providing an opportunity for the program to market itself as having met the National Standards and therefore, differentiate itself from other programs.
○ stimulating the program through the application process to critically examine itself and make needed changes and improvements.
○ providing a mechanism for cost-effective peer review and consultation by some of the most respected diabetes educators in the country, and
○ providing primary referral sites for American Diabetes Association Affiliates to refer patients for diabetes education.

To apply for Recognition you will need to obtain an application and *Meeting the Standards Manual* from the American Diabetes Association, Recognition Program, 1660 Duke Street, Alexandria, VA 22314, (800) 232-3472, ext. 214.

Completed applications with supporting documentation must be sent to the ADA Recognition Program along with the current processing fee. The application will be reviewed by an expert panel of diabetes educators, and if approved, the program is recognized for 3 years.

RESOURCES

Psychosocial

Alogna M: Perception of severity of diabetes and health locus of control in compliant and noncompliant diabetic patients. *Diabetes Care* 3:533–44, 1980.

Bandura A: *Social foundations of thought and action: A social cognitive theory.* Englewood Cliffs, NJ, Prentice Hall, 1986.

Becker MH (Ed.): *The Health Belief Model and Personal Health Behavior.* Thorofare, NJ, Charles B. Slack, 1974.

Becker MH, Janz N: The health belief model applied to understanding diabetes regimen compliance. *Diabetes Educator* 11:41–47, 1985.

Brink SJ (Ed.): *Pediatric and Adolescent Diabetes Mellitus.* Chicago, Year Book Medical Publishers, 1987. Includes discussion of developmental factors, disease factors, and a range of clinical issues (e.g., drugs, alcohol) concerning type I diabetes in children and adolescents.

Edelstein J, Linn MW: Locus of Control and the Control of Diabetes. *Diabetes Educator* 13:51–54, 1987.

Edelwich J, Brodsky B: *Diabetes: Caring for Your Emotions as Well as Your Health.* Reading, MA, Addison Wesley, 1986. For patients and professionals, provides explanation of the range of emotional responses normal for patients with diabetes and the impact on overall health.

Follansbee D: Assuming responsibility for diabetes management: What age? What price? *Diabetes Educator* 15: 347–52, 1989. Summary of empirical studies documenting the impact of parental involvement in children's diabetes management through puberty.

Hurley CC, Shea CA: Self-efficacy: Strategy for enhancing diabetes self-care. *Diabetes Educator* 18:146–50, 1992.

Kurtz MS: Adherence to diabetes regimens: empirical status and clinical applications. *Diabetes Educator* 16:50–55, 1990.

Maiman L, Becker M: Scales for measuring health belief model dimensions: a test of predictive value, internal consistency, and relationships amoung beliefs. *Health Educ Monographs* 5:215–31, 1977.

Register C: *Living With Chronic Illness: Days of Patience and Passion.* New York, Bantam, 1987. Discusses impact of chronic disease on the spouse relationship and how family members can cope in positive ways with the increased stress of living with chronic illness.

Rubin RR, Biermann J, Toohey B: *Psyching Out Diabetes: A Positive Approach to Your Negative Emotions.* Los Angeles, Lowell, 1992.

Wooldridge KL, Wallston KA, Graber AL, Brown AW, Davidson P: The releationship between health beliefs, adherence, and metabolic control of diabetes. *Diabetes Educator* 18:495–500, 1992.

Nutrition

American Diabetes Association: Position Statement: Nutrition recommendations and principles for people with diabetes mellitus. *Diabetes Care* 17:519–22, 1994.

Cooper, N: *The Joy of Snacks.* Minneapolis, Chronimed, 1991.

Eating Healthy Foods. Alexandria, VA, Am. Diabetes Assoc., and Chicago, Am. Dietetic Assoc., 1988. An introduction to meal planning, especially helpful with low-literacy patients.

Ethnic and Regional Food Series. Alexandria, VA, Am. Diabetes Assoc., and Chicago, Am. Dietetic Assoc. Information about cultural food habits and healthy but traditional modifications. Now available: Mexican-American, Jewish, Chinese, Hmong American, Philippino, Cajun Creole, Southern Fare, Navajo, and Alaska Native.

Exchange Lists for Meal Planning. Alexandria, VA, Am. Diabetes Assoc., and Chicago, Am. Dietetic Assoc., 1995. Colorful charts, helpful tips on good nutrition, and an introduction to the Exchange Lists for your patients.

Franz MJ: *Exchanges for All Occasions,* 3rd ed. Minneapolis, Chronimed, 1993.

Franz MJ, Horton ES, Bantle JP, Beebe CA, Brunzell JD, Coulston AM, Henry RR, Hoogwerf BJ, Stacpoole PW: Technical review: Nutrition Principles for the management of diabetes and related complications. *Diabetes Care* 17:490-5–18.

Meal Planning Approaches for Diabetes Management: Chicago, Am. Dietetic Assoc., 1994. Professional guide to alternate meal plan approaches.

Month of Meals Series. Alexandria, VA, Am. Diabetes Assoc. Meal planning made easy with 28 days of breakfasts, lunches, and dinners. Five books, each with a different focus.

Nutrition Guide for Professionals: Diabetes Education and Meal Planning. Alexandria, VA, Am. Diabetes Assoc., and Chicago, Am. Dietetic Assoc., 1988. Information on creating meal plans using the Exchange Lists and complete data bases of nutrients.

Pregnancy

Jovanovic-Peterson L (Ed.): *Medical Management of Pregnancy Complicated by Diabetes,* 2nd ed. Alexandria, VA, Am. Diabetes Assoc., 1995. Vital information for the obstetrician, primary-care physician, dietitian, and educator.

Diabetes and Pregnancy: What to Expect. Alexandria, VA, Am. Diabetes Assoc., 1992. A valuable resource for educators and their patients with diabetes who are considering pregnancy.

Gestational Diabetes: What to Expect. Alexandria, VA, Am. Diabetes Assoc., 1992. A comprehensive guide for patients and educators.

Foot, Skin, and Dental Care

Diabetic Foot Care. Alexandria, VA, Am. Diabetes Assoc., 1990. Guidelines for a successful foot-care program for patients written for health-care professionals.

Type I Diabetes

Baum JD, Kinmonth AL: *Care of the Child with Diabetes.* Edinburgh, U.K., Churchill Livingstone, 1985.

Betschart J: *It's Time to Learn About Diabetes: A Workbook on Diabetes for Children.* Minneapolis, Chronimed, 1991.

Brink SJ: *Pediatric and Adolescent Diabetes Mellitus.* Chicago, Year Book Medical Publishers, 1987.

Chase HP: *Understanding Insulin Dependent Diabetes,* 7th ed. Denver, Children's Diabetes Foundation, 1992.

DCCT Research Group: The effects of intensive treatment of diabetes in the development and progression of long-term complications in insulin dependent diabetes mellitus. *N Engl J Med* 329:977–86, 1993.

Drash AL: *Diabetes Mellitus in the Child and Adolescent.* Chicago, Year Book Medical Publishers, 1987.

Jackson RI, Guthrie RA: *The Physiological Management of Diabetes in Children.* New York, Elsevier Science Publishing Company, 1986.

Kelnar CJH: *Childhood and Adolescent Diabetes.* London, Chapman and Hall, 1995.

McArthur RG: *Children Have Diabetes too. Learning Together as a Family,* Calgary, Alberta Children's Hospital, 1984.

Moyniham P, Balik B, Eliason S, Haig B: *Diabetes Youth Curriculum: A Toolbox for Educators.* Wayzata, MN, International Diabetes Center, 1988.

Santiago JV (Ed.): *Medical Management of Insulin-Dependent (Type I) Diabetes Mellitus,* 2nd ed. Alexandria, VA, Am. Diabetes Assoc., 1994. An update of the comprehensive *Physician's Guide to Insulin-Dependent (Type I) Diabetes Mellitus* for the entire health-care team.

The Take-Charge Guide to Type I Diabetes. Alexandria, VA, Am. Diabetes Assoc., 1994. The best resource book for anyone with type I diabetes.

Travis, LB: *An Instructional Aid on Insulin Dependent Diabetes Mellitus,* 9th ed. Austin, TX, Century Business Communications, Inc., 1993.

Travis LB, Brouhard BH, Schreiner BJ: *Diabetes Mellitus in Children and Adolescents.* Philadelphia, W.B. Saunders, 1987.

Type II Diabetes

Branch LG, Meyers AR: Assessing physical function in the elderly. *Clinics in Geriatric Medicine,* 3:29–51, 1987.

Ciocon JO, Potter JF: Age-related changes in human memory: normal and abnormal. *Geriatrics* 43(10):43–48, 1988.

Folstein MF, et al: The Mini-Mental Health Exam. *JAMA,* 185:914–19, 1963.

Petzinger, R A: Diabetes aids and products for people with visual or physical impairment. *The Diabetes Educator,* March/April 121–38, 1992.

Raskin P (Ed.): *Medical Management of Non-Insulin-Dependent (Type II) Diabetes Mellitus,* 3rd ed. Alexandria, VA, Am. Diabetes Assoc., 1993. An update of the comprehensive *Physician's Guide to Non-Insulin-Dependent (Type II) Diabetes Mellitus* for the entire health-care team.

Type II Diabetes: Your Healthy Living Guide. Alexandria, VA, Am. Diabetes Assoc., 1992. The best resource book for anyone with type II diabetes.

General

Buyer's Guide to Diabetes Supplies. Alexandria, VA, Am. Diabetes Assoc. A yearly reprint from *Diabetes Forecast* comparing features on everything from insulin to glucose meters to injection aids.

Clinical Practice Recommendations. Alexandria, VA, Am. Diabetes Assoc. A yearly supplement to *Diabetes Care* containing all current American Diabetes Association medical position and consensus statements and technical reviews.

Davidson JK: *Clinical Diabetes Mellitus: A Problem-Oriented Approach,* 2nd ed. New York, Thieme Medical Publishers, 1991.

Diabetes Forecast. Alexandria, VA, Am. Diabetes Assoc., monthly consumer magazine.

Etzwiler DD, Franz MJ, Hollander P, Joynes JO: *Learning to Live WELL with Diabetes.* Minnetonka, MN, International Diabetes Center, 1991.

Funnell MM, Haas LB: Technical Review: National Standards for diabetes self-management programs. *Diabetes Care* 17:100–116, 1995.

Haire-Joshu D (Ed.): *Management of Diabetes Mellitus: Perspectives of Care Across the Life Span.* St. Louis, Mosby-Year Book, 1992.

Kahn CR, Weir GC: *Joslin's Diabetes Mellitus,* 13th ed. Philadelphia, Lea & Febiger, 1994.

Lebovitz HE (Ed.): *Therapy of Diabetes Mellitus and Related Disorders,* 2nd ed. Alexandria, VA, Am. Diabetes Assoc., 1994. The comprehensive guide to diabetes treatment.

Meeting the Standards: A Manual for Completing the American Diabetes Association Application for Recognition. Alexandria, VA, Am. Diabetes Assoc., 1991, or in press. Assistance in having your diabetes education program recognized by American Diabetes Association.

Rifkin H, Porte D (Eds.): *Diabetes Mellitus: Theory and Practice,* 4th ed. New York, Elsevier Science Publishing Company, 1990.

OTHER SOURCES OF INFORMATION AND MATERIALS

AMERICAN ASSOCIATION OF
DIABETES EDUCATORS
(800) 338-3633
(312) 644-2233
444 N. Michigan Ave
Suite 1240
Chicago, IL 60611-3901

AMERICAN DIABETES ASSOCIATION
(800) 232-3472
1660 Duke Street (703) 549-1500
Alexandria, VA 22314

AMERICAN DIETETIC ASSOCIATION
(800) 366-1655 Nutr. Hotline
(800) 877-1600
216 West Jackson Blvd.
Suite 800
Chicago, IL 60606-6995

ARMCHAIR FITNESS VIDEOS
(800) 453-6280
CC-M Productions
8510 Cedar Street
Silver Spring, MD 20910

BECTON DICKINSON CONSUMER
PRODUCTS
(800) 237-4554
One Becton Drive
Building #2
Franklin Lakes, NJ 07417-1883

BOEHRINGER MANNHEIM
CORPORATION
(800) 858-8072
9115 Hague Rd.
P.O. Box 50100
Indianapolis, IN 46250-0100

CHRONIMED, INC.
(800) 444-5951
(612) 541-0239
Ridgedale Office Center
Suite 250
13911 Ridgedale Dr.
Minneapolis, MN 55305

DISETRONICS MEDICAL SYSTEMS, INC.
(800) 688-4578
(612) 551-1941
13005 16th Avenue North
Suite 500
Plymouth, MN 55441

ELI LILLY AND COMPANY
(800) 545-5979
(317) 276-2000
Lilly Corporate Center
Indianapolis, IN 46285

HOME DIAGNOSTICS, INC.
(800) 342-7226
(908) 542-7788
51 James Way
Eatontown, NJ 07724

INTERNATIONAL DIABETES CENTER
(612) 927-3393
13911 Ridgedale Dr.
Minnetonka, MN 55447

INTERNATIONAL DIABETES
FEDERATION
32-2/647-4414
40 Rue Washington
1050 Brussels, Belgium

JOSLIN DIABETES CENTER
(617) 732-2415
Communications Office
One Joslin Place
Boston, MA 02215

JUVENILE DIABETES FOUNDATION
(800) 223-1138
432 Park Ave., South
16th Floor
New York, NY 10016

LIFESCAN, INC.
(800) 227-8862
(408) 263-9789
1000 Gilbraltar Drive
Milpitas, CA 95035-6312

MILES, INC. (BAYER)
(800) 348-8100
P.O. Box 70
Elkhart, IN 46515

MINIMED TECHNOLOGIES
(800) 933-3322
12744 San Fernando Rd.
Sylmar, CA 91342

NATIONAL DIABETES INFORMATION
CLEARINGHOUSE
(301) 468-2162
Box NDIC
9000 Rockville Pike
Bethesda, MD 20892

NOVO NORDISK PHARMACEUTICALS,
INC.
(800) 727-6500
(609) 987-5800
100 Overlook Center
Suite 200
Princeton, NJ 08540

THE UPJOHN COMPANY
(800) 253-8600
(616) 323-4000
7000 Portage Road
Kalamazoo, MI 49001

The mission of the American Diabetes Association is to prevent and cure diabetes and to improve the lives of all people affected by diabetes.

The American Diabetes Association (ADA) is the nation's leading voluntary health organization dedicated to diabetes research, information, and advocacy. Through the efforts of state affiliates, local chapters, and thousands of volunteers in more than 800 communities across the United States, ADA carries out this mission, educating and building public awareness about diabetes.

PROFESSIONAL SECTION MEMBERSHIP

As a member of ADA's Professional Section, you access an important network of 11,000 professionals involved in all aspects of diabetes health care —from diabetes treatment and education to diabetes research.

ADA provides a wide range of services and benefits to its professional members, including discounted registration fees for scientific meetings and education programs at the local and national levels; a subscription to one of ADA's professional journals; discounts on the entire library of ADA journals and books; listing in the Professional Section Membership Directory; council membership; a free subscription to Professional Section News, ADA's quarterly member newsletter; and the latest ADA Clinical Practice Recommendations.

Journal Subscriptions

DIABETES

The world's most cited journal in the field of diabetes research. Features major scientific papers related to the molecular, biochemical, and cellular aspects of diabetes. 12 issues/yr.

DIABETES CARE

This monthly clinical research journal presents the latest clinical findings related to diagnosis, diet, exercise, monitoring, drug therapy, complications, and management of diabetes. Includes analysis and commentary on what the latest findings mean for you and your patients. 12 issues/yr.

DIABETES REVIEWS

World-renowned diabetes investigators review specific topics in their fields and discuss the clinical significance of their research. Each issue is devoted to a single topic and explores the hottest issues in a convenient format for the busy clinician to keep up-to-date on what's truly new in research. 4 issues/yr.

CLINICAL DIABETES
Newsletter geared toward professionals with busy schedules. Presents in-depth reviews on important topics in diabetes treatment, plus medical and legal case studies and digests of current research. 6 issues/yr.

DIABETES SPECTRUM
Concise, ready-to-use information for diabetes educators and counselors. Translates the latest clinical findings into practical strategies, techniques, and materials you can use immediately to help your patients. 6 issues/yr.

DIABETES FORECAST
ADA's magazine for patients and their families features advice on diet, exercise, and other lifestyle changes, plus the latest developments in new technology and research. It is a valuable tool for patient education.

For more information about membership and subscriptions, contact:

AMERICAN DIABETES ASSOCIATION
Customer Service Department
1660 Duke Street
Alexandria, VA 22314

To order, call (800) 232-3472 or (703) 549-1500.
Or mail in the order form on page 64.

THE ADA CLINICAL EDUCATION SERIES ON CD-ROM   NEW!
The first all-in-one database of diabetes treatment information. Includes: Medical Management of Type I Diabetes; Medical Management of Type II Diabetes; Therapy for Diabetes Mellitus and Related Disorders, 2nd Ed.; Medical Management of Pregnancy Complicated by Diabetes, 2nd Ed.; plus ADA's Clinical Practice Recommendations 1995. It's all on one compact disc, allowing for quick searches of key terms or phrases across all titles. It also features a "hypertext link" giving you instantaneous browsing between text, references, and illustrations. If you need assistance, technical experts are available to help. System requirements: Macintosh - 68020 or greater processor, System 7.0 or greater, 2MB RAM (4MB recommended); Windows - 386 or 486 processor (486 recommended), Windows 3.1 or greater, 4MB RAM. 1995. #PCDROM1
Nonmember: $225.00; Member: $179.50

INTENSIVE DIABETES MANAGEMENT   NEW!
An all-inclusive "how to" on implementing tight diabetes control in your practice. Written by a team of experts with first-hand DCCT experience, this valuable guide provides you with the practical information you need. Contents: The Team Approach, Education, Rationale for Intensification, Multiple-Component Insulin Regimens, Monitoring, Nutrition, Psychological Support and Behavioral Issues, Follow-Up and Preventive Care Guidelines, Alternative Insulin Delivery Systems, Complications and Adverse Effects, and Resources. Softcover; approximately 112 pages. #PMIDM Nonmember: $37.50; Member: $29.95

HANDBOOK OF DIABETES AND EXERCISE   Summer 1995!
The first comprehensive guide to prescribing exercise as a therapy. Endorsed by the American College of Sports Medicine, this valuable book examines the physiological effects of exercise and its metabolic benefits for patients with diabetes. It also delves into dietary management, insulin adjustment, and behavioral issues. Softcover; approximately 350 pages. #PMHDE
Nonmember: $49.95; Member: $39.95

MEDICAL MANAGEMENT OF INSULIN-DEPENDENT (TYPE I)
DIABETES, 2ND EDITION
formerly: *Physician's Guide to Insulin-Dependent (Type I) Diabetes*
The DCCT proved that complications such as neuropathy, nephropathy, and retinopathy can be halted, or prevented, with proper diabetes management. This book helps you help your patients improve their diabetes management providing instruction on all issues impacting type I diabetes, including: blood glucose regulation, nutrition, exercise, blood pressure, and blood lipid levels. 1994. Softcover. #PMMT1 Nonmember: $37.50; Member: $29.95

MEDICAL MANAGEMENT OF NON-INSULIN-DEPENDENT (TYPE II)
DIABETES, 3RD EDITION
formerly: *Physician's Guide to Non-Insulin-Dependent (Type II) Diabetes*
This new book will give you the tools you need to diagnose and treat type II diabetes and other forms of glucose intolerance. Includes: revised diagnosis and classification criteria, updated information on pathogenesis, new strategies for achieving better metabolic control, new information on preventing and treating complications, as well as ADA's new nutrition recommendations and standards of medical care. NIDDM. 1994. Softcover. #PMMT2
Nonmember: $37.50; Member: $29.95

THERAPY FOR DIABETES MELLITUS AND RELATED DISORDERS, 2ND EDITION
Put the knowledge of more than 50 diabetes experts right at your fingertips! Updated to reflect DCCT findings, each chapter focuses on a different aspect of diabetes and its complications, presenting a concise, practical approach to treatment. Chapters include: DCCT: Significance & Implications; Rationale for Management of Hyperglycemia; Role of the Diabetes Educator; Nutrition Management; Metformin; Antihypertensive Therapy; Noninvasive Cardiac Testing; Chronic Renal Failure; Dyslipidemia; and much more. 1994. Softcover; 384 pages. #PMTDRD2 Nonmember: $34.50; Member: $27.50

MEDICAL MANAGEMENT OF PREGNANCY COMPLICATED
BY DIABETES, 2ND EDITION
Just updated with the new ADA Nutrition Recommendations! A must-read for anyone involved in treating women with type I, type II, or gestational diabetes! This concise, yet comprehensive guide takes you through every aspect of pregnancy and diabetes, from prepregnancy counseling to postpartum follow-up. Provides precise protocols for treatment of both pre-existing and gestational diabetes. Tabbed and well indexed for easy access to important information. 1995. Softcover; 136 pages. #PMMPCD Nonmember: $37.50; Member: $29.95

DIABETES EDUCATION GOALS   NEW!
Features the most up-to-date advice on how to assess, plan, and evaluate patient education and counseling programs, including the newly revised content areas recommended by the National Diabetes Advisory Board. Divided into sections on IDDM, NIDDM, and gestational diabetes, the book highlights both short-term and continuing goals. It also features sections devoted to age-sensitive considerations and approaches for educating patients with special challenges to learning. More than a series of checklists, this valuable guide focuses on the education process and emphasizes assessing the unique needs of each patient. A vital addition to your library! 1995. Softcover; 64 pages. #PEDEG Nonmember: $21.95; Member: $17.50

MAXIMIZING THE ROLE OF NUTRITION IN DIABETES MANAGEMENT   NEW!
This book discusses the role of medical nutrition therapy (MNT) in diabetes management, integrating medical, nutritional, and behavioral sciences. The focus is on the implications of the DCCT for nutritional management of type I and type II diabetes. Topics include: exercise, insulin regimens, oral hypoglycemic agents, blood glucose monitoring, and diabetes complications. 1994. Softcover; 64 pages. #PMNDMB Nonmember: $21.95; Member: $17.50

ADA 1994 NUTRITION RECOMMENDATIONS: A LECTURE PROGRAM
These color slides present an in-depth discussion of ADA's new nutrition guidelines, covering topics such as the goals of medical nutrition therapy for type I and type II diabetes, and recommendations on protein, carbohydrates, and fiber. Includes talking points for slides and copies of the ADA nutrition position statement and technical review. 21 color slides. #PMNDMSS Nonmember: $60.00; Member: $50.00

DIABETES: 1995 VITAL STATISTICS   Fall 1995
Our ever-popular book of diabetes facts and figures has been revised to include the most up-to-date information available. You'll find new information on prevalence and incidence by age and race, diabetes risk factors, diabetes in minorities, complications, mortality, use of health care, costs, treatment, and more. Extensive charts and graphs clarify important information. Perfect for researchers, diabetes educators, and anyone interested in the latest diabetes data. 1995. Softcover; 72 pages. #PMDVS95 Nonmember: $18.50; Member: $14.75

CLINICAL PRACTICE RECOMMENDATIONS 1995   NEW!
Stay on top of the diabetes treatment recommendations from the American Diabetes Association. This supplement to *Diabetes Care* features all current ADA position and consensus statements related to clinical practice. Topics include: screening, standards of medical care, exercise, pancreas transplantation, food labeling, self-monitoring, neuropathy, lipid disorders, and more. It also contains the recently revised "National Standard for Diabetes Self-Management Education Programs." 1995. Softcover; 104 pages. #PJSCPR95
Nonmember: $12.50; Member: $10.00

CARDIOVASCULAR RISK FACTOR MANAGEMENT: A LECTURE PROGRAM
This 3-hour program focuses on diabetes and its complications as risk factors for atherosclerotic vascular disease. Covers epidemiology, pathophysiology, assessment, and treatment for each risk factor. Includes case study discussion and presenter's script. 1993. 92 color slides. #PMCEP3SS
Nonmember: $250.00; Member: $200.00

RESOURCES ORDER FORM

Title		Qty.	Price	Total
CD-ROM Clinical Education Series	#PCDROM1	____ @	$ _____ each =	$ _____
Intensive Diabetes Management	#PMIDM	____ @	$ _____ each =	$ _____
Handbook of Diabetes and Exercise	#PMHDE	____ @	$ _____ each =	$ _____
Medical Management of Type I Diabetes, 2nd Edition	#PMMT1	____ @	$ _____ each =	$ _____
Medical Management of Type II Diabetes, 3rd Edition	#PMMT2	____ @	$ _____ each =	$ _____
Therapy for Diabetes Mellitus, 2nd Edition	#PMTDRD2	____ @	$ _____ each =	$ _____
Medical Management of Pregnancy Complicated by Diabetes, 2nd Edition	#PMMPCD	____ @	$ _____ each =	$ _____
Diabetes Education Goals	#PEDEG	____ @	$ _____ each =	$ _____
Maximizing the Role of Nutrition in Diabetes Management	#PMNDMB	____ @	$ _____ each =	$ _____
1994 ADA Nutrition Recommendations: A Lecture Program	#PMNDMSS	____ @	$ _____ each =	$ _____
Diabetes: 1995 Vital Statistics	#PMDVS95	____ @	$ _____ each =	$ _____
Clinical Practice Recommendations 1995	#PJSCPR95	____ @	$ _____ each =	$ _____
Cardiovascular Risk Factor Management	#PMCEP3SS	____ @	$ _____ each =	$ _____

Shipping & Handling
Up to $30.00.................$3.00
$30.01–$50.00..............$4.00
Over $50.00 ....8% of order

Publications Subtotal: $ _____
VA Residents Add 4.5% Sales Tax: $ _____
Shipping & Handling (based on subtotal): $ _____
Grand Total: $ _____

SHIP TO:
Name _____
Addres _____
City/State/Zip _____

PH39502

Payment enclosed (check or money order) OR
Charge my: ☐ VISA ☐ MC ☐ AMEX
Account #_____
Signature _____ Exp. Date_____

Allow 2–3 weeks for shipment. Add $3.00 to shipping & handling for each additional shipping address. Add $15 to shipping & handling for each international shipment. Foreign orders must be paid in U.S. funds, drawn on a U.S. bank. Prices subject to change without notice.

Mail to: American Diabetes Association
             1970 Chain Bridge Road
             McLean, VA 22109-0592

APPLICATION FOR PROFESSIONAL MEMBERSHIP

(please print)

Name _____

Title _____ Organization/Institution_____

Address _____

City _____ State _____ Zip _____

Phone (_____) _____ Is this your ☐ Home or ☐ Office?

Education: Degree _____ Specialty _____ Date Earned _____

Degree _____ Specialty _____ Date Earned _____

Primary Area of Focus ☐ Clinical Practice ☐ Research ☐ Education ☐ Industry

PROFESSIONAL SECTION MEMBERSHIP DIRECTORY INFORMATION

Please check your specialty or specialties (up to 3) for your Directory listing:

☐ Administration (AD)
☐ Biochemistry (BC)
☐ Cardiology (CA)
☐ Dentistry (DO)
☐ Dermatology (DE)
☐ Education (ED)
☐ Epidemiology (EP)
☐ Adult Endocrinology (EN)
☐ Exercise Physiology (EX)
☐ Family Practice (FP)
☐ General Practice (GP)

☐ Geriatrics (GE)
☐ Internal Medicine (IM)
☐ Immunology (IU)
☐ Metabolism (ME)
☐ Nephrology (NE)
☐ Neurology (NR)
☐ Nursing (NS)
☐ Nutrition (NU)
☐ Obstetrics/Gynecology (OG)
☐ Ophthalmology (OP)
☐ Optometry (OT)

☐ Orthopedics (OR)
☐ Osteopathy (OS)
☐ Pathology (PT)
☐ Pediatric Endocrinology (PN)
☐ Pediatrics (PE)
☐ Pedorthic Management (PR)
☐ Pharmacology (PA)
☐ Pharmacy (PM)
☐ Physical Therapy (PX)
☐ Physiology (PY)
☐ Podiatry (PO)

☐ Psychiatry (PS)
☐ Psychology (PC)
☐ Public Health (PH)
☐ Research (RE)
☐ Social Work (SW)
☐ Surgery (SU)
☐ Urology (UR)
☐ Other:
_____
_____
_____

Please check one of the following locations:

☐ Hospital
☐ HMO
☐ Public Health
☐ Private/group practice

☐ Pharmaceutical/
Manufacturing
☐ Pharmacy
☐ University/Acedemic

☐ Nursing Home
☐ Private Research Center
☐ Home Health
☐ Government

☐ Other:
_____

FREE COUNCIL MEMBERSHIP

Please check your selection(s). Professional Section members receive *one free* Council membership. Additional Council Membership are available for $25 each.

☐ Council on Complications (TT)
☐ Council on Diabetes in Pregnancy (BB)
☐ Council on Diabetes in Youth (EE)
☐ Council on Behavioral Medicine and Psychology (PP)
☐ Council on Education (SS)

☐ Council on Foot Care (RR)
☐ Council on Epidemiology and Statistics (CC)
☐ Council on Clinical Endocrinology, Diabetes & Metabolism (SS)
☐ Council on Exercise (XX)

☐ Council on Health Care (DD)
☐ Council on Nutritional Sciences and Metabolism (AA)
☐ Council on Molecular, Cellular & Biochemical Aspects of Diabetes (MM)

MEMBERSHIP CATEGORY/DUES INFORMATION

Please check appropriate membership category and journal selections. Physicians must select Category I.

	Category I	Category II
Regular	☐ $125	☐ $ 50
In-Training	☐ $ 65	☐ $ 25
International.................................	☐ $180	☐ $ 65
International In-Training..............	☐ $118	☐ $ 40

If you choose:
Category I
Please select one
☐ *Diabetes*
☐ *Diabetes* plus *Abstract Book*
(Add $10 U.S., CAN, MEX/$18 International to dues)
☐ *Diabetes Care*

Category II
members automatically receive *Diabetes Spectrum*

APPLICATION FOR PROFESSIONAL MEMBERSHIP—CONTINUED

ADDITIONAL JOURNAL SUBSCRIPTIONS

	Regular	International**
Diabetes (monthly)	☐ $75	☐ $130
Abstract Book (annual) (for 1995 Scientific Sessions)	☐ $10	☐ $18
Diabetes Care (monthly)	☐ $75	☐ $130
Diabetes Reviews (quarterly)	☐ $45	☐ $65
Diabetes Spectrum (bimonthly)	☐ $15	☐ $30
Diabetes Forecast (monthly)	☐ $12	☐ $37
Clinical Diabetes (bimonthly)	☐ $15	☐ $21

**Includes all members outside the U.S., Canada and Mexico. Prices reflect a charge for expedited delivery service.

I am enclosing:

☐ A. $ _____ for a ☐ New ☐ Renewed Membership

☐ B. $ _____ for publications

☐ C. $ _____ for _____ additional council(s)

☐ D. $ _____ for 7% GST (*Canadian members only*: applies to total of A, B, & C)

TOTAL AMOUNT $_____.

☐ Payment enclosed (check or money order)

☐ Charge my: ☐ VISA ☐ MC ☐ AMEX

Account #_____

Signature _____ Exp. Date_____

Questions? Call ADA Customer Service at 1-800-232-3472, ext. 343 or (703) 549-1500, ext. 343. Or fax to (703) 549-6995.

The portion of membership dues set aside for publications is as follows:

Category I: Diabetes or Diabetes Care $75 **Category II:** Diabetes Spectrum $15

Please allow 7–9 weeks for order processing.

Mail to: American Diabetes Association
Professional Section Membership
Department 0028
Washington, DC 20073-0028

Managing Investor Relations

Strategies and Techniques

Managing Investor Relations

Strategies and Techniques

Joseph J. Graves, Jr.

DOW JONES-IRWIN
Homewood, Illinois   60430

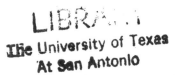

© DOW JONES-IRWIN, 1982

ISBN 0-87094-346-4
Library of Congress Catalog Card No. 82–71348

Printed in the United States of America

1 2 3 4 5 6 7 8 9 0 MP 9 8 7 6 5 4 3 2

To my wife, Millie,
for support, patience, and understanding.

Foreword

Over the past two decades, investor relations, perhaps more so than any other corporate function, has experienced a significant upgrading. In earlier days, the financial relations specialist prepared news releases on quarterly results, wrote and made certain the quarterly report to stockholders was in the mail on the agreed-on date, and most critical, suffered through the preparation of the annual report. The same person sometimes, but not all that often, was called upon to write speeches for presentations to security analyst groups. Rarely did the financial public relations person hold face-to-face meetings with security analysts, then mostly regarded as the exclusive domain of the chief financial officer or his duly appointed, numbers-oriented representative.

The financial relations specialist was the communications technician—the person who put words on paper and was the interface with the typesetter and the printer.

But times have changed and the role of the financial or investor relations specialist has changed. Still the communicator, the investor relations person (nowadays as likely to be female as male) contributes to both policy and strategy in relationships with the total financial community. It makes little difference that the function may report to the chief financial officer rather than the chief public relations officer. The function is now appropriately recognized in the corporate hierarchy befitting the importance of its mission.

Moreover, there has been a gratifying expansion in the scope of the job. No longer is it the primary mission of the financial relations officer to "put out a release." The job starts with an analysis of the corporation itself and its positioning vis-à-vis other corporations against which it will be measured by the financial community. It involves a careful analysis of the market for its securities and present and potential investors, employing sophisticated research techniques.

It brings into being a strategy that reconciles the needs of the marketplace with the objectives of the corporation. And it implements programs to reach target audiences with key corporate messages. All the while it fulfills SEC and New York Stock Exchange obligations and observes the myriad of legal restraints governing the disclosure of sensitive information.

Most certainly, this informative and comprehensive book on investor relations could not have been written 20 years ago, or even 10. The investor relations function was not nearly so developed as to encompass the broad range of activity which Joe Graves so ably sets forth in this, the most complete and up-to-date book on the investor relations function. As a contributor to and as a chronicler of the now-recognized and appreciated role of investor relations, Joe Graves merits the respect and gratitude of his highly skilled associates who link America's corporations with the world of investors who furnish the wherewithal that assures their very existence. It merits the attention not only of investor relations specialists but even more so, senior corporate officers whose principal responsibility is the financial well-being of the corporation.

Harold Burson

Preface

In 1980, a respected financial publication stated that one of the problems in discussing financial communications is the lack of information on the subject. With 30 years of experience in the field, backed by bulging boxes of resource material, I found the statement to be incredibly untrue.

So why would a respected publication make the statement? An intensive investigation on my part produced the answer: There has never been a single source that brought the information together. I immediately began the arduous and methodical task of poring through my files and the resource works of other experts in the field.

Now, for the first time, the diverse opinions of numerous thought leaders in financial communications and the findings of dozens of surveys on the major facets of financial communications are brought together in one document. There is one very important, marked difference between my book and other attempts to explain financial communications in various publications.

Rather than a dull, stereotyped ABC listing of what to do, I have included coverage of a wide range of activities that have worked and not worked on various audiences in the marketplace. I have also drawn profiles on the overall market and its numerous segments. *Thus, the advice given in this book is not merely what to do but why to do it.*

The result is a highly informative and useful handbook with all of the successes, failures, and foibles, directing you, the reader, in how I and other experts have done it, why we have done it, and what will work for you.

Thanks to Barbara Allamian, Patricia Conerty Clarke, L. James Lovejoy, Ellen Steininger, and Joanne Tremulis for all of the research and other chores.

Joseph J. Graves, Jr.

Contents

and suppliers; and setting up the plan, which covers design, copy, photography, your role in the process, and how to schedule the plan flow.

Chapter 11—Corporate Advertising, 243

What a vague and indefinite art we practice! Corporate advertising, still in its infancy compared with other communications techniques, is veiled in a shroud of mystique. The reasons why are given along with the history of corporate advertising; its numerous definitions; the various viewpoints, including those of the professional, management, the Street, and trade; who is responsible for it; its inner workings; the three Cs; preparing for the message; what you say; and pumping the P/E.

Other contents: the role of advocacy; how much is spent on corporate advertising; the best media in which to use it; and the effectiveness of corporate advertising.

Chapter 12—Meetings, 281

Financial analysts say they want their face-to-face sessions to be strictly business, but do they mean it? Here are descriptions of rather "unusual" meetings which analysts really enjoyed.

Other contents: the amount of time management devotes to meetings; the contents of meetings; the types of programs; the number of society visits by management; the visits analysts make; the number and types of meetings the professionals attend; what the professionals like to hear; how to stage successful meetings, as related by the experts; and detailed plans for a successful meeting.

Chapter 13—On the Offense in Troubled Times, 311

The old expression "The best defense is a good offense" is very applicable to the corporate raid. For the company that wants to remain independent, there is advice on the historical record and the defense and battle plan. The defense and battle plan consists of three sections: yardstick to measure vulnerability; long-range preventive measures; and specific measures to combat an offer. Also included: offering yourself up for marriage; the odds of success today; how companies are prepared or unprepared; and whether there should even be a defense.

Chapter 14—How to Organize Your Communications, 324

Being a good manager is a fundamental step toward doing your job in the most professional manner. To do so, you must overcome the Neanderthal thinking of some managements. Investor relations, born in the go-go days of the yo-yo stock market, has had a troubled history. Compare yourself with the typical investor relations manager on age, experience, education, activities, and salary. Also discussed are in-house versus outside counsel, including a list of the largest communications counselors; organizing the communications function by type of company; and the search for the "optimum."

CHAPTER ONE

The Market Constituency

More and more of U.S. industry is coming to be owned by banks, pension funds and other large financial institutions, and less and less by individual investors. The result is a profound change in American capitalism—and in the market for common stocks.[1]
U.S.News & World Report, July 18, 1977

At least 7 million shareholders have defected from the stock market since 1970, leaving equities more than ever the province of giant institutional investors.[2]
Business Week, August 13, 1979

The NYSE's 1980 Shareownership Survey disclosed a dramatic resurgence of shareownership in the United States between mid-1975 and mid-1980.[3]
New York Stock Exchange Fact Book, 1981

GLOOM, DOOM, AND—CHEER!

The 4.6 million shareholders who entered the stock market from 1975 to 1980 raised the total to 29.8 million individuals for the beginning of the 1980 decade. While this number was short of the record 30.8 million individuals in the market in the early 1970s, it was a dramatic increase of 18.1 percent.

Why the wide disparity between what leading business publications were predicting and what actually happened, especially since the predictions were supported by hosts of economic and investment professionals? Did it exist because the publications were relying on the conventional wisdom that the public would not come back to equities

---

[1] "Who Owns American Industry? The Big Shift Underway," *U.S.News & World Report*, July 18, 1977, p. 70. Copyright 1977, U.S.News & World Report, Inc.

[2] "The Death of Equities," *Business Week*, August 13, 1979, p. 54. Reprinted from the August 13, 1979 issue of *Business Week* by special permission, © by McGraw-Hill, Inc., New York, N.Y. 10020. All rights reserved.

[3] Barbara Wheeler, *New York Stock Exchange Fact Book*, 1981, p. 47.

at least until the economics were right again—and they did not see normalcy in the economy for the foreseeable future?

To communicate to the market, you must have a basic understanding of what the market is. To understand why it acts and reacts is a science that often puzzles experts. But some of the forces at work will be explained, along with an in-depth report on who owns corporate America.

U.S.News & World Report was relying on a group of experts, its Economic Unit, when it drew these conclusions:

> More people than ever before have a stake in the stock market, but the interests of most are reflected through the financial institutions that represent them and now do the great bulk of the actual buying and selling of shares.
>
> Fewer people are involved directly in the market through ownership of stocks in their own names. From the high-water mark of 31 million in 1970, the number of shareholders has fallen to little more than 25 million at latest count—and it may be even smaller now.
>
> The big institutions now own so much of the stock of leading corporations that they are finding it more difficult to buy or sell these well-known stocks without driving prices sharply up or down. As a result, there is a growing interest—among individuals and more recently among the institutions, too—in finding smaller companies that are growing and well managed and whose shares have not yet been gobbled by big investors.[4]

"There is concern over what the swift shift in ownership of American industry will lead to in the future. There's every reason to believe this shift will continue," *U.S.News & World Report* concluded with a low degree of optimism.[5]

Business Week saw the problem in a different way. It saw a mass exodus from the market by institutions. The publications bleakly noted:

> And now the institutions have been given the go-ahead to shift more of their money from stocks—and bonds—into other investments. If the institutions, who control the bulk of the nation's wealth, now withdraw billions from both the stock and bond markets, the implications for the U.S. economy could not be worse. Says Robert S. Salomon, Jr., a general partner in Salomon Bros., "We are running the risk of immobilizing a substantial portion of the world's wealth in someone's stamp collection."[6]

---

[4] "Who Owns American Industry?", p. 70.

[5] Ibid., p. 71.

[6] "The Death of Equities," p. 54.

Business Week added:

> Even institutions that have so far remained in the financial markets are pouring money into short-term investments and such "alternate equity" investments as mortgage-backed paper, foreign securities, venture capital, leases, guaranteed insurance contracts, indexed bonds, stock options, and futures. At the same time, individuals who are not gobbling up hard assets are flocking into money market funds to nail down high rates, or into municipal bonds to escape heavy taxes on inflated incomes. Few corporations can find buyers for their stocks, forcing them to add debt to a point where balance sheets seem permanently out of whack. On Wall Street, the flight from stocks has forced firms to push alternative investments hard— thereby drawing still more money from the stock market.[7]

Reasons for Fleeing the Market

It was said in the late 1970s that only the elderly who did not understand the changes in the nation's financial markets, or who were unable to adjust to them, were sticking with stocks. Numerous reasons were given for the flight from the market. One was that the end of fixed stock market commissions had thinned the ranks of firms that sold stocks and had reduced the profit from selling stocks for virtually all firms. It was apparent that new rules had developed and that some of the old rules no longer applied.

One rule whose demise helped do the stock market in could be summed up thus: By buying stocks, investors could beat inflation. Stocks were a reasonable hedge when inflation was low. But they proved helpless against the awesome inflation of the 1970s. People no longer think of stocks as an inflation hedge, and they are right. Since 1968, according to a study by Salomon Brothers, stocks have appreciated by a compound annual rate of 3.1 percent, while the consumer price index has surged by 6.5 percent. By contrast, gold, diamonds, and single-family housing rose in price far faster than stocks.

The biggest ogre was inflation, according to many sources. Part of the rationale for this view was that during periods of rapid inflation profits fall because most businesses cannot raise prices quickly enough to keep up with costs. Profit gains are largely illusory because inflation makes them look rosier than they actually are. Experience, too, has taught investors that inflation leads to an economic downturn that will wreck corporate profitability and stock prices. This happened in 1974, when a deep recession followed the last burst of double-digit inflation. Investors will jump from stocks to bonds or other investments to nail down high rates. Inflation also prompts corporations to sell debt because it is tax deductible and can be paid off in cheaper dollars. What-

---

[7] Ibid.

ever caused it, the institutionalization of inflation—along with structural changes in communications and psychology—killed the U.S. equity market for millions of investors, *Business Week* concluded.

Today, the old attitude of buying solid stocks as a cornerstone for one's life savings and retirement has simply disappeared, along with the inflation hedge concept, in the minds of some. Said one U.S. executive, "Have you been to an American shareholders' meeting lately? They're all old fogies. The stock market is just not where the action's at."

The Gloom versus Reality

How did the gloom and doom compare with what actually happened from the late 1970s well into the 1980s?

The NYSE study noted that a resurgence of institutional and individual investor confidence in equities had made 1980 a bonanza year for the New York Stock Exchange. Average daily volume set a record of 44.9 million shares, easily surpassing the previous record of 32.2 million shares. Aggregate volume came to 11.4 billion shares, producing an extraordinary turnover rate of 36 percent. Trading volume measured in dollars increased 57 percent to a record $375 billion.

Volume records in other equity markets were also broken. The American Stock Exchange broke its record volume set in 1968. Regional exchanges continued to expand, while over-the-counter trading exploded with heavy interest in new equity issues.

Leading this surge was the entry of 6½ million shareholders into the market for the first time. Their median age of only 36 years had a dramatic effect on the overall median age of investors. It was 46 years in 1980, compared with 53 years in 1975, marking the lowest overall median age since at least the early 1950s, when it was 51 years.

As I have noted, the wide disparity between what leading business publications were predicting and what actually happened may have arisen because the publications were relying on the conventional wisdom that the public would not come back to equities until the economics were right again.

There is a question of whether or not conventional wisdom was a fact or a rationalization by academicians, congressmen, and government regulators whose anti-savings and anti-investment persuasion made it impossible for most companies to raise equity capital. There were full up and down economic cycles during the 1950s and 1960s when the market was gaining an average of 1 million new investors each year. There also were full up and down economic cycles in the 1970s when the market was losing close to a million investors every year. The difference between the two periods was not simple economic conditions.

Triggering the flight from the market was the Tax Reform Act in 1969. By raising the capital gains tax rate to 49 percent, the act threw risk-reward ratios out of kilter. This worsened when Congress and the SEC made it unprofitable for brokerage firms to provide small investors with the broad range of equities research they needed. These federal policies were enacted at a time when business really needed help in trying to build stronger shareholder bases. It is interesting to note that individual investors have returned to the market since 1978 when the taxes on capital gains came down at the demand of both business and investors.

What Influences a Stock?

The turnaround because of legislative attitudes is important, but it is also necessary to analyze stocks because stocks are influenced by many factors other than the fundamental nature of a company.

Approximately one third of a stock's price movement is accounted for by market influence, one third by industry group influence, and one third by earnings and company fundamentals. A stock with poor earnings can be dragged up by favorable market and group influences, or a stock with good earnings can be dragged down by unfavorable market and group trends.

For example, I noticed that the performance of railroads would pull up or drive down the stock prices of Trans Union Corporation and other tank car leasing companies even though there was little relationship between car leasing and railroad operations. By leasing to shippers and not doing business with railroads, Trans Union had an annual growth rate of 12 percent for 12 years, as compared to the ups and downs of railroads, but it was still under the strong influence of railroad stock pricing.

Sometimes the market just ignores every communications device used to promote interest in a stock because the price-earnings multiple of the stock is being adjusted to come back into line with the market. Such trends can dominate a stock for a long period of time, sometimes years. One example is Baxter Travenol. Its earnings grew consistently in excess of 20 percent per year, and its dividend was raised at least once a year for more than 10 consecutive years. However, the stock was priced 25 percent lower in the 1980s than in the early 1970s. The problem was that Baxter was one of the nifty-50 institutional favorites in the early 1970s, when it had a price-earnings multiple of 80. Ten years later its price was 14 times earnings, and there was no promotion the company could use to change it.

Stocks run through cycles that take them from low relative valuation and low investor interest to high relative valuation and high investor interest and down again. Week-to-week movements can be influenced, but generally little change can be made against a tidal movement from overvaluation to undervaluation once it is under way. Often a swing to one extreme will be followed by an equal, but opposite, swing, so it is important to know where the stock of your company fits in its ownership cycle at any given time.

Effects on the Market

Many people believe that the market is primarily determined by economic trends and political developments. While these are important, the availability and cost of money, the psychology of investors, and a sense of history are more important.

The financial community may be confused because the stock market today is marching to a different drummer. Long-term trends in the economy, the stock market, and business cycles are distorted and out of synchronization. Causing the distortion are the effects of long economic cycles related to inflation and overinflated credit, the overvaluation of common stocks during the post–World War II bull market that ended in the late 1960s, and the change in preference from stocks to bonds and other investments by institutional investors in the 1970s.

The economy and the stock market are thought to be in transition from one stage of development to another. The underlying conclusion is that this transition reflects a basic background of profound change. The economy is going from supergrowth to a period of slow growth whose duration is unknown. The stock market has been trying to adjust to changes in the economy and to correct the excesses in valuation created in the enthusiastic 1960s. But people, relying on 1950 and 1960 models, are having problems as the environment of the market changes because traditional business cycle analysis is inadequate and even shortsighted.

But transition periods are not unique in stock market history, and this may be one of the weak links in the efforts of business publications to position the stock market in the late 1970s. Transition occurred in the early 1920s, the mid-1930s, and the late 1940s. In each case, an inconsistent stock market confused investors, yet each transition led to a new major up cycle in stocks. Transition means uncertainty, and this, in turn, breeds investor apathy. Some feel that we are in such a phase now. When the transition will end is debatable because of the apparent lack of progress in the major averages. But there are investors who believe that stocks will remain one of the most attractive investment alternatives for many years.

These investors base their conclusion on the idea that since fewer investable funds have been allocated to stocks, these are at attractive prices for any rise. Once the majority of institutions that are still putting minimal new money into equities while holding large cash reserves realize that stocks are undervalued, these institutions will enter the market with renewed vigor. The potential shift of funds from pension funds, insurance companies, and alternative investments is enormous. Thus, the case for a big rise in stock prices becomes persuasive.

There were complete cycles of themes in the evolution of investor psychology from post-World War II to the early 1970s. The themes ranged from conservative to high-risk aggressive themes. Early themes were conservative. There was yield based on total return and asset orientation. This was followed in the late 1950s by the emergence of growth themes involving utilities and foods. Within a decade, high-risk growth themes began to emerge with no particular emphasis on yield or assets. The pinnacle of risk taking was reached with the end of the cycle following the big decline in 1973 and 1974. By then, the theme was growth at any cost. Based on history, the cycle will repeat and aggressive attitudes toward stock ownership will develop again. Eventually, growth will again command a premium. The question is when?

WHO OWNS CORPORATE AMERICA?

While the debate flourished over the death or life of the securities market and the role of the individual investor, *Fortune* was making an in-depth study and forecast for another segment of the financial community—the 25 largest securities firms:

Its forecast: "Before it's finished, the securities business, like the accountants, may be dominated by a 'Big Eight.'"[8]

The Securities Industry

The action since "Mayday," May 1, 1975, when unfixed commission rates on stock transactions came into being, raises images of the old gasoline price wars that used to decimate the ranks of service stations. *Fortune* noted:

> The securities industry has been engaging in "commission-rate wars" on institutional trades, and these too have led to battlefield casualties. The new price competition has all but wiped out one class of firm, the small institutional broker whose main selling point is the research it does on stocks. It has helped extinguish some fine old Wall Street names—White, Weld, for example, which has just been bought by Merrill Lynch. It has encouraged large firms to merge with their own kind and to acquire smaller firms, on the assumption that size will help them deal with this rugged new environment.[9]

In the early 1960s, the number of New York Stock Exchange member firms reached a high of 681. For a while after that, the Exchange population fell slowly, and then, with the arrival of Wall

[8] Carol J. Loomis, "The Shakeout on Wall Street Isn't Over Yet," *Fortune*, May 22, 1978, p. 59. Copyright © 1978 by Time, Inc.

[9] Ibid.

Street's "back office" problems in the late 1960s, it dropped with a rush as the more inefficient firms were forced to liquidate or merge. Two recessions, ever-rising costs, and a declining stock market subsequently clobbered the Street's profits and accelerated the trend. Still more amalgamations resulted from the efforts of many larger firms to go "full service" by acquiring smaller operations with complementary product lines. Between the end of 1968 and Mayday in 1975, the number of NYSE member firms declined from 646 to 505, an average loss of more than 20 firms a year. By the early 1980s, it had shrunk below the 450 level.

Also taking its toll was pricing on institutional trades which eliminated some competitors, most notably a flock of "research" firms having little in the way of other business, such as retail trading, underwriting, or money management, to cushion the shocks. In the era of fixed rates, such firms made extraordinary returns on capital. After Mayday, their problem became one of survival.

With most research firms having accepted merger counsel from the moon, *Fortune* said,

> The institutional business is primarily in the hands of broad-based firms that mutter a lot about "hanging in there" and "being a survivor" and somehow making do in a world still plainly characterized by overcapacity. Basically, these firms expect a continuing shakeout and, by means of it, an eventual return of the institutional business to profitability. Contemplating this golden future, each firm is naturally eager not to get shaken out itself in the meantime. To survive, however, requires it to extract maximum revenues from other parts of its business—and sets up a few more reasons for merging.
>
> At most Wall Street firms these days, hopes about getting those revenues rest on retail business—i.e., individual investors. The particular obsession of most firms is building the size of the sales forces that tap the retail market. If all the firms that would like to acquire more salesmen managed to get all they wanted, the assembled army would be just about large enough to elect a U.S. president.[10]

Many of the leading securities firms cherish their present character and hope to avoid change. (See Table 1–1 for data on *Fortune*'s Big 25 in securities.) Among these are investment bankers that do not want to merge with retail wire houses, partnerships that would like to cling to their clubby ways, and a collection of firms that cannot quite imagine themselves as the junior partner in a merger. Asked an executive at E. F. Hutton, "Do you imagine now that we are going to step out and hyphenate the name?"

The top of the industry also includes a large number of publicly owned companies whose permanent capital might stave off merger for a long time—perhaps even if merger were wise. One can only specu-

---

[10] Ibid., p. 61.

Table 1-1

The *Fortune* Big 25 in securities

THE BIG 25: A LIST YOU'VE NEVER SEEN BEFORE

RANK	COMPANY	SECURITIES REVENUES ($000) 1977	1972	TOTAL CAPITAL ($000) 1977	RANK	1972	RANK	EQUITY CAPITAL ($000) 1977	RANK	1972	RANK	BROKERAGE OFFICES 1977	1972	EMPLOYEES 1977	1972
1	MERRILL LYNCH & CO. INC.[1]	633,566	575,600	645,867	1	464,256	1	545,867	1	444,256	1	365	245	22,539	20,662
2	DEAN WITTER REYNOLDS ORGANIZATION INC.[2]	286,495	136,570	157,853	4	82,361	4	151,035	3	63,578	6	223	82	8,640	4,638
3	THE E.F. HUTTON GROUP INC.[3]	243,723	119,593	174,276	3	82,281	5	123,152	4	59,853	8	201	97	6,741	4,003
4	LOEB RHOADES, HORNBLOWER & CO.[4]	223,410	78,587	120,000	6	80,103	7	97,500	6	65,903	4	161	29	5,646	1,907
5	PAINE WEBBER INC.[5]	206,632	114,468	117,561	8	80,251	6	82,861	9	63,581	5	136	77	5,124	3,947
6	BACHE GROUP INC.[6]	189,391	130,000*	152,325	5	123,501	3	121,439	5	104,241	2	166	113	6,298	5,500
7	SHEARSON HAYDEN STONE INC.[7]	134,250	41,616	84,043	11	29,798	20	49,164	14	22,118	19	128	28	4,137	1,600
8	GOLDMAN, SACHS & CO.	122,250	99,626	117,600	7	77,000	8	92,600	7	62,000	7	14	11	1,615	1,462
9	KIDDER, PEABODY & CO. INC.	120,000*	70,000*	81,011	12	46,027	13	67,213	10	41,499	11	50	38	2,500	1,700
10	LEHMAN BROTHERS KUHN LOEB INC.[9]	112,671	59,096	75,600	15	40,835	16	49,100	15	23,300	18	10	9	1,554	1,248
11	SMITH BARNEY, HARRIS UPHAM & CO. INC.[8]	110,000*	70,000*	61,250	18	46,991	11	33,971	20	23,322	17	90	18	3,132	1,398
12	BLYTH EASTMAN DILLON & CO. INC.[10]	104,737	45,000	85,051	9	40,900	15	52,943	13	24,700	16	43	39	2,495	1,250
13	DREXEL BURNHAM LAMBERT GROUP, INC.[11]	99,367	51,472	75,659	14	41,704	14	39,362	17	20,269	20	34	16	2,311	1,237
14	SALOMON BROTHERS[12]	92,802	75,725	191,700	2	130,700	2	161,950	2	100,700	3	11	11	1,431	1,090
15	MORGAN STANLEY & CO. INC.	82,361	27,326	61,500	17	19,600	22	57,700	11	15,600	21	6		1,100	440
16	THE BECKER WARBURG PARIBAS GROUP[13]	76,800	54,340	67,462	16	30,278	19	41,130	16	28,393	14	14	12	2,043	1,324
17	FIRST BOSTON, INC.	73,427	46,512	84,164	10	56,770	10	84,164	8	56,770	10	18	13	1,187	715
18	THOMSON McKINNON INC.	71,745	41,000	46,480	19	28,522	21	16,780	23	9,995	24	91	55	2,478	1,653
19	DONALDSON, LUFKIN & JENRETTE, INC.[14]	69,139	28,495	76,741	13	64,140	9	53,891	12	58,240	9	17	7	1,526	649
20	A.G. EDWARDS & SONS, INC.[15]	57,353	29,200	35,000	22	16,787	23	34,425	19	14,668	22	126	65	1,898	1,260
21	BEAR, STEARNS & CO.	55,600	41,000	45,500	20	37,500	17	37,500	18	37,500	12	10	8	1,100	783
22	OPPENHEIMER & CO., INC.	41,506	43,207	28,936	24	46,514	12	11,855	24	34,759	13	5	2	1,200	700
23	L.F. ROTHSCHILD, UNTERBERG, TOWBIN[16]	39,820	23,491	40,963	21	30,400	18	31,763	21	26,909	15	13	12	915	750
24	INTER-REGIONAL FINANCIAL GROUP, INC.[17]	37,247	22,568	29,548	23	16,268	24	19,843	22	11,552	23	40	20	1,029	522
25	MOSELEY, HALLGARTEN & ESTABROOK, INC.[18]	33,342	11,020	15,439	25	5,752	25	7,340	25	3,330	25	31	16	812	433
	TOTAL	3,317,634	2,035,512	2,671,529		1,719,239		2,164,548		1,417,036		2,003	1,026	89,451	60,921

[1]1977 data include White Weld Holdings, Inc., acquired in April 1978. [2]1977 data are for the fiscal year ended August 31 and combine Dean Witter Organization Inc. and Reynolds Securities International Inc., which merged in January this year. [3]1972 data are for Dean Witter & Co. Inc. [4]1977 data include California Windsor, a life-insurance company acquired in December. [5]1977 data combine Loeb, Rhoades & Co. and Hornblower, Weeks, Noyes & Trask, Inc., which merged in January this year. 1972 data are for Loeb, Rhoades & Co. [6]1977 data are for the fiscal year ended September 30 and include Mitchell, Hutchins, Inc., acquired in May. 1977 [7]1977 data are for the fiscal year ended July 31 and include Shields Model Roland Holding Corp., acquired in May. 1977. 1977 data are for the fiscal year ended June 30 and include Faulkner, Dawkins & Sullivan, Inc., acquired in August last year. 1972 data are for CBWL-Hayden Stone Inc. [9]1977 securities-revenue data are for the fiscal year ended September 30 and combine Lehman Brothers and Kuhn, Loeb & Co., which merged in December last year. 1972 data are for Lehman Brothers. [10]1972 data are for Blyth & Co. Inc. [11]1972 data are for Burnham & Co. Inc. [12]All data are for the fiscal year ended September 30 [13]1977 data are for the fiscal year ended October 28. 1972 data are for A. G. Becker & Co. Inc. [14]1977 data include Pershing & Co. and Wood Struthers & Winthrop Inc., both acquired in December. 1977 [15]1977 financial data are for the fiscal year ended February 28. 1978, and, except for securities revenues, are preliminary [16]1977 data are for the fiscal year ended September 30 and include C. E. Unterberg, Towbin. [17]1977 data are for Dain, Kalman & Quail. Inc. [18]1972 data are for F. S. Moseley & Co. *FORTUNE estimate, based on known data for other recent years

Source: Carol J. Loomis, "The Shakeout on Wall Street Isn't Over Yet," *Fortune*, May 22, 1978, p. 61.

Credit: *Fortune* Magazine Art Department/Bob Weiss Associates, Inc.

late as to the eventual shape of the industry. One hypothesis put forth by Paine Webber is that the industry may shake down into a "Big Eight," but accommodating a sizable number of smaller specialist and regional firms—somewhat in the mode of the accounting profession. Most of the Big Eight would be fully integrated firms whose very size would make them capable of standing toe to toe with their institutional customers.

Stocks Have Wide Ownership

While there is concern about the decline of the small shareholder, the concentration of stocks in funds, and the impact of these developments on corporate America, there is evidence of considerable dispersion of ownership of U.S. companies.

Leading the list of owners are American Telephone & Telegraph, with more than 3 million investors, and General Motors, nearly 1.2 million investors (see Table 1–2).

The answer to who owns American business is a key—perhaps the best there is—to understanding the U.S. economic system. In one way or another, almost every American owns American business. The long-term growth of sharowner population and stock market volume is important because the future of the securities markets, as we know them today, depends on the continued participation of the individual shareholder.

Despite increasing activity by institutions, the NYSE expects that individuals will continue to hold the majority of the shares listed on the Exchange in the foreseeable future. Incidentally, of the 1,540 common stocks listed on the NYSE in the early 1980s, the top 50 issues accounted for 41 percent of the value of all common shares listed (see Table 1–3).

For those investors who look for income, American industry has produced an excellent record of payouts. As evidence of the longevity of the dividend records for all NYSE common stocks, see Table 1–4.

The "Stock Market Elite," as tracked annually by *Financial World* magazine, shows companies that have paid dividends for more than 50 years (see Table 1–5).

While these records are impressive, there have been financial institutions with even longer records. Bank of New York Company, Inc., and First National Boston Corporation, for example, have paid annual dividends since 1784. Among other early leaders are Industrial National Corporation, 1791; Citicorp and First National State Bancorporation, 1813; Chemical New York Corporation, 1827; First Pennsylvania Corporation, 1828; Morgan (J. P.) & Co., Inc., 1840; and Chase Manhattan Corporation, 1848.

Table 1–2
NYSE companies with the largest number of common
shareholders of record, early 1981

Company	Shareholders
American Tel. & Tel.	3,026,000
General Motors	1,191,000
Int'l Business Machines	737,000
Exxon Corp.	697,000
General Electric	524,000
General Tel. & Electronics	486,000
Texaco, Inc.	394,000
Sears, Roebuck	350,000
Ford Motor Co.	346,000
Southern Co.	345,000
American Electric Power	338,000
Gulf Oil	312,000
Mobil Corp.	272,000
Commonwealth Edison	269,000
Pacific Gas & Electric	261,000
Philadelphia Electric	253,000
RCA	252,000
U.S. Steel	248,000
Standard Oil of California	247,000
Detroit Edison	242,000
Consolidated Edison	237,000
Eastman Kodak	234,000
Tenneco, Inc.	232,000
Public Service Elec. & Gas	231,000
International Tel. & Tel.	214,000
du Pont de Nemours	213,000
Niagara Mohawk Power	211,000
Chrysler Corp.	209,000
Atlantic Richfield	203,000
Northeast Utilities	196,000
Southern California Edison	193,000
Standard Oil (Indiana)	188,000
Ohio Edison	183,000
Virginia Elec. & Power	183,000
Westinghouse Electric	176,000
Middle South Utilities	175,000
Consumers Power	172,000
BankAmerica	171,000
Union Electric	169,000
Union Carbide Corp.	164,000
Occidental Petroleum	161,000
Long Island Lighting	160,000
Pennsylvania Power	157,000
General Public Utilities	151,000
Columbia Gas System	144,000
Pan American World Airways	140,000
Bethlehem Steel	139,000
Transamerica Corp.	138,000
Duquesne Light	138,000
Greyhound Corp.	137,000

Barbara Wheeler, *The New York Stock Exchange Fact Book,*
1981, p. 35.

Table 1-3
50 leading stocks in market value, December 31, 1980 (in millions)

Company	Listed shares	Market value
Intl'l Business Machines	584.1	$ 39,648
Exxon Corp.	453.2	36,540
American Tel. & Tel.	740.6	35,457
Standard Oil (Indiana)	304.3	24,308
Schlumberger, N.V.	200.7	23,483
Shell Oil	308.9	17,993
Mobil Corp.	212.6	17,167
Standard Oil of California	171.1	17,020
Atlantic Richfield	236.3	15,037
General Electric	231.5	14,177
General Motors	297.3	13,415
Texaco, Inc.	274.3	13,132
Eastman Kodak	161.6	11,269
Halliburton Co.	118.0	9,854
Gulf Oil	211.9	9,245
Phillips Petroleum	154.4	9,074
Standard Oil (Ohio)	120.8	8,697
Getty Oil	88.5	8,134
Union Oil of California	173.5	7,742
Union Pacific	96.0	7,557
Conoco, Inc.	113.5	7,417
Teledyne, Inc.	32.3	6,985
Minnesota Mining & Mfg.	118.0	6,962
Dow Chemical	202.0	6,489
Merck & Co.	75.9	6,432
Johnson & Johnson	61.9	6,172
du Pont de Nemours	146.6	6,155
Tenneco, Inc.	118.4	6,142
Sun Ço.	123.3	6,009
Procter & Gamble	82.7	5,698
Morris (Philip), Inc.	124.8	5,396
Hewlett-Packard Co.	60.0	5,367
SmithKline Corp.	66.5	5,317
Superior Oil	26.6	5,257
Xerox Corp.	84.3	5,045
Caterpillar Tractor	86.5	5,017
Sears, Roebuck	325.3	5,002
Raytheon Co.	44.5	4,894
Eli Lilly	75.8	4,820
Reynolds (R. J.) Inds.	104.4	4,761
American Home Products	168.4	4,737
BankAmerica	147.8	4,471
Weyerhaeuser Co.	128.6	4,389
Digital Equipment	45.9	4,360
Marathon Oil	61.5	4,354
Boeing Co.	97.6	4,318
Dresser Industries	79.7	4,263
General Tel. & Electronics	154.8	4,199
Coca-Cola Co.	124.0	4,138
Cities Service	84.7	4,025
Total	8,305.9	$497,540

Source: Barbara Wheeler, *New York Stock Exchange Fact Book*, 1981, p. 36.

Table 1–4
Dividend record

	Number of stocks	
Number of consecutive years dividends paid	*Quarterly record*	*Annual record*
100 or more	5	33
75 to 99	33	79
50 to 74	137	203
25 to 49	493	499
20 to 24	87	57
20 years or more	755	871
10 to 19	171	167
Less than 10*	614	502
Total	1,540	1,540

* Includes nonpayers and stocks with no quarterly records.
Source: Barbara Wheeler, *New York Stock Exchange Fact Book, 1981*, p. 28.

Table 1–5
Stock market elite

	Dividends	
Company	*Year incorporated*	*Paid since*
Abbott Laboratories....................	1900	1926
Allied Chemical	1920	1887
American Brands	1904	1905
American Can	1901	1923
American Elec. Pwr.	1906	1909
American Express	1965	1870
American Home Prods.	1926	1919
American Natural Res.	1964	1904
American Tel. & Tel.	1880	1881
AMF, Inc.............................	1900	1927
Anchor Hocking	1928	1914
Archer-Daniels-Midland	1925	1927
Atlantic City Elec.....................	1907	1919
Baltimore G. & E.	1906	1910
Beneficial Corp.	1929	1929
Blue Bell	1962	1923
Borden, Inc...........................	1899	1899
Boston Edison	1886	1890
Burroughs Corp........................	1886	1895
Central Hudson G. & E.	1926	1903
Chesebrough-Pond's	1880	1883

Table 1–5 (continued)

	Dividends	
Company	Year incorporated	Paid since
Cincinnati Bell	1873	1879
Cincinnati G. & E.	1837	1853
Cleveland Elec. Illum.................	1892	1901
Coca-Cola Co.........................	1886	1893
Columbus & So. Ohio E................	1906	1927
Combustion Engr.	1912	1911
Commonwealth Edison	1887	1890
Consolidated Edison	1884	1885
Consumers Power	1910	1913
Continental Group....................	1853	1854
Conwood Corp.	1900	1903
Corning Glass Works	1875	1881
CPC Int'l	1906	1920
Dart & Kraft	1980	1924
Credithrift Fin'l	1927	1930
Dayton P. & L.	1911	1919
DeLuxe Check Print.	1920	1921
Detroit Edison	1903	1909
Diamond Int'l	1881	1882
Duke Power	1917	1926
du Pont (E. I.)........................	1903	1904
Eastman Kodak.......................	1901	1902
Enserch Corp.........................	1926	1926
Exxon Corp...........................	1882	1882
Fisher Scientific	1902	1907
GATX Corp.	1916	1919
General Electric	1892	1899
General Foods	1922	1922
General Mills	1928	1898
Gillette Co.	1901	1906
Heinz (H. J.)	1900	1911
Heller (W. E.) Int'l...................	1919	1921
Hercules, Inc.	1912	1913
Honeywell, Inc.	1927	1928
Household Finance	1925	1917
Interco, Inc...........................	1911	1913
Int'l Bus. Mach.	1911	1916
Jefferson-Pilot	1968	1913
Johnson & Johnson	1887	1905
Kansas G. & E.	1909	1922
K mart Corp.	1912	1913
Kellogg Co.	1922	1923
Kroger Co.	1902	1902
Lilly (Eli)	1901	1885
Macy (R. H.) & Co.	1919	1927
Marsh & McLennan	1923	1923
May Dept. Strs.	1910	1911
Melville Corp.	1916	1916
Nabisco, Inc.	1898	1899

Table 1–5 (*concluded*)

Company	Dividends Year incorporated	Dividends Paid since
Nalco Chemical	1928	1928
National Fuel Gas	1902	1903
National-Standard	1907	1916
National Steel	1929	1907
New Eng. Tel. & Tel.	1883	1886
NL Industries	1891	1906
Norfolk & Western	1896	1901
Oklahoma G. & E.	1901	1908
Pacific G. & E.	1905	1919
Owens-Illinois	1907	1907
Pacific Lighting	1886	1909
Pennwalt Corp.	1850	1863
Peoples Drug Strs.	1928	1927
Pfizer, Inc.	1900	1901
Philadelphia Elec.	1902	1902
Philip Morris	1919	1928
Procter & Gamble	1890	1891
Public Service (Colo.)	1906	1907
Public Service E. & G.	1903	1907
Rexnord, Inc.	1892	1894
Reynolds (R. J.) Indus.	1899	1900
Richardson-Merrell	1933	1922
Safeway Strs.	1926	1927
San Diego G. & E.	1905	1909
Shell Trans. & Trading	1897	1898
Southern Calif. Ed.	1909	1909
Standard Oil (Calif.)	1911	1912
Stanley Works	1852	1877
Sterling Drug	1901	1902
Tampa Electric	1899	1900
Trans Union	1891	1914
Travelers Corp.	1863	1864
UGI Corp.	1882	1885
Union Carbide	1917	1918
Union Electric	1922	1906
Union Oil of Calif.	1890	1916
Union Pacific Corp.	1897	1900
United Illuminating	1899	1900
U.S. Gypsum	1901	1919
U.S. Tobacco	1911	1912
Universal Leaf Tobacco	1918	1927
Upjohn Co.	1909	1909
Washington Gas Light	1849	1852
Westvaco Corp.	1899	1892
Woolworth (F. W.) Co.	1911	1912
Wrigley (Wm.) Jr. Co.	1910	1913

Source: "The Stock Market Elite," *Financial World*, January 15, 1981, p. 65. Copyright © 1981 by Macro Communications, Inc. Reprinted by permission of *Financial World*.

WHO INVESTS IN AMERICA?

U.S.News & World Report said that the big increases in stock ownership came because the pension funds, insurance companies, and bank trusts together acquired more than one fourth of all corporate stock. The pension reform law, however, forced the trustees of pension funds to diversify their holdings. Many of them put a larger part of their new money into corporate and U.S. government bonds. Some analysts think that one reason why the stock market became so sluggish is that pension funds became less eager buyers of stock. Mutual funds, meanwhile, became net sellers of stocks in order to take care of investors who redeemed their shares.

The Standard & Poor's Corporation (S&P) Stock Guide seemed to underscore the degree to which the institutions were becoming the major owners of the country's best-known firms. The figures below represent the portion of the companies' outstanding shares owned by banks, investment companies, and insurance companies. If pension funds had also been included, the percentages in many instances would have been much higher.

Company	*Percent*
AMP	61
IBM	34
General Motors	26
Xerox	39
K mart	46
Caterpillar Tractor	44
International Paper	44
J. C. Penney	44
McDonald's	45
Deere & Co.	40
Digital Equipment	57
Texas Instruments	47
Alcoa	53
Upjohn	45
Raytheon	48
Philip Morris	43

U.S.News & World Report asked, "Does the growing role of the institutions mean that a handful of financial executives are going to call the shots for most of American industries in the years to come?"[11]

Not necessarily, for two reasons.

---

[11] "Who Owns American Industry?", p. 71.

First, large holders are numbered in the hundreds or thousands, so that they cannot really speak with one voice to the management of the firm whose stock they own. Standard & Poor's, for example, indicated that nearly 1,400 institutions held IBM shares. At the bottom of the S&P list of companies with wide institutional ownership, 162 institutions held stock in Air Products & Chemicals and Illinois Power.

Second, many of the large holders are reluctant to give the appearance of dictating to corporate managers. If they become unhappy about a company's performance, they would prefer to just quietly sell their holdings rather than raise a fuss that might attract unfavorable attention to the stock. That could cause its price to drop so that they would lose money before they could unload it.

The Individual

A NYSE shareownership survey conducted during 1975 revealed that almost one out of five shareowners (18.1 percent) had left the stock market since early 1970. Individual shareowners numbered 25.3 million and included one out of six adult Americans in mid-1975. However, by the beginning of the 1980s, the number was near the 30 million level, suggesting that the difficult days of the early 1970s were behind (see Table 1–6).

The nearly 30 million shareowners held shares in some 11,000 publicly owned corporations and investment companies. They traded 15.5 billion shares with a trading value of $476 billion. The average size of a trade was 845 shares. The average shareowner's income rose from $13,500 in early 1970 to $19,000 in 1975 and to about the $30,000 level by the early 1980s, pretty much in line with changes in purchasing power.

Further, the NYSE estimates that more than 100 million Americans are indirect owners whose savings are invested, in part, in savings banks, pension funds, insurance companies, and other financial institutions, which, in turn, invest in stocks. For example, by the end of 1980, the assets of the 1,000 largest employee benefit systems stood at $472 billion, according to a survey by *Pension & Investment Age*.[12]

The top 100 funds accounted for 65.8 percent of the assets of the top 1,000. Of those top 100 funds, 55 were corporate funds, 42 were public employee funds, 2 were union funds, and the last was the United Nations Joint Staff Fund. The money was flowing to investments overseas and investments in real estate, call options, financial futures, venture capital partnership, and gold, as well as investments in stock.

The top funds/sponsors (assets in $ millions) were:

---

[12] Reprinted with permission from the January 1981 issue of *Pensions & Investment Age*. Copyright © 1981 by Crain Communications Inc.

18

1.	AT&T Bell System Cos.	$31,100
2.	California Public Employees	18,055
3.	General Motors	14,123
4.	N.Y.C. Employees/Teachers	13,474
5.	N.Y. State Common.	13,308
6.	N.Y. State Teachers	7,914
7.	N.J. Division of Invest.	7,570
8.	General Electric	7,184
9.	Ford Motor Co.	6,442
10.	U.S. Steel & Carnegie	5,540
11.	Texas State Teachers	5,300
12.	IBM Corp.	5,200
13.	Wisconsin Investment Board	5,015
14.	E. I. du Pont de Nemours	4,930
15.	Ohio Teachers	4,742
16.	Ohio Public Employees	4,561
17.	Michigan State Employees	4,559
18.	North Carolina Employees	4,470
19.	Exxon Corp.	4,339
20.	Minnesota Investment Board	4,122
21.	Florida Retirement System	4,000
22.	Pennsylvania School Employees	3,968
23.	Washington Public Employees	3,126
24.	Western Conf. of Teamsters	3,110
25.	General Telephone & Electronics	3,000
26.	Sears	3,000

Institutional Investors

The NYSE study shows that in 1975 institutional investors held $230.5 billion worth of NYSE stocks, or 33.6 percent of the $685.1 billion total market value of all NYSE issues (see Table 1-7).

Life insurance companies held $21.9 billion worth of common stocks. These holdings accounted for 3.1 percent of the market value of all NYSE-listed stocks. The holdings of NYSE-listed common stocks by nonlife insurance companies were worth $11.3 billion, or 1.7 percent of the total value of all NYSE issues.

Open-end investment companies held $35.2 billion worth of NYSE-listed stocks, representing 5.1 percent of all issues. Closed-end investment companies held $5.4 billion worth, which represented under 1 percent of the value of all NYSE-listed issues.

The largest holders of NYSE stocks were private and public pension funds. Their combined holdings were worth $105 billion. Holdings of private pension funds stood at $82.2 billion, and those of public pension funds stood at $22.8 billion. Both represented record-high holding levels, and, combined, they accounted for 15.3 percent of the market value of all NYSE-listed stocks and for 46 percent of the total value of all institutional holding in NYSE issues.

Nonprofit institutions—foundations, educational endowments, and all others—held a total of $22.1 billion worth of NYSE stocks. Finally,

Table 1–6
Highlights of eight NYSE shareowner surveys

	1952	1956	1959	1962	1965	1970	1975	1980
Number of individual shareowners (000s)	6,490	8,630	12,490	17,010	20,120	30,850	25,270	29,840
Number owning shares listed on NYSE (000s)................	n.a.	6,880	8,510	11,020	12,430	18,290	17,950	23,520
Adult shareowner incidence in population	1 in 16	1 in 12	1 in 8	1 in 6	1 in 6	1 in 4	1 in 6	1 in 5
Median household income	$7,100	$6,200	$7,000	$8,600	$9,500	$13,500	$19,000	$27,750
Number of adult shareowners with household income:								
Under $10,000 (000s)	n.a.	n.a.	9,340	10,340	10,080	8,170	3,420	1,720
$10,000 and over (000s)	n.a.	n.a.	2,740	5,920	8,410	20,130	19,970	25,410
Number of adult female shareowners (000s)	3,140	4,620	6,350	8,290	9,430	14,290	11,750	13,530
Number of adult male shareowners (000s)	3,210	4,020	5,740	7,970	9,060	14,340	11,630	14,030
Median age	51	48	49	48	49	48	53	46

n.a. = Not available.
Source: Barbara Wheeler, New York Stock Exchange Fact Book, 1981, p. 47.

Table 1–7
Estimated holdings of NYSE-listed stocks by selected institutional
investors (billions)

Type of institution	Year-end				
	1949	1965	1973	1974[r]	1975[r]
U.S. institutions					
Insurance companies					
Life	$ 1.1	$ 6.3	$ 20.0	$ 16.3	$ 21.9
Nonlife	1.7	10.1	16.4	10.4	11.3
Investment companies					
Open-end	1.4	29.1	38.5	27.1	35.2
Closed-end	1.6	5.6	5.9	4.0	5.4
Noninsured pension funds					
Corporate and private	0.5	35.9	82.1	58.2	82.2
State and local govern-					
ment................	*	1.4	19.6	15.9	22.8
Nonprofit institutions					
Foundations	2.5	16.4	21.5	16.9	22.1
Educational endowments	1.1	5.9	7.7	5.5	7.2
Other	1.0	7.7	9.5	6.6	8.7
Common trust funds	*	3.2	5.8	4.7	6.1
Mutual savings banks	0.2	0.5	2.1	1.7	2.3
Subtotal..............	$11.1	$122.1	$229.7	$167.7	$225.4
Foreign institutions†					
Investment, insurance,					
and miscellaneous					
cosigners	—	—	—	3.3	5.1
Total	$11.1	$122.1	$229.7	$171.0	$230.5
Market value of all NYSE-					
listed stock	$76.3	$537.5	$721.0	$511.1	$685.1
Estimated percentage held by					
institutional investors	14.5%	22.7%	31.8%	33.4%	33.6%

[r] = Revised estimates.
* Less than $50 million.
† Not included are foreign banks, brokers, and nominees. This institutional
group held an estimated $12.0 billion of NYSE-listed stocks at year-end 1974 and
$18.5 billion at year-end 1975. Miscellaneous institutions consist of pension funds
and other employee benefit funds or trusts.
Source: Barbara Wheeler, *New York Stock Exchange Fact Book, 1981*, p. 50.

foreign institutions held a record $5.1 billion worth. This accounted for
2.2 percent of all institutional holdings in NYSE issues and for under 1
percent of the mid-1970s total market value of NYSE stocks.

How Do Investors Follow the Market?

In 1966, the NYSE established the NYSE Common Stock Index to
provide a comprehensive measure of the market trend for the benefit

of the many investors concerned with general market price movements. The index was also designed to provide a valuable statistical yardstick for professional analysts, brokers, and other students of the market.

Covering all common stocks listed on the Exchange, the index reflects the trend in stock prices day to day, hour to hour, and even minute to minute. The composite index and its net change from the previous day's close are printed on the ticker tape every half hour, along with the actual dollars and cents change in the average price of all common stocks. Four subgroup indexes—industrial, transportation, utility, and finance—and their net changes appear on the tape every hour on the hour.

Composite and subgroup closing indexes and net changes are printed at the end of the day, along with the range for the day.

The price indexes are based on the aggregate market value of NYSE common stocks, adjusted to eliminate the effects of capitalization changes, new listings, and delistings. The procedure used is to weigh the price of each stock by the number of shares listed. The aggregate market value, which is the sum of the individual market values, is then expressed in relation to the base period market value; in this index, December 31, 1965, equals 50.

Changes in capitalization, new listings, and delistings are handled by adjusting the base period value accordingly. For example, if a new issue is listed, the base value is increased, so that addition of the current market value does not distort the index values.

Historically, the composite index is available on a weekly basis from January 7, 1939, to May 28, 1964 (having been linked to the SEC index), and on a daily closing basis from May 28, 1964, to the present. The four subgroup indexes are available from December 31, 1965, on a daily closing basis.

CHAPTER TWO

The Parameters of the Professionals

UNDERSTANDING THE PROFESSIONAL

Communicating with the investment professional would be a simple task if all investment professionals were clones, sterile in thought and motivation, and if they operated in a constantly level market. The facts are that none of these is true. How then can you communicate with diverse audiences in an ever-changing market?

Considerable evidence is available through numerous studies to determine how and why the professional becomes interested in a company, how research is secured and used, the techniques of the "big hitters," the role of the professional recommendation in customer decision making, the magic of MPT, where business is conducted, what investors think of the professionals, the "ideal" broker, how investors rank characteristics of the professional and the brokerage firms, the importance of the individual in choosing a brokerage firm, and what the professional looks for in management.

The data provide guideposts to help you understand how the professional thinks, acts, and does business. While each professional is different, the material builds a profile of the average professional. From this, you can begin planning your corporate strategies, which precede the development of your communications plan. To understand the professional of today, let us look backward briefly at the professional and the recent market environment.

The Changing Environment

Once upon a time . . .

There was a realmdom, known as Wall Street, that reached over all of the land. Sitting on the throne was King Financial Analyst I. The strength of his ruling power was wisdom of research.

Alas, as time came to pass, the throne was weakened by plague,

22

pestilence, and apathy. The king saw other fiefdoms shrink, merge, or disappear. His followers mysteriously disappeared by the millions. The king looked in his magic mirror and knew that he was as wise as ever, but the burdens of research were so heavy that his followers were doing their own thing.

So, too, with the modern-day financial analyst. He has seen the number of analysts shrink so that instead of enjoying the luxury of following a handful of companies, he now follows 45 companies in five industries. And although his techniques and analysis have improved greatly over the past decade, the entire analytic process has been slowed by the sheer burden of numbers.

He has encountered other troubles along the way. He has seen himself shunted from industry to industry, and his followers have undergone pangs of expansion, contraction, and expansion. It was not unusual for a transportation analyst to be assigned to ecology in the late 1960s and early 1970s only to be back in transportation today.

The analyst's legions of individual investors soared past a record 30 million in the early 1970s, plummeted to 25 million in the middle of the decade, and are back to near 30 million today. In the late 1960s, these individual investors relied heavily on the professional advice of the financial analyst, but surveys conducted a decade later indicated that 44 percent of them were relying on their own judgment and that only 27.4 percent were relying on financial advisers. Also impacting on the financial analyst was the so-called two-tier stock market that emerged in the early 1970s. Volumes and price-earnings ratios (P/E ratios) soared for institutional favorites, but "second-tier" companies watched the P/E ratios plummet.

In response to this challenge, investor relations professionals began to break away from the traditional circles of influence in the investment community, addressing instead two new audiences that became the hot buttons of the 1970s: regional brokerage firms and broker salespersons—the registered reps. The next logical step for investor relations was an emphasis on regional money centers, where a more receptive ear might be found for a solidly performing smaller company that failed to make the nifty-50 list of institutional favorites. At the same time, regional financial communities became more powerful and more sophisticated. Local banks expanded, and, of particular interest to investor relations, much of this expansion occurred in portfolio management functions.

Meanwhile, investment research capabilities across the country were cut drastically during the two major market slumps of the 1970s. Investor relations professionals responded with another effort to maintain interest in their companies: direct communications with the broker sales force. This, in effect, bypassed the shrinking investment research community.

How the Professional Becomes Interested in You

Research department heads and broker sales managers at the nation's leading regional brokerage firms said that, first, both analysts and brokers were always interested in a potentially good investment prospect, whether or not the firm was in their geographic region. Second, they said that research department sponsorship was essential before direct communications to the broker sales force could really be effective. Third, they said that the analyst might become interested in a company through the efforts of the investor relations officer or through communications but that in order to form a solid impression of the company, the analyst wanted to meet the chief executive officer one-on-one. Then, the broker sales managers might call for staff meetings with the CEO.

Fourth, both analysts and brokers stressed the importance of tuning communications efforts to each audience. Analysts want the basics—fundamental analysis techniques prevail. Sales managers stressed marketability, saying that their reps needed a tight definition of who the company was, where it was going, and why.

Most research heads said they would follow any company that had good investment potential, regardless of its size, location, or other considerations. Of those analysts having "cutoff" points on the size of a company they would follow, about a half dozen pointed to annual sales levels that ranged from $50 million to $300 million. Some required a minimum level of earnings—from $1 million to $7 million; others said that a minimum float ranging from 50,000 to 4 million shares was essential. The research heads reported that broker salespersons followed their firm's research recommendations closely, so that without research department sponsorship, going direct to the broker was a big waste of time.

The broker sales forces in the regional firms agreed that they generally followed the lead of research in choosing companies to pursue. But they picked their favorites from among these on the basis you would expect from a salesperson—marketability. "We go where the money is," was a sentiment expressed in many ways. Retail salespeople don't spend a lot of time learning about a company, simply because they don't often get the opportunity to discuss a particular stock in depth. "Usually, we get a minute or two on the phone to spark interest, and if it's not there, we're through," said an Atlanta sales manager. "So, obviously, regional presence, a good float, active trading, visibility, and a solid performance record are all keys."

Meeting the basic criteria of the investment professional does not guarantee that you will be followed. You must determine the interest in your industry, how your performance measures against that of others in your industry, and why you currently are or are not being followed.

Your chief financial and chief communications officers can do this in a relatively brief time by contacting 6 to 10 analysts in your industry. The information will help you determine the communications needs of your company. On the other hand, not meeting the criteria does not necessarily mean you should not communicate. Your strategy could be to cultivate current shareholders or to concentrate directly on key brokers in your geographic area.

Securing Research

Surveys, however, were to show that not everyone was marching to the tune of the analyst "piper." A 1978 survey of stockbroker registered representatives conducted by Lowengard & Brotherhood and Marketing Services, Inc., showed that while 89 percent of the reps utilized their firm's own research report, 78 percent also used investor advisory services, 73 percent used company annual and interim reports; 53 percent used other firms' research reports; 41 percent used newsletters; and 32 percent used company 10-Ks.[1]

Newsletters read to keep registered representatives informed were: *Professional Tape Reader,* 14 percent; *Value Line,* 12 percent; *United Business Service,* 8 percent; *Indicator's Digest,* 5 percent; *Kiplinger Letter, Dow Theory,* and *Standard & Poor's Trendline,* 4 percent; *Babson's Chartist* and *Argus Research,* 3 percent; and *Speculator, Market Logic, Professional Investor, RHM Survey, Tillman Survey, McGraw-Hill,* and *Smart Money,* 2 percent. Others receiving mention were *Equity, Personal Finance, Granville, O.T.C. Newsletter, Wall Street Digest,* and *Financial Weekly.*

Research by me for Trans Union Corporation revealed an interesting tangent. My study showed that the majority of stockbroker representatives do not conduct their own research and are content to rely on recommendations from the firm. The top performers—"the big hitters"—however, *do* rely on their own research. They tend to look for companies in low P/E industries that demonstrate superiority to competitors.

The segments of the spectrum in which the broker views his role were expressed well in the Trans Union survey:

Broker 1

I work both sides of the Street. I manage some of my own accounts and do securities analysis as well. I do not consider a broker's communications needs all that dissimilar to an analyst's. Both groups seek essentially the same type of information. But there may be a slight difference in detail.

A broker is looking for timely material. By this, I mean all the interim

---

[1] *Study of Stockbroker Registered Representatives in New England, 1978,* Lowengard & Brotherhood and Marketing Services, Inc., Hartford, Conn.

quarterly statements, the annual report, and news releases on significant corporate developments. I do not see any differentiation between any analyst's decision-making process versus a broker's. All the analyst is doing is helping the registered representative. In many respects, the analyst is the conduit between the broker's client and the company.

Broker 2

I do very little research on my own; my business is selling to individuals. I use no information from companies unless I request it. Our research department provides us with all the information I would require on a particular company. Usually, I do not even look at annual reports. All unsolicited mail is thrown out—no matter how clever it is. My only other information comes through casual exchange with other brokers.

If I go to a broker meeting twice a year, that is a lot. These meetings are not really informative. The companies' job is to make themselves look good. This positive image does not reflect the true picture. Occasionally, though, they bring up new angles. None of the brokers I know go to these meetings unless they are extremely interested in a company.

The analysts are really the ones who recommend companies. Analysts with a good following are read by everyone—and everything they recommend gets visibility. Also, if a friend suggests a company that my analysts don't follow, I mention it to them before I advise my clients to buy. About 80 percent of my customers rely on me for a buy decision.

Broker 3

I have been on the Street for 27 years. I deal basically with the retail investor. Most of my business revolves around five or six wealthy clients. I do not have discretionary accounts. When I first started on the Street, my work was largely service oriented. I was always sending annual reports and press releases to clients. Now I am more of an order taker. About half my clients make their investment decision before calling me.

Broker 4

I generally use three informational sources for background research. First, I consult the *Professional Tape Reader.* This is a broker service our firm subscribes to. It provides technical and statistical stock information. If a particular stock looks interesting, I will then read the Standard & Poor's tear sheet. Finally, if I have definite interest, I will get the company's annual report from the library. Earnings trends, recognized products, and capitalization are the main factors I weigh in investment decision making. I prefer smaller capitalization growth situations to the blue chips.

What Professionals Read

The registered representative is influenced by media advertising, just as the financial analyst is (see Chapter 11).

The top reference source is *The Wall Street Journal,* with 79 percent of the registered representatives saying that they have investigated a company after reading advertising in that medium. This was followed by *Barron's*, 62 percent; *Business Week*, 53 percent; and *Registered Representative*, 48 percent. Other publications mentioned by the registered representatives were *Forbes*, 15 percent; *OTC Review/Chronicle*, 7 percent; *Dun's Review* and *Security Trader's Handbook*, 4 percent; and *Financial World*, 2 percent.[2]

What other communications vehicles turn on the registered representative? One survey used the reverse method to determine what vehicles the registered representative considered least valuable. The least valuable vehicle was direct mail, at 51 percent. A distant second was press releases, at 15 percent, which suggests that the registered representative has neither the desire nor the time to pore over direct mail. Ranking low on the reverse list, and thus suggesting high readership, were annual reports, 8 percent; quarterly reports, 4 percent; and dividend news and luncheons, 3 percent.

The Wall Street Journal, according to numerous studies, continues to be read regularly by virtually every investment professional. *Business Week* is next, followed by *Fortune* and *Barron's*. Each of these publications is read regularly by roughly equal proportions of analysts and portfolio managers (see Table 2–1).

Table 2–1
Publications read regularly

	Analysts	Portfolio managers
The Wall Street Journal	99%	99%
Business Week	82	78
Fortune	64	59
Barron's	60	68

Source: Eugene E. Heaton, Jr., "Current Practices and Attitudes in the Investor Relations Field," *Investor and Financial Relations, 1980 State of the Art Report* (New York: Opinion Research Corporation, December 3, 1979), p. 79. Copyright © 1979, Opinion Research Corporation.

Opinion Research Corporation (ORC) says that when it looks at analysts and portfolio managers, it finds some sizable differences between them in the value they attach to different information sources. Both groups say they find two sources highly useful—*the annual report* and *company presentations* (see Table 2–2). These are, in effect, the big guns—the sine qua non—of corporate investor relations, the ones that need your best people and talents.

---

[2] Ibid.

Table 2–2
"Most useful" information sources

	Analysts	Portfolio managers
Annual report	94%	91%
Company presentations	77	84

Source: Eugene E. Heaton, Jr., "Current Practices and Attitudes in the Investor Relations Field," *Investor and Financial Relations, 1980 State of the Art Report* (New York: Opinion Research Corporation, December 3, 1979), p. 76. Copyright © 1979, Opinion Research Corporation.

Beyond these two sources, the differences between the two groups begin to emerge. For example, analysts consider various types of company-oriented written material more useful than do portfolio managers. It's the analyst's job to dig deeply, and he or she needs this more detailed information to get the job done. Thus, quarterly reports, 10-Ks and supplementary materials always rate higher with analysts than with brokers.

When it comes to various types of personal contact—such as informal personal contacts with corporate representatives or visits to the company—analysts give these methods of communicating more importance than do portfolio managers (see Table 2–3). The portfolio man-

Table 2–3
"Most useful" information sources

	Analysts	Portfolio managers
Handling of inquiries	55%	30%
Informal contact, information from company representatives	55	29
Time and attention during visits	48	18

Source: Eugene E. Heaton, Jr., "Current Practices and Attitudes in the Investor Relations Field," *Investor and Financial Relations, 1980 State of the Art Report* (New York: Opinion Research Corporation, December 3, 1979), p. 77. Copyright © 1979, Opinion Research Corporation.

ager just has too many companies to keep track of, too many other things to do, to devote as much time to maintaining personal contact as the analyst does.

On the other hand, portfolio managers are at least somewhat more oriented than analysts toward *secondary* sources of information, such as the opinion of other investment professionals, industry research reports, and articles about companies in the media—though it's important to note that the first two sources are quite important to analysts as well (see Table 2–4).

Table 2–4
"Most useful" information sources

	Analysts	Portfolio managers
Opinion of other analysts	66%	75%
Industry research reports	63	73
Articles about company in news media..................	36	49

Source: Eugene E. Heaton, Jr., "Current Practices and Attitudes in the Investor Relations Field," *Investor and Financial Relations, 1980 State of the Art Report* (New York: Opinion Research Corporation, December 3, 1979), p. 78. Copyright © 1979, Opinion Research Corporation.

These data suggest that the way to influence portfolio managers is by influencing those analysts whose views count in the investment community. This may bring us right back to square one—make sure the portfolio manager has the basic information available, but concentrate most heavily on the analyst.

This material suggests at least a three-tier approach with written materials. They are direct mail consisting of the annual and quarterly statements along with other pertinent corporate information, financial and corporate news to the major business publications, and a mailing list for secondary financial publications and newsletters.

How the Big Hitters Do It

Back in the mid-1960s, Edgerton Welch decided his family-controlled Citizens Bank & Trust Company in Chillicothe, Missouri, needed a trust department. Today, his tiny $6 million fund ranks first among all bank- and insurance-managed funds, with an enviable average return of 34.1 percent for a five-year period. *Forbes* reported that his method is simplicity itself.[3] He begins by reading the *Value Line Investment Survey.*

He looks to see which stocks are ranked highest for year-ahead performance. Then, Welch checks to see which industry groups Value Line likes. If the service is bullish on both an industry and a particular

---

[3] "He's Got a Little List," *Forbes*, March 30, 1981, pp. 47–50. Copyright © 1981 by Forbes, Inc.

30

company in it, he becomes even more interested. Next, he checks *E. F. Hutton's Master List.* If this gives its top rating to a top *Value Line* selection, then Welch is likely to buy it. He checks to make sure that earnings estimates project annual growth of at least 25 percent for the next few years. He chats with a couple of Kansas City, Missouri brokers he trusts; with his son, William, the bank's president; and with Ed Douglas, a bank officer. From all of this he develops a consensus. But he makes every final decision himself.

Another self-researcher is Melvin Daum of Bay Harbour Islands, an affluent Miami suburb. On a little makeshift bulletin board above Daum's desk, there's a newspaper clipping whose headline reads, "What the Airlines Are Really Worth." The clipping contains vital financial information about 10 major U.S. airlines—everything from current market valuations of their stock to per share appraisals of what their jet planes and other assets would probably bring if they were sold. The airline data are just one of countless research tools that Daum, an account executive and vice president of Dean Witter Reynolds, uses to select stocks, reported *Registered Representative.*[4] He scans business publications daily for information with investment overtones.

By finding undervalued securities and recommending them to his clients, Daum has become one of the elite of the brokerage business—a $1 million producer. He does his own research from stacks of material, but usually he can just look at something and decide whether it's worth further digging into. He likes low-P/E stocks, wanting to know more about what they might earn in the future than about what they have earned in the past. If he can get a good yield and good prospects along with the low P/E, so much the better.

Another big hitter, Stephen H. Karelitz of Boston, does 100 percent of his own research and has a very simple approach to each potential new investment—he must sell himself first. "I do my own homework," he states. "My prime criterion is that an investment must be good enough for me to put my own money into it. If you are willing to sign the check and put your own money on the line, it's very easy to sell your clients." He has turned in gross production in excess of $1.5 million to become the top stockbroker for Shearson Hayden Stone.

Registered representatives in New England ranked their "own" research highest, at 29 percent, as the most important source of information on which to base a "buy" decision.[5] Other sources on which these registered representatives based buy decisions were *Value Line* and *Standard & Poor's,* 14 percent; annual reports, 12 percent; sales, earn-

---

[4] "Big Hitters: How They Do It—Why They Do It," *Registered Representative,* September–October 1979, pp. 18–29. Copyright © 1979 by Plaza Publishing Company, Inc.

[5] *Study of Stockbroker.*

ing trends, and future prospects, 9 percent; security analysts' opinions, 8 percent; company 10-K's, 5 percent; and the company itself, 4 percent. Receiving miscellaneous mentions were product innovations, the *E. F. Hutton Buy List*, personal contacts, *Mitchell's Reports*, officers of the company, *Moody's Service*, and the *Dow Tape*.

These representatives said that in conducting their research they were influenced by their own firm's research reports, by investment advisory services such as Standard & Poor's, by advertising in *The Wall Street Journal*, by meetings that their own firm sponsored, and by public companies' annual and interim reports.

The representatives admitted that they were influenced by advertising, which was remarkable because most investment people have a hard time admitting such influence. The survey also revealed that editorial matter in their favorite business media exerted a strong influence on the investment recommendations of these representatives.

The Professional Recommendation

More than three quarters of the New England representatives felt that more than half of their sales were based on their recommendations rather than their customers' independent decisions. Almost all of the representatives felt that their recommendations accounted for at least one quarter of their customers' buy decisions (see Table 2–5).

Table 2–5
Recommendation of representative versus customer's decision in stock purchase determination

	Percent of stock sales			
	10–25	*26–50*	*51–75*	*76–100*
Recommendation by rep or his firm	2%	21%	37%	40%
Decision of customer	52	40	6	2

Base: 211.
Source: *Study of Stockbroker Registered Representatives in New England, 1978*, Lowengard & Brotherhood and Marketing Services, Inc., Hartford, Conn.

A little more than two thirds of the representatives sampled had considerable or complete discretion in recommending stock purchases to customers (see Table 2–6).

The communications environment today is fractured. In the early 1970s, the investor relations executive talked to the security analyst and the security analyst talked to the rest of the world. This neat package no longer exists. With the decline of Wall Street, there is no

Table 2-6
Discretion allowed by firms in suggesting stocks
to customers

Degree of discretion	Percent
Complete discretion	39%
Rough guidelines provided	29
Some leeway allowed	18
Must stay with firm's buy list	14
Execute only	—
	100%

Base: 211.
Source: *Study of Stockbroker Registered Representatives in New England, 1978*, Lowengard & Brotherhood and Marketing Services, Inc., Hartford, Conn.

longer a body of security analysts to pass on the information. There are at least four segments: individual shareholders, registered representatives, portfolio managers, and security analysts. Although the market is drawing back investors, it will never return to its old system. To reach the segmented market, the current communications situation is information overload. The average annual report tripled in volume in the 1970s. Some financial analysts have even complained that information suffocation is making the job of stock evaluation tougher.

Enter the Magic of MPT

Into the vast minefield of stock evaluations, in the late 1970s, came the great panacea that would professionalize stock selections. It was called MPT—modern portfolio theory. The chief uses of MPT are to evaluate portfolio diversification, to implement an "active" strategy for returns superior to those provided by a "passive" strategy, to identify specific stocks for inclusion in the portfolio, and to monitor portfolio performance.

MPT research indicates that on average only about 22 percent of stock price behavior reflects a company's own performance; the rest is attributable to market influence and to industry and other stock group trends. Data disclosed by MPT research explain what kinds of corporate performance, financial policies, and communications affect stock price behavior and in what way. Also, MPT is supposed to show how and why individual stocks behave as they do and how and why individual stocks are perceived as belonging to groups.

Supporters of MPT claim that it has provided a tangible impetus to investor relations. Their reasoning is that as a result of MPT chief executives and investor relations managers have begun to impose the same planning discipline that prevails among the more established line functions. Increasingly, investor relations programs have been supplanted by strategies, including the establishment of goals and objectives based on careful research and analysis. In the process, investor relations is becoming capable of measurement and evaluation, and the benefits accruing to a true professional are becoming the lot of the investor relations practitioner: more independence in the job, increased stature within the senior management group, and greater opportunity for promotion to other staff and line jobs.

Rather than being a detective in the minfield, however, MPT appears to be more like a dud. The use of MPT is quite fractionated with only 20 percent of analysis or portfolio managers reporting that their institutions use MPT in all of their portfolios. About 50 percent of them say MPT is not used at all, and based on their input, there is no sign of a strong trend toward wider use of MPT. Less than 10 percent of the professionals in institutions now not using MPT say that their institutions are planning to use it in the future. Besides being a fad, institutions view it as costly because of computer facilities required. But the biggest reason for some not to use it is that MPT does not equal human judgment. It is not surprising, then, that MPT has had little impact on presentations to the investment community. Only 7 percent of the professionals believed that there had been a change; 80 percent said that there had been no change; and 13 percent were not sure. The result of self-research by brokers and individuals has prompted changes in the traditional ways in which information flows from a company to the marketplace, says Anthony D. Hughes, executive vice president financial relations, Burson-Marsteller, and international public relations firm.

Figure 2–1 indicates the traditional flow under which the analyst was king. Figure 2–2 shows the flow now in existence.

The ORC study confirms that there is an increased trend toward direct contact with brokerage firms and registered representatives by companies. Among the professionals, 83 percent believe that such a trend exists. Surprisingly, 94 percent of them consider it a positive development, especially for smaller companies that are likely to be overlooked unless they take the initiative, companies with new products that the investment community should be informed about, highly diversified companies that are complicated to follow, and companies operating in a rapidly changing business environment.

Where Business Is Conducted

Investing is a telephone business. More than two thirds of the investors prefer to do business by telephone compared with less than one third for personal contact, mail, and telegram. While slightly more than

34

Figure 2-1
Diagram A

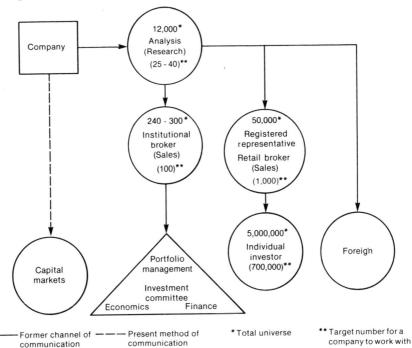

————— Former channel of   — — — Present method of   * Total universe   ** Target number for a
communication   communication   company to work with

one half of the investors usually conduct their business from work, approximately 40 percent conduct business from home. This creates an interesting insight of the investor. While less than 10 percent do business in the broker's office, they consider the location of the broker's office very important. According to one survey I read, more than 90 percent of the investors choose a brokerage office near their place of work or home. They apparently want the security of knowing the broker is nearby if needed.

The fact that brokers do much of their business over the telephone or away from the office affects the types of communications that you should provide them. Because brokers are too busy to read reams of material and have only seconds to sell your company over the telephone, massive pieces of literature such as the annual report are taboo. Brokers much prefer a flash card—a 3-by-5-inch card with new, pertinent information about your company.

What Investors Think of Professionals

A study of the NYSE suggests that the closer the relationship is between the broker and the investor, the more highly the broker is

Figure 2–2
Diagram B

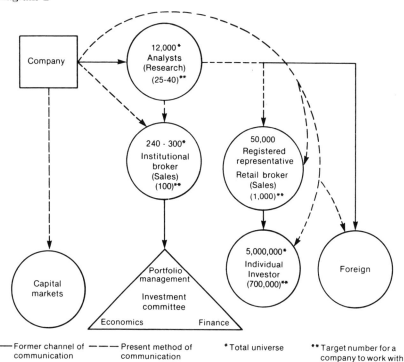

———— Former channel of   — — — Present method of   * Total universe   ** Target number for a
            communication   communication   company to work with

regarded by the investor.[6] Investors who had not made any trades
during the prior year gave brokers generally, only a 44 percent favorable rating but gave their own broker a 78 percent favorable rating.
Those who had made one to five trades gave brokers generally a 40
percent rating and gave their own broker 79 percent. The heavy trader
gave his own broker an 81 percent favorable rating but thought more
favorably of brokers generally, giving them a 56 percent favorable
rating.

Characteristics Important to the Investor

The *most important* characteristics of brokerage firms are (1) honesty, (2) financial stability, (3) accurately handled transactions, and (4)
well-trained brokers. All of these characteristics are basic aspects of
any business relationship, not characteristics peculiar to the securities
industry. This shows that the business basics of the securities industry
are not unique. The characteristics considered to be at the second level
of importance include specific brokerage *services* that do reflect the

[6] *Public Attitudes toward Investing* (New York: NYSE, 1978).

unique character of the securities business—good research, a better chance to make money, a wide range of services, and experts available for consultation. This identifies areas for performance and distinction. Of *least* importance are customer education and the availability of financial planning services, characteristics generic to financial services but not unique to securities investments.

Who Is the Ideal Broker?

Investors see the "ideal" broker as an honest, knowledgeable service agent who provides them with information and fulfills orders but does not pressure them. The "ideal" broker is *not* seen as a professional on whom investors in general could (or would) rely for investment advice, financial planning assistance, or education about investing. This may be both the cause and the result of the small number of delegators in the investor population and of the large number of mutual decision makers who feel that they cannot (or do not wish to) rely completely on their broker.

The picture of the broker as a communication and service coordinator for individual investors is found in Greenwich Research Associates (GRA) studies dealing with institutional investors. GRA's surveys show that institutional investors want salespeople representing their important research brokers to facilitate the communication of their firm's research. They do not look to the salesperson to "add value" by applying their judgment of value or prices.

The Professional or the Firm?

In response to rising competition from the larger national firms, Piper Jaffray & Hopwood, Inc., a Minneapolis-based regional investment firm, undertook a major study to determine what motivates investors to do business with a particular brokerage firm.[7] Hundreds of interviews with customers (Piper's and others) uncovered several surprising facts. The sample comprised 525 investors who were interviewed on a geographic basis, so that most of the sponsoring firm's market area was represented in the sample. The sample was drawn with an approximate 50–50 split between high- and low-commission customers.

One not-so-surprising finding was that customer loyalty hinges primarily on the qualities of the individual broker, not on the reputation of the firm. The majority said that they were first and foremost interested in finding—and keeping—a broker who would listen to them and understand their financial needs. Asked how they decided

---

[7] "How Loyal Are Your Clients?" *Registered Representative*, May 1980, pp. 82–83. Copyright © 1980 by Plaza Publishing Company, Inc.

where to take their business, those interviewed gave responses that were 70 percent broker related and only 30 percent company related. The key findings were that *investors want to deal with a responsive and attentive person* who will handle requests efficiently and rapidly and who exhibits a high degree of interest in the customer's account. Investors regard financial strength and experience in their investment interests as the most important characteristics of the brokerage firm. However, they rank the importance of both of these firm-related characteristics below the importance of the representative.

A key question dealt with the relative importance of the firm versus the registered representative when choosing a brokerage house. The responses strongly favored the representative, by about 70 to 30 in most cases. This finding seems to confirm the belief that the broker is the key factor in what happens between the firm and its clients. In fact, based on the 70–30 response spread, the broker is the company in the eyes of many customers.

This finding also seems to run counter to the marketing strategies adopted by several national brokerage houses whose advertising emphasizes their reputation, skills, and strength. If the finding is valid, then it seems logical to assume that a firm can make a larger impact on potential customers by advertising the quality of its representatives. An overemphasis on the firm itself probably would not make much of an impression on the typical investor, who is looking for individualized service.

Investors were also asked to rank particular characteristics of the registered representative in terms of overall importance. "Responsiveness" was clearly viewed as the single most important characteristic of the representative by both customers and prospects. Rated as an "absolutely essential" characteristic by 72 percent of the customers and 60 percent of the prospects, "responsiveness" far outdistanced the runner-up, "shows importance of your business." This characteristic was defined as feeling that the broker wants you as a customer, that your business is important. It is worth noting that the top two characteristics are personal attributes, not business-oriented traits.

Representative characteristics rated as least important were business oriented. Only 34 percent of the customers and 25 percent of the prospects rated "knows many investment areas" as absolutely essential. Only 32 percent of the customers and 23 percent of the prospects rated "makes recommendations based on your best interests" as absolutely essential.

In general, the specific characteristics of the firm were ranked as less important than those of the representative. However, among both customers and prospects there was a wide variation in the importance attributed to the characteristics of the firm. For instance, among customers 69 percent rated "financial strength" as absolutely essential.

The Professional Looks at Management

Mark J. Appleman, publisher of the *Corporate Shareholder*, turned the microscope away from how the investment professional is viewed to how the professional views corporate management.[8] He surveyed 1,440 financial analysts in eight metropolitan areas: Boston, Hartford, New York, Philadelphia, Pittsburgh, Providence, Rochester, Washington, D.C., and Wilmington. Appleman said that you might come to feel about the process of judging management the way one seasoned congressman did about the legislative process: With laws and sausages, he declared, it is better not to know how they are made.

The least equivocal of Appleman's major findings was also the most ambivalent. Among those surveyed, 9 out of 10 gave the greatest weight to financial results. The implication, that management is as effective as the company was successful in the past reporting period, gives a 180-degree twist to the dictum that a company is only as good as the people running it. In short, 90 percent of financial analysts profess a positive predilection for putting the quantitative cart before the qualitative horse—and the remaining 10 percent see the sequence as reasonably congruous.

This apparent headstand, moreover, is but the first of several eyebrow raisers uncovered by Appleman's survey. Investment professionals split down the middle in their assessment of the importance of specific criteria usually regarded as fundamental to management evaluation. For instance, only a modest majority (58 percent) said that they gave greatest weight to capital generation and corporate growth strategy (56 percent). A somewhat slimmer majority fully accepted as obligatory the four cardinal measures of management. Marketing and innovativeness both rated "highest priority" with 53 percent of the respondents, but the other two measures, management of people and the personal integrity and fairness of top officers, came in at an even 50 percent.

Although on the whole purely objective readings on management were accorded greater levels of priority than were subjective criteria, the preferences indicated were quite underwhelming in both categories. Acknowledged utilization of even fundamental criteria was spotty. Thus: a mere 46 percent of the respondents gave a "highest priority" rating to consistency of financial practices and capital structure with stated company goals; 43 percent gave highest priority to consistency of corporate aims and financial practices with shareowners' interests, while 13 percent gave the same standard low priority; and communication of performance targets within economic, industry,

---

[8] Mark J. Appleman, "How Professionals View Corporate Management," *Corporate Shareholder*, February 11, 1981, pp. 2–3. Copyright © 1979 by Corporate Shareholder, Inc. Material may not be reproduced or redistributed without written permission.

political, and regulatory contexts rated higher priority with 25 percent and low priority with an offsetting 27 percent.

On the subjective side, the strongest showing was made by management turnover/pattern of tenure, which rated highest priority with 38 percent. But trading pattern of top officers buying/selling company stock turned out to be highest priority with only 12 percent and low priority with 58 percent. Personal impressions rated highest priority with 33 percent, low priority with 18 percent. And compensation ratio of number 1 and number 2 executive showed up as highest priority with less than 2 percent and low priority with 50 percent.

The study sample duplicated as closely as possible that used for a 1979–80 survey by *The New York Times*, which among other things, confirmed that for nearly 9 out of 10 analysts in the same area, the most important criterion for judging a particular company was "quality of management." While there was a limit to the statistical findings, Appleman said that this did not hold true for the possible interpretations. Based on his insights acquired over a period of 20 years from working with analysts both on the Street and from the corporate side, Appleman felt that certain observations were inescapable.

First, it is easier to discern a CEO's direct impact on a mid-range company than on a large one, where middle management tends to place its imprint on programs. Second, it is easier to quantify top-executive effectiveness in a retailing company, where the time lag between management decisions and operating results may be annual or seasonal, than in, say, a mining company, where this year's operating results may reflect commitments of capital and human resources made 10 to 15 years earlier, possibly by a previous management team. Third, when nearly all analysts lean on corporate financial results as a measure of management—while at the same time contending that management is the cause and financial results in the effect—this is not out of doublethink or professional schizophrenia. By training and personal bent toward the statistical, analysts are not too well equipped to practice what they profess about management appraisal. Fourth, many analysts may pretend to be less than human—that is, less influenced by subjective factors than other humans—because they feel that the dignity, and possibly the survival, of their profession call for a computer-like posture. Analysts claim to be impervious to nonobjective influences, such as their gracious or shabby treatment by a particular management or their experience with a company's advertising, public relations, and investor relations communications. Finally, investment professionals are less shaky about their evaluations when these concern companies with managements that take responsibility for establishing the scale of values on which they expect to be weighed and measured and that communicate those objectives to the financial community.

CHAPTER THREE

The Individual Investor

The typical individual investor is a little old lady in tennis shoes who uses the Ouija board for counseling.
Anonymous

WHAT IS THE INDIVIDUAL INVESTOR ALL ABOUT?

To identify shareholder attitudes and opinions, the Burson-Marsteller public relations firm conducted numerous surveys, many of them for me, among varied individual investor audiences from which it created a composite shareholder. Drawing such a composite is a necessary corporate strategy prior to communications planning. As with the investment professional in Chapter 2, it is important to know the makeup of the individual investor so that you will know *what* to communicate as well as to *whom*. The information in this chapter helps profile the individual investor as Chapter 2 profiled the investment professional.

The firm noted that several questions permitted multiple responses, resulting in tabulations, in some instances, in excess of 100 percent. Nevertheless, the surveys made it possible to draw up a profile of the individual investor with interesting and significant implications.

Buying Decision

A significant portion of the investors surveyed—44.1 percent—reported using their own judgment in selecting appropriate investments. This figure is made more meaningful by the substantially lower portion, 27.4 percent, whose share purchases were based on the recommendation of financial advisers. The 27.4 percent figure ties in closely with the 25 percent figure the investment professionals mentioned in Chapter 2. About 60 percent more individuals use their own judgment for investment selection than use the recommendation of professional advisers. This information should have particular rele-

40

vance for professional advisers. Two immediate questions come to mind:

1. How significant an influence, if any, were financial advisers in developing the individual's purchase decision?

2. Are investment advisers gaining or losing in their efforts to market their services? What has the trend been over the past few years, and, more important, what does this imply for the future profitability and viability of investment advisers?

The one major surprise was the high ranking of the "other" category—in which 11.8 percent cited various nonbusiness reasons for acquiring shares while friends and relatives recommended the stock in 14 percent of the purchases (see Table 3–1). Only 5.6 percent of the respondents reported using financial publications as the basis for their decision. From these results, it can be assumed that published material fails to influence people, consciously or unconsciously, to a significant degree. An attempt to isolate possible feedback effects between published material and investor opinion-decision development would be extremely valuable. Unfortunately, such effects could not be determined through the surveys under study. However, possible feedback reactions notwithstanding—the impact of financial publications was significantly low.

The survey results are significant to your communications plan. If, for example, you have been relying heavily on publicity, is this a proper target in view of the low rating of financial publications? On the other hand, the role of your publicity may be merely to bring your company name to the attention of the investor for a decision to be made later. The results do indicate, however, that a multifaceted communications program will be necessary to reach the financial adviser, the financial press, and the individual investor. A more detailed discussion on information sources appears later in this chapter.

Since such a large number of individual investors claim to make their own decisions, it will be helpful for you to know the approach they use in evaluating securities. The most common method is the fundamental approach, in which the investor has a personal need for and a personal standard of return on the investment. The second most common approach is a fundamental and technical approach, in which considerable study is made of the particular investment to go along with the personal need. The pure technical approach is used very seldom.

Investment Objectives

For strategy planning, it is necessary for you to know why investors invest, so that you can plan your communications accordingly. Income with growth, for example, was the primary investment objective of the

Table 3–1
On whose recommendation did you buy the stock?

	Financial adviser		Financial publication		Friends/ relatives		Own judgment		Other		Total share- holders
	Number	Percent	Number	Percent	Number	Percent	Number	Percent	Number	Percent	Number
Survey 1	1,310	23.5	325	5.8	850	15.3	2,480	44.5	605	10.9	5,570
Survey 2	380	30.6	55	4.4	233	18.7	397	32.0	178	14.3	1,243
Survey 3	2,237	32.7	320	4.7	1,086	15.9	1,981	30.0	1,214	17.8	6,838
Survey 4	303	31.9	56	5.9	133	14.0	386	40.6	73	7.7	951
Survey 5	4,304	27.8	940	6.1	922	6.0	8,013	51.7	1,306	8.4	15,485
Total	8,231	27.4	1,696	5.6	3,224	10.7	13,257	44.1	3,376	11.2	30,087
Average....		29.3		5.4		14.0		39.8		11.8	

Source: Burson-Marsteller Surveys.

majority of respondents (see Table 3–2). If you can meet that objective, your job has been simplified. If not, you will have to determine whether you can fulfill the other objectives, which, in order, were growth, income, and safety. It is important to realize that, by using their own judgment, investors have succeeded in properly matching their investment goals with appropriate opportunities. Based on the average company profile, in terms of risk, dividend yield, and growth, shareholders have selected issues which—on average—have a 10.7 percent estimated growth rate. The average risk factor, as measured by the beta coefficient, is 0.99—with a 4.9 percent dividend yield. On average, the growth-income classification fits the stated objectives of approximately 50 percent of the respondents as well as the typical investment character of those companies participating in the surveys. It is interesting to note, because companies are often under a misapprehension on this point, that only 11.9 percent selected their stock for income, since a 4.9 percent dividend yield is not overly attractive in light of other available risk/reward investment opportunities (see Table 3–3).

Five percent reported that they were specifically interested in performance safety. Considering that the average safety factor (as measured by Value Line's investment ranking) is 2.4 out of a possible 1 to 5 range, it is likely that safety-oriented investors would prefer a ranking more closely approaching 1.

The most important stated investment goal for individual investors is long-term gain, which is followed by current income and intermediate-term gain.

While these surveys accurately portray the motivations behind the decision making of the individual investor, three college professors were curious about the basis for the motivations. Several years ago, their curiosity led them to an in-depth study of the behavioral patterns of individual investors. The study, as reported in the *Journal of Business*, was conducted by Wilbur G. Lewellen, professor of management, Purdue University; Ronald C. Lease, associate professor of finance, University of Utah; and Gary G. Schlarbaum, associate professor of management, Purdue University.[1]

They addressed empirically the matter of the portfolio decision processes of the individual equity investor. Their objectives were to identify the systematic patterns of investment behavior exhibited and to appraise the rationality of those patterns—that is, were the patterns internally consistent and did they fit with reasonable a priori notions with regard to appropriate responses to risk, liquidity, and personal tax considerations?

---

[1] Wilbur G. Lewellen, Ronald C. Lease and Gary G. Schlarbaum, "Patterns of Investment Strategy and Behavior among Individual Investors," *Journal of Business*, 1977, pp. 297–332. Copyright © 1977 by the University of Chicago Press.

Table 3–2
What is your primary investment objective?

	Income		Growth		Income and growth		Safety		Other		Total share-holder responses
	Number	Percent	Number	Percent	Number	Percent	Number	Percent	Number	Percent	
Survey 1.........	915	18.0	950	18.7	2,815	55.5	280	5.5	115	2.3	5,075
Survey 2.........	184	14.8	228	18.3	723	58.0	112	9.0	0	0	1,247
Survey 3.........	639	10.0	1,022	16.0	4,665	73.0	1,022	16.0	64	1.0	7,412
Survey 4.........	64	7.1	251	27.6	533	58.7	42	4.6	18	2.0	908
Survey 5.........	1,340	9.5	4,570	32.5	7,077	50.4	733	5.2	337	2.4	14,041
Total	3,142	11.0	7,021	24.5	15,813	55.0	2,189	7.6	534	2.0	28,683
Average		11.9		22.6		59.0		8.1		1.5	100%

Source: Burson-Marsteller Surveys.

Table 3–3
Important company characteristics

	Beta	Safety ranking*	Yield†	Growth rate‡
Survey 1	0.65	2	4.6%	10.5%
Survey 2	0.95	3	6.7	6.5
Survey 3	0.90	2	5.6	11.5
Survey 4	1.0	2	4.0	8.5
Survey 5	1.45	3	3.7	16.5
Average	0.99	2.4	4.9	10.7

* Based on Value Line's Standard.
† Current dividend yield.
‡ Value Line's estimated 1974–76 to 1979–81 earnings per share growth rate.
Source: Burson-Marsteller Surveys.

The investor group consisted of a sample of approximately 1,000 persons drawn from the customer clientele of a large national retail brokerage house. It comprised individuals who had accounts open with the firm over a six-year period, and it was stratified geographically to match the composition of the total population of U.S. common shareholders. Among the most startling messages to emerge from the data was the fact that investment behavior is very much a direct and systematic function of personal circumstances. The researchers said that a number of statistically significant socioeconomic cross-sectional patterns were observable, that the same key independent variables show up reliably in connection with quite a broad spectrum of investment phenomena, that the directions of the influence of these variables are stable and internally consistent, and that these effects are revealed equally by each of several analytic approaches and are generally in accord with what seem to be logical behavioral scenarios.

The dominant elements are investor age, income level, and sex, essentially in that descending order of importance. These characteristics override occupation, material status, family size, and educational background as significant influences. The latter attributes make an occasional modest contribution to the explanation of differences in investment style and strategy, but they are notable largely for the rarity of their impact. As for the impact of age on investment goals, the older the investor, whether male or female, the less was his or her reported interest in short-term capital gains (see Table 3–4).

The concern about dividends, on the other hand, increases with age but diminishes with family income level. At all income levels, greater age produces greater relative interest in dividends (see Table 3–5).

46

Table 3–4
Short-term capital gains as a portfolio goal versus
investor age (cross-classification analysis)

	Goal importance rating				
Investor age	1	2	3	4	Total
Male investors					
Under 45	.25*	.30	.26	.19	1.00
45–54	.37	.27	.23	.13	1.00
55–64	.58	.20	.14	.08	1.00
65 and over	.65	.23	.07	.05	1.00
Probability of independence less than .0001.					
Female investors					
Under 45	.28	.32	.28	.12	1.00
45–54	.48	.30	.09	.13	1.00
55–64	.71	.17	.05	.07	1.00
65 and over	.72	.18	.05	.05	1.00
Probability of independence equals .0015.					

* I.e., 25 percent of male investors below age 45 rate short-term capital gains "1" in importance on a scale of 1 to 4, where the rating categories are: 1—irrelevant, 2—slightly important, 3—important, and 4—very important.

Source: Wilbur G. Lewellen, Ronald C. Lease, and Gary G. Schlarbaum, "Patterns of Investment Strategy and Behavior among Individual Investors," *Journal of Business*, 1977, pp. 297–332. Copyright © 1977 by the University of Chicago.

These patterns not only complement the patterns for the short-term capital gains ratings but also appear to be reasonable reactions to personal tax, liquidity, and career cycle considerations. When an individual enjoys a substantial annual income, he or she should have less need for additional immediate cash returns from an investment portfolio, and the heavy tax burden imposed on those returns would further reduce their attractiveness. As an individual passes peak employment earnings years and moves toward and into retirement, however, it seems appropriate to shift the portfolio toward income securities as a means of offsetting an earnings loss. Thus, major revisions in dividend importance ratings occur beginning at age 55.

Two investment goal alternatives in the survey, long-term and intermediate-term appreciation, exhibited no comparable sensitivity to personal circumstances. The consistency with which the former was highly rated as an objective permitted little scope for discerning patterns. The latter showed some variation across investor groups, but in neither a systematic nor a statistically significant manner. When asked about the performance criterion used in assessing their investment suc-

Table 3–5
Dividend income as a portfolio goal versus investor age and income
(cross-classification analysis)

	Goal importance rating			
	1	2	3	4
Age versus dividend goal importance				
Investor age (years)				
Under 45	.35	.38	.18	.09
45–54	.27	.39	.25	.09
55–64	.10	.28	.29	.33
65 and over	.05	.18	.23	.54
Income versus dividend goal importance				
Investor family income				
Under $15,000	.10	.22	.22	.46
$15,000–$24,900	.18	.28	.27	.27
$25,000–$49,999	.19	.28	.27	.26
$50,000 up	.22	.46	.20	.12
Age versus dividend goal importance, by income bracket				
Investors with incomes below $15,000				
Under 45	.29	.33	.17	.21
45–54	.21	.47	.15	.18
55–64	.10	.21	.30	.39
65 and over	.04	.13	.21	.62
Investors with incomes between $15,000 and $24,999				
Under 45	.31	.43	.18	.08
45–54	.30	.36	.26	.08
55–64	.14	.26	.32	.28
65 and over	.04	.12	.25	.59
Investors with incomes between $25,000 and $49,999				
Under 45	.36	.31	.23	.10
45–54	.27	.33	.29	.11
55–64	.08	.24	.30	.38
65 and over	.08	.21	.24	.48
Investors with incomes of $50,000 and over				
Under 45	.43	.43	.11	.03
45–54	.30	.46	.19	.05
55–64	.07	.43	.22	.28
65 and over	.04	.54	.27	.15

Source: Wilbur G. Lewellen, Ronald C. Lease, and Gary G. Schlarbaum, "Patterns of Investment Strategy and Behavior among Individual Investors," *Journal of Business*, 1977, pp. 297–332. Copyright © 1977 by the University of Chicago.

cess, 42 percent of the respondents indicated that one of the major public indexes—the DJIA, NYSE, or the S&P 500—was selected. Another 45 percent reported that they had a personal standard of return which was an amalgam of experience, evidence, and concepts of "fair" yield. The remainder employed scattered measures.

Age was also a determinant of risk taking (see Table 3–6). The results were consistent with the portfolio goal ratings, in that age and

Table 3–6
Expressed investment risk-taking desires versus investor age (cross-classification analysis)

	Scaled desire to take risks				
Investor age	1	2	3	4	5
Under 45	.20	.18	.17	.27	.18
45–54	.20	.18	.17	.28	.17
55–64	.29	.24	.12	.23	.12
65 and over	.33	.26	.17	.15	.09

Source: Wilbur G. Lewellen, Ronald C. Lease, and Gary G. Schlarbaum, "Patterns of Investment Strategy and Behavior among Individual Investors," *Journal of Business*, 1977, pp. 297–332. Copyright © 1977 by the University of Chicago.

risk taking were inversely related, with the major shifts again taking place at age 55.

The investment tactics employed within the sample displayed a richer variety of demographic differences than did the goals toward which the several subgroups were aiming, so that distinctions between male and female investors became apparent (see Table 3–7). The areas of information gathering and decision making are illustrations. In general, male investors claimed to do considerably more of their own investment analysis, spending more time and money on that activity than did female investors. Women tended to rely heavily on their broker's advice for portfolio decisions and to maintain a given level of dependence on their broker.

The study reveals that at all ages the proportion of female investors who designated "broker advice" the primary source of their security selection decisions was well above that of their male counterparts. Male investors, correspondingly, were less sanguine than female investors in a direct rating of the value of their broker's counsel, were substantially more entranced by the usefulness of paid external research services, and spent more time in evaluating information to reach decisions.

Table 3–7
Investment analysis and investor demographics
(cross-classification analysis)

Primary security selection approach versus age and sex

| | Primary approach to analysis | | |
Investor age	Funda-mental, technical, or both	Rely on broker advice	Other
Male investors			
Under 55 .... .71	.71	.20	.09
55–64 .... .71	.71	.17	.09
65 and over .... .75	.75	.11	.14
Probability of independence = .0192			
Female investors			
Under 55 .... .56	.56	.35	.09
55–64 .... .52	.52	.36	.12
65 and over .... .55	.55	.34	.11
Probability of independence = .9778			

Rating of value of investment information, by sex

| | | Information useful | | |
Source of information	Never	Occa-sionally	Gen-erally	Always
Broker				
Males .... .07	.07	.32	.41	.20
Females .... .07	.07	.23	.43	.27
Probability of independence = .0712				
Research service subscriptions				
Males .... .23	.23	.45	.21	.11
Females .... .31	.31	.54	.10	.05
Probability of independence = .0001				

Time spent per month on investment analysis and decision making, by sex

| | Time spent (hours) | | | |
Sex	0–5	5–10	10–20	Over 20
Males	.51	.19	.14	.16
Females	.68	.16	.10	.06

Source: Wilbur G. Lewellen, Ronald C. Lease, and Gary G. Schlarbaum, "Patterns of Investment Strategy and Behavior among Individual Investors," *Journal of Business,* 1977, pp. 297–332. Copyright © 1977 by the University of Chicago Press.

Table 3–8
Ranking of financial goals by degree of importance

	Total	Stock owners
"Very" or "fairly" important to majority of households		
Income/normal expenses	91%	85%
Keeping up with inflation	88	85
Protection for family	87	86
Income/retirement	87	85
Personal control of assets	82	84
Improved standard of living	78	70
Estate for spouse/children	74	70
Tax minimization	67	67
Purchase of home	65	55
Guaranteed fixed return	62	61
Children's college expense	59	55
Liquidity—cash or equivalent	54	59
"Very" or "fairly" important to minority of households		
Long-term capital appreciation	47	61
Fun/challenge	45	41
Minimal downside risk	42	45
Maximum leverage from available funds	40	49
Quick profits	31	28
Savings/investing for big-ticket expenditure	27	30
Diversification	24	39
Action—frequent trading	12	10

Public Attitudes toward Investing (New York: NYSE, 1978), p. 10.

A study by the New York Stock Exchange agrees (see Table 3–8). The study states:

> Younger and less affluent financial decision makers do not stress the same goals as their older and more affluent counterparts. Those under 35 and those with incomes below $15,000 give much greater importance to income for normal expenses, improving their standard of living, and buying a home than do other groups. Younger people are also more concerned than their elders with college expenses, the personal challenge of investing, short-term profits, accumulating money for large expenditures, and minimizing taxes.
>
> Households with incomes above $25,000 put above-average emphasis on capital appreciation, minimizing taxes, minimizing downside risk, maximizing leverage, and diversification of investments. A majority of financial decision makers regard three investment vehicles as most appropriate for meeting their own financial goals—life insurance, cash savings, and real estate other than one's own home. (see Table 3–9.)

Table 3–9
Investment vehicles viewed as best meeting most important financial goals

Goal	Vehicle (percent of household)
Protection for family	Life insurance (57%)
Income/normal expenses	Real estate other than home (22%), savings certificate (19%)
Income/retirement	Life insurance (25%), savings certificate (22%), real estate other than home (19%)
Keeping up with inflation	Real estate other than home (32%)
Personal control of assets	Savings certificate (25%), real estate other than home (24%)
Purchase of home	Savings certificate (21%), real estate other than home (20%)
Estate for spouse/children	Life insurance (47%), real estate other than home (26%)
Improved standard of living	Real estate other than home (30%)
Children's college expenses	Savings certificate (35%), life insurance (26%)
Tax minimization	Real estate other than home (24%)
Guaranteed fixed return	Savings certificate (21%), life insurance (20%)

Public Attitudes toward Investing (New York, NYSE, 1978), p. 11.

The most widely held investment vehicles, in addition to one's own home, are those perceived as involving the smallest element of risk— life insurance, various types of fixed-income savings, and other real estate (see Table 3–10). Treasury bills and municipal bonds are rated low risk but are not widely held—possibly because most financial decision makers are not very familiar with them. Common stock, considered moderate in risk, is ranked 6th riskiest of 20 vehicles.

Holders of listed common stock are likely to have a number of other investments. Nearly all have life insurance, a passbook savings account, and their own home or apartment. Smaller, but significant, numbers have U.S. savings bonds or savings certificates, participate in an employee savings plan, and own other real estate or such tangibles as gems or art. Another 25 percent also hold unlisted common stock, preferred stock, or stock mutual funds. One third of those who own real estate other than their home also hold listed common stock; half as many hold unlisted common stock, preferred stock, or stock mutual funds.

Since common stock only rates ninth as an investment vehicle, the challenge which should be addressed is how to tap some of the assets from more popular vehicles. This would require some profound analy-

52

Table 3–10
Ownership of investment vehicles

	Percent of households	
	Own now	Owned once
Life insurance	92%	4%
Passbook savings account	86	4
Own home	83	3
U.S. savings bonds	47	22
Employee savings plan	34	12
Savings certificate	34	8
Real estate other than home	30	9
Tangible investments	29	2
Common stock (listed)	27	11
Employee profit-sharing plan	25	10
Ownership in private company	19	10
Investment retirement account	16	1
Stock mutual funds	11	9
Annuity	10	2
Unlisted common stock	9	8
Preferred stock	9	5
Long-term U.S. bonds	6	5
Municipal bonds	5	5
Convertible securities	5	5
U.S. Treasury bills	5	4
Corporate bonds	5	3
Tax-free mutual funds	3	1
Tax shelters	2	2
Money market mutual funds	2	1
Options	1	2
Warrants	1	2
Commodity contracts	1	1

Public Attitudes toward Investing (New York: NYSE, 1978), p. 12.

sis and thinking. For instance, is the flow of millions of investors in and out of the market under variable economic conditions due to the conditions themselves? Is it due to other investments offering higher yield or greater safety? Is it due to government regulations? Or is it due to the failure of managements to sell and keep confidence in the stock market? Does human behavior suggest that there is a trace of truth in each of these possibilities? Perhaps, understanding why investors leave the marketplace may be helpful. The biggest reason for withdrawal, according to the NYSE, is the search for safer, less risky investments (20 percent). Other reasons given were: put money in other investments such as real estate, 20 percent; suffered a loss when the market went down, 14 percent; needed money, 14 percent; faced major household expenses, such as college education, 7 percent; and have less to invest now, 7 percent. Personal financial situations thus appear to be strong reasons as compared to the large factors impacting on the market.

An even larger group than those investors who abandoned the stock market consists of those people who have never entered it. Their reasons, as determined by the NYSE, are interesting: 36 percent said they could not afford it; 28 percent said it was too risky; 17 percent said they were not interested; 16 percent needed money for other purposes; and 13 percent lacked knowledge of the stock market. Other than needing money for other purposes, the stated reasons suggest to me that American industry has failed to convince or educate millions of new investors on the benefits of stock investment.

How the Investor Keeps Informed

The overwhelming source of investment information is the broker. It is interesting that the broker is the key information source even though the majority of investors claim that they make their own decisions. This would suggest that communications to the broker are a necessity. While banks and investment literature follow far behind the broker, it should be noted that nearly one fourth of general public investors rely on a different, nonmarket institution, namely banks, for investment advice. The "mind penetration" of investors is something to be closely watched, from a communications viewpoint, as the nature of industry competition changes.

Types of Communication Desired

On the average, the communications most welcomed by shareholders are annual reports, 73.1 percent, and quarterly reports, 60.9 percent (see Table 3–11). Indeed, shareholders expect and are justifiably entitled to the perennial statement and review of company progress, or the

Table 3–11
Type of communication desired

	Annual report	Quarterly report	Form 10-K	Speeches by company officials	Important press releases
Survey 1	70.2%	67.6%	11.6%	25.7%	36.4%
Survey 2	77.2	51.8	14.2	23.5	38.7
Survey 3	72.9	60.0	14.8	26.3	35.0
Survey 4	72.0	64.0	7.0	22.0	34.0
Average	73.1	60.9	11.9	24.4	36.0

Source: Burson-Marsteller Surveys.

lack of it, with supporting explanations. However, is the desire for typical quarterlies the result of need or habit? Quarterly reports are generally unaudited. This diminishes their relative value. In addition, and more important, such reports tend to reflect short-term secular trends in business activity and therefore are best interpreted in light of the broader corporate outlook.

Of the respondents to the Burson-Marsteller surveys, one out of three wished to receive important press releases. Approximately one quarter of the respondents expressed a desire to receive summaries of speeches made by corporate officials to financial analysts. Significantly fewer wished to receive their company's 10-K report. Since the desire of shareholders for more and sophisticated information seems to be increasing, it is somewhat surprising that so few wanted to see such a valuable document as the 10-K. After all, the 10-K is widely regarded as the single most important information source available on any company. I suspect that its poor readership is due to the fact that in most companies the 10-K is still in the hands of accountants and lawyers who succeed in making it more tedious than footnotes. One contribution that could be made by the communications department is to make the 10-K readable through better presentation of material.

Areas of Special Interest in Annual Reports

Though few investors base their final investment decision on the annual report alone, most investors do find the annual report valuable in leading them toward that decision. Their interest in the various aspects of annual reports is along the following order of priority: financial statements, 40.6 percent; operational review, 32.6 percent; and shareholder letters, 26.8 percent (see Table 3–12). The combined results of financial statements and operational review, 73.2 percent, point to a substantial and possibly increasing interest, knowledge, and sophistication on the part of shareholders. There is obviously a desire to get more deeply involved with business investments—which, for most investors, are an important depository for their hard-earned dollars. That desire is probably the result of poor stock performance over the past few years and of uncertainties about the future performance of stocks.

Business Publication Reading

More than three quarters of the combined shareholders reported reading business and financial publications on a regular basis (see Table 3–13). Investors apparently are attempting to increase their level of business knowledge, keep close tabs on their investments, and search for new investment potentials. Market vicissitudes and uncer-

Table 3-12

What is of particular interest to you in annual report?

	Financial statements		Shareholder letters		Operational review		Total shareholders
	Number	Percent	Number	Percent	Number	Percent	
Survey 1	2,575	40.1%	1,645	25.6%	2,200	34.3%	6,420
Survey 2	700	45.5	293	19.0	546	35.5	1,539
Survey 3	2,875	42.9	2,237	33.3	1,598	23.8	6,710
Survey 4	496	41.4	255	21.3	448	37.4	1,199
Survey 5	3,742	38.6	2,416	24.9	3,545	36.5	9,703
Total	10,388	40.6	6,846	26.8	8,337	32.6	25,571
Average		41.7		24.8		33.5	

Source: Burson-Marsteller Surveys.

Table 3–13
Do you regularly read business and financial publications?

	Yes		No		Other/no answer		Total
	Number	Percent	Number	Percent	Number	Percent	Number
Survey 1	3,450	68.0%	1,625	32.0%	0		50
Survey 2	666	75.6	149	16.9	66	7.5%	881
Survey 3	11,113	79.1	2,760	19.7	168	1.2	14,041
Total	15,229	76.1	4,534	22.7	234	1.2	29,997
Average		74.2		22.9		2.9	100%

Source: Burson-Marsteller Surveys.

tainties are undoubtedly among the reasons for this effort since these readers reported that they did not, in fact, use business and financial publications as the basis for their ultimate investment decisions.

Sources of information by individual investors in Advisory Committee on Corporate Disclosure survey are shown in Table 3–14.

Is There a Model Investor?

No one has yet pushed the magic button on a computer and said, "Voilà, here is the perfect investor." Considerable information on the characteristics of the average investor has been gathered through studies of various investor segments that have been conducted at different times. While the weightings may vary by degree, common threads run through the foregoing studies.

My observations are that the average investor, drawn from the general population, is the male head of a household, married, a homeowner, moderately affluent, well educated and a professional or manager in his middle years (see Table 3–15).

Characteristics of the typical investor as developed by Professors Lewellen, Lease, and Schlarbaum varied in weighting by percentages, but the largest percentages were in my average range (see Table 3–16).

The percentages of the SEC study also vary, but the same general groupings occur (see Table 3–17).

Investors describe themselves as belonging to different categories—or segments—based on their needs, wealth, or investing styles. The largest proportion of investors see themselves as *mutual decision makers*, persons who work closely *with* their brokers in making investment decisions. The next largest groups are the *delegators*, persons who are too busy with their own careers to spend time on their investments and who therefore *rely* heavily and exclusively on their brokers to make the investment decisions; the *novices*, persons whose investment philosophy has not yet crystallized; the *individualists*, persons who say they make all their investment decisions themselves; and, finally, the *traders*, persons who are interested primarily in short-term gains.

Investor—Large or Small?

The final questions are: (1) How small an investor do you want investing in your company? (2) Is he or she worth it?

If you want a broad base of individual shareowners, you have to cope with an extensive and expensive shareowner relations program. At one company I worked for, I determined that it cost more to annually service one share of stock than the stock was selling for at the time. With the cost of servicing versus the cost of money, it was determined

Table 3-14
Value ranking of information types direct and street name investors combined

Types of information	Extremely useful		Moderately useful		Not very useful		Not useful at all		No opinion		Total		No response
	Number	Percent	Number	Percent	Number	Percent	Number	Percent	Number	Percent	Number	Percent	Number
Charts or statistics of security prices	697	18	1,539	41	689	18	358	9	516	14	3,799	100	630
Financial statement data, balance sheet, income statement, etc.	1,999	50	1,436	36	254	6	101	3	205	5	3,995	100	437
Company's own assessment of its *future* business prospects	1,107	28	1,879	47	597	15	178	5	203	5	3,964	100	466
Outside assessment of *the company's future* business prospects	1,440	37	1,655	42	358	9	157	4	290	8	3,900	100	521
Future economic outlook of industry of which company is a part	2,188	58	1,420	38	173	4	0		0		3,781	100	438

Charts displaying *the company's* earnings and sales over recent years	1,489	38	1,701	43	443	11	130	3	201	5	3,964	100	464
Information about general business outlook in the U.S. economy	1,196	30	1,826	46	587	15	141	4	207	5	3,957	100	470
Information about year-to-year changes in *the company's* financial statement items	1,436	36	1,690	43	479	12	129	3	225	6	3,959	100	471
Information about quality of *the company's* management	2,112	54	1,076	28	364	9	122	3	218	6	3,892	100	533
Charts or tables displaying key financial ratios of *the company*	746	19	1,476	39	868	23	311	8	431	11	3,832	100	599
Information about *the company* product—nature of product, potential markets	1,744	44	1,608	41	306	7	103	3	192	5	3,953	100	475
Recent investment activities of large institutions	563	14	1,295	33	1,006	26	557	14	523	13	3,944	100	685
Miscellaneous other	220	31	71	10	13	2	9	1	399	56	712	100	43

Individual Investor Opinion Survey, Advisory Committee on Corporate Disclosure, Securities and Exchange Commission, 1977.

Table 3–15
Characteristics of the average investor

Median income	$32,600
Professional/managerial occupation	74%
College graduate.....................	71
Own home	86
Married	87
Dependent children..................	51
Male	90
Median age.........................	51 years

that holdings under 25 shares were inefficient, so the company offered to buy holdings under that amount. An even larger question than the cost of servicing a broad base of shareowners is whether, in fact, such a base provides any market stability, or even whether it provides a defense against takeovers.

Surprisingly, given the extent of market sophistication, hard empirical proof is tough to obtain. In fact, it does not appear to exist. I have been unable to find any quantitative studies as to the advantages or disadvantages of having a large base of small, individual shareholders other than my own experience on servicing costs. Yet, the traditional wisdom—that it pays to have a diversified base of owners—has been accepted by most companies. This is reflected in a survey conducted by a proxy solicitation firm. The survey found that a substantial majority of companies consider the ideal percentage of individual holders to be 75 percent or more.

The logical reasons for this view might appear to include: depth and breadth of market; ability to withstand a tender offer; deconcentration of voting control held by financial institutions; purchase of more shares by individuals (trading up) over time; loyalty of individuals, who see themselves as investors and not traders; product loyalty of individuals—they buy more of the company's product than do non-shareholders and institutional holders; individuals' support of company on political issues; and popular support by individuals—economics aside, no large corporation can afford the social pressures that will build up against it if its shares are not broadly distributed.

But the contrary corporate finance officer may venture these points in rebuttal: you'll never get enough individuals to sop up all the institutional holdings; it takes less time and effort to convince a sophisticated investor to reject a tender offer than it takes to reach all the "little guys" throughout the land; institutions don't vote shares—they recognize that their shareholder role is to be passive owners, not active managers; no study has been done on whether oddlot holders turn into

Table 3–16
Characteristics of the investor—Lewellen,
Lease, and Schlarbaum study

Characteristic	Percent
Age	
Under 21	Less than 1
21–34	3
35–44	12
45–54	29
55–64	26
65 and over	30
Sex	
Male	80
Female	20
Family income	
Under $5,000	2
$5,000–$9,999	8
$10,000–$14,999	15
$15,000–$19,999	13
$20,000–$24,000	18
$25,000–$49,999	26
$50,000 and over	18
Education	
Less than high school	11
High school graduate	12
Some college	23
BA/BS	31
Graduate degree	23
Occupation	
Professional/technical	27
Manager/proprietor	29
Clerical/service	7
Craftsman/laborer	3
Farm owner/farm laborer	2
Not employed	32

Wilbur G. Lewellen, Ronald C. Lease, and Gary G. Schlarbaum, "Patterns of Investment Strategy and Behavior among Individual Investors," *Journal of Business*, 1977, pp. 297–332. Copyright © 1977 by the University of Chicago Press.

round lot holders over time; and there is no evidence that an individual shareholder will buy more of a company's product than a nonshareholder.

Shareholder support for company positions is fragile at best. As *Barron's* editor Robert Bleiberg has noted, shareholder turnover on the

62

Table 3–17
Characteristics of the investor—SEC study

	Number	Percent
Education completed		
Attended or graduated		
elementary school	143	3
One to three years high school	235	5
Graduated high school	680	16
One to three years college	812	19
Graduated college	1,196	27
Some postgraduate work,		
master's degree, Ph.D. or		
equivalent, etc.	1,289	30
	4,355*	100%

* Excludes nonindicating responses.

Gender		
Male	3,287	78
Female	906	22
Total	4,193*	100%

* 236 respondents failed to indicate gender.

Age		
Under 21	29	0*
21–24	32	0*
25–34	291	7
35–44	438	10
45–54	737	17
55–64	1,246	29
65–74	1,078	25
75 and older	516	12
Total	4,367†	100%

* Actual percentage is 0.7 percent.
† Excludes 52 nonindicating responses.

Family income		
Under $5,000	66	1
$5,000–$9,999	183	4
$10,000–$14,999	369	9
$15,000–$24,999	972	23
$25,000–$49,999	1,609	38
$50,000–$99,000	757	18
$100,000–$499,000	312	7
$500,000 and over	13	0†
Total	4,281*	100%

* 150 respondents failed to indicate family income or gave multiple answers.
† Actual percentage is 0.3 percent.

Source: Individual Investor Opinion Survey, Advisory Committee on Corporate Disclosure, Securities and Exchange Commission, 1977.

New York Stock Exchange in 1976 was 23 percent, and "a constituency that is constantly changing, ever-shifting, so to speak, is scarcely the most solid foundation on which to build."

You can resolve the issue to some degree by conducting your own research among the individual shareholders of your company. Your communications department can determine why those shareholders bought the stock in the first place and whether they are candidates for additional stock purchases; whether those shareholders buy more of your product than do nonshareholders (by comparing their dollar purchases with your product's general standing in the marketplace); whether your individual shareholders pay more attention to company product ads than do nonshareholders; and how your costs of producing and mailing to small shareholders in terms of the size of their holdings compare with the costs you incur to satisfy the *information* needs of large shareholders. Frequent meetings with large shareholders, for example, may be expensive.

What it may come down to is a matter of individual company preference. I have heard impassioned pleas for the role of the small investor through the years. They go like this:

> The small investor is traditionally the most highly motivated producer of economic wealth in our society. It is from the small investor that our work ethic stems, along with the sense of frugality that requires us to save today for tomorrow's needs.

> Over the long pull, if the small investor can't make money in the market, the United States will run out of investment capital for new plants and equipment, research that generates new technology, and funds for corporate expansion. The whole system will wind down to a deep depression.

> Institutions add little to capital formation. They are basically dealers in secondhand securities. They generate a lot of stock sales volume but no capital for industry and very little profit for the securities industry. Their only loyalty is to the investment committee's batting average, not the companies behind the stock.

> It is the small investor who buys the new equity issues that industry needs for its growth and that Wall Street must have to stay solvent.

> It is the small investor who buys the stock of the smaller companies that do pay big dividends.

> It is the small investor who buys the highly speculative start-up situations.

> It is the small investor who reinvests dividends into more shares of the company's stock. It is only the small investor who shows any investment loyalty.

But to all of these pleas, the basic question remains: Where is the proof of the pudding?

Investor Concerns

The 75 percent of companies that want small individual sharehold-ers, for whatever reason, must be prepared to deal with their concerns. Georgeson & Co. has said that shareholders have numerous concerns—129 to be exact (see Figure 3–1). Your research can deter-mine which of these concerns are priorities for you.

Figure 3–1
Checklist of stockholder concerns—1982

I. *Investor relations*
   A. Proxy and voting
      1. Availability of management for stockholder contact and discus-sion.
      2. Related party disclosures: names of large holders with whom the company conducts business where there is a potential con-flict of interest, e.g., law firms, banks, insurance companies.
      3. Role of institutional holders in formulating corporate policy.
      4. Analyst recommendations in proxy voting.
      5. Identity of largest holders not included in proxy statement.
      6. Omission of stockholders' proposals from proxy statements.
      7. Opportunity for a stockholder to respond to management pro-posals.
      8. Handling of unmarked proxies.
      9. Secret ballot.
      10. Cumulative voting rights.
      11. Voting results of last year's meeting.
      12. Price at which company may be for sale.
   B. Dividend policy and security information
      1. Dividend policy.
      2. Dividend reinvestment plan (intention to shift to original issue plan if favorable tax legislation is passed).
      3. Availability of dividend reinvestment plan for IRAs, etc.
      4. Stock repurchases.
      5. Stock dividend/stock split.
      6. Analysts, portfolio managers and brokers who follow the stock.
   C. Annual report and annual meeting
      1. Availability of transcript of annual meeting.
      2. Time and location of annual meeting.
      3. Inclusion of 10-K in annual report package.
      4. Cost of annual report.
      5. Post meeting report.
      6. Presence of auditors at annual meeting.
II. *Corporate governance*
   A. Directorship policies and activities
      1. Responsibility of directors to community and public at large.
      2. Director compensation.
      3. Retirement/separation policy for directors.

Figure 3–1 (*continued*)

---

    4. Reports to stockholders on board meetings.
    5. Attendance at directors' meetings.
    6. Nominating procedure for directors.
    7. Women/minorities on the board.
    8. Frequency of directors' meetings.
    9. Directors as stockholders.
    10. Staggered board.
    11. Outside versus inside directors.
    12. Procedure for determining management compensation.
    13. Perquisites, especially use of corporate aircraft and lodging facilities and loans to officers.
    14. Policy on committees.
    15. Function of committees.
    16. Composition of committees.
    17. Public policy committee.
    18. Disclosure of bylaw changes.
  B. Corporate matters
    1. Current investigation of company by regulatory agency.
    2. Status of pending stockholder suits.
    3. Report on internal controls.
    4. Procedures to prevent improper use of corporate assets.
    5. Responsibilities of corporate counsel.
    6. Client/attorney relationship.
    7. Presence of company counsel on board.
    8. Disagreements with auditors.
    9. Lobbying activities.
    10. Legal fees.
    11. Audit fees.
    12. Public relations and advertising expenditures.
    13. Employment of auditors as management consultants.
    14. Policy on ensuring independence of auditors.
    15. Labor problems.
    16. Compliance with Foreign Corrupt Practices Act.
    17. View toward amending the FCPA.
III. *Public Affairs*
  A. Government relations
    1. Involvement in South Africa, Panama, Libya, etc.
    2. Trade with communist nations.
    3. Domestic political contributions.
    4. Political action committee.
    5. Employment of former government employees.
    6. Products (particularly nuclear) and services for military use.
    7. Foreign political considerations.
    8. Conflicts with regulatory authorities.
    9. Investment in or imports from countries with human rights problems.
    10. Tax incentives for investors.

Figure 3-1 (*continued*)

---

     11. Arab boycott.
- B. Community relations
  1. Criteria for corporate contributions.
  2. Use of increased corporate deduction for contributions.
  3. Noncash contributions to institutions, universities, and other organizations of higher education.
  4. Control over corporate social activity.
  5. Social objectives of corporations.
  6. Environmental/ecological concerns.
  7. Industrial hazards such as waste, nuclear power, safety, etc.
  8. Nuclear power as an energy source.
  9. Policy on plant closings, notice to community, etc.
  10. Redlining.
  11. Increased employment opportunities/job training for disadvantage of youth.
- C. General
  1. Social criteria for pension fund investments.
  2. Disclosure of socially significant information.
  3. Role of corporation in public affairs.
  4. Truth in advertising.
  5. Energy conservation measures.
  6. Investments/spending to influence sales.
  7. Refusal to do business on ethical grounds.
  8. Equal pay for work of equal value.
  9. Written affirmative action plan.

IV. *Financial management*
- A. Financial reporting
  1. Impact of Economic Recovery Tax Act of 1981.
  2. Inflation accounting.
  3. Assessment of income versus cash flow.
  4. Estimated plant age.
  5. Actual expenditures for replacement of productive capacity versus expansion.
  6. Bonds-for-stock swaps.
  7. Tax benefit sales/purchases.
  8. Apportionment of working capital.
  9. Liquidity of the company.
  10. Adequacy of capital resources.
  11. Availability of and company policy toward forecasts and forward-looking information.
  12. Trends in profitability.
  13. Debt structure.
  14. Impact on earnings of stock appreciation rights.
  15. Effect of LIFO adjustment.
  16. Effective tax rate.
  17. Local/state taxes, including "severance."
  18. Deferred taxes.

3 / The Individual Investor   67

Figure 3-1 (*concluded*)

---

      19. Contingency tax liabilities.
      20. Debt repayment.
      21. Currency losses/gains under new standard.
      22. Cost of government regulations.
      23. Impact of wage/price guidelines.
      24. Loss operations.
      25. Operating capacity.
      26. R&D expenses.
      27. Contingency legal liabilities.
      28. Product liability insurance.
      29. Pension liability.
      30. Effect of accelerated depreciation.
   B. Financial policy
      1. Dependence on financial institutions.
      2. Management of real estate assets.
      3. Goals for financial ratios.
      4. Capital spending program.
      5. Acquisition program.
      6. Financing philosophy: equity versus debt, potential dilution of common stock.
      7. Responsibility for financial statements.
      8. Management of international currency.
V. *Business management*
   A. Operations
      1. Inflation-fighting program.
      2. Energy conservation and efficiency.
      3. Product safety.
      4. Pricing policy.
      5. Unit shipment rate.
      6. International operations and risk exposure.
   B. Human Resources
      1. Management advancement/succession.
      2. Wage/compensation policies.
      3. Labor relations.
      4. Level of unionization of work force.
      5. Incentive programs.
      6. Antidiscrimination program.
      7. Occupational health and employee rights.

Source: "Checklist of Stockholder Concerns," Georgeson & Co. Inc., New York, 1982.

CHAPTER FOUR

The Securities and Exchange Commission and Stock Exchanges

THE TIGHT SHIP OF REGULATION

Financial communications have been more the result of regulation than of desire. In those instances where there were no communications, such organizations as the Securities and Exchange Commission (SEC) and the stock exchanges set minimal standards of disclosure. Similar regulations were enacted to ensure accuracy.

Communications is not the only aspect of the financial community to be regulated. To protect the investor, virtually every aspect of the securities business has become subject to extensive regulation and scrutiny. To illustrate, before a new security may be offered to the public, the issuer and the underwriters must comply with a number of federal and state laws. Before a brokerage firm or a sales representative can offer services to the public, another series of legal requirements must be met. Even after a firm or an individual has qualified to do business with the public by meeting entrance and capital requirements, trading activities and business practices are subject to strict rules and guidelines.

The responsibility for administering and enforcing these regulations is shared by government agencies and industry organizations. To ensure the integrity of their respective markets, the National Association of Securities Dealers (NASD) and the various securities exchanges regulate and monitor the business activities of their members in cooperation with the various state securities commissions, the Municipal Securities Rulemaking Board, the Federal Reserve Board, and the SEC. The basic framework of regulation is provided by federal statutes that were initially enacted in 1933 and 1934 and were subsequently amended on several occasions to expand the scope of regulation.

The Securities Act of 1933 regulates the underwriting and distribution of corporate securities by providing for the registration of securities offerings with the SEC and by requiring appropriate disclosure of all material facts to ensure that prospective investors receive informa-

68

tion which will enable them to make intelligent investment decisions. The Securities Exchange Act of 1934 gives the SEC authority to regulate the sales practices of securities brokers and dealers, and to oversee the procedures and governance of the exchanges and the over-the-counter market. The antifraud provisions of the 1933 and 1934 acts authorize the SEC to curb fraudulent schemes and manipulative activity.

The Investment Company and Investment Advisers acts of 1940, also subsequently amended, build upon this framework. The Investment Company Act imposes regulations dealing with the organization and operation of mutual funds and the distribution of their securities. The Investment Advisers Act requires investment advisers to register with the SEC and to comply with guidelines concerning their activities.

Most states have legislation pertaining to the sale of securities. These statutes, often referred to as *blue-sky laws*, are administered and enforced by the various states. While the laws vary by state, blue-sky legislation generally requires that dealers in securities be licensed, that securities originally offered for sale be *qualified* or registered with the proper state authorities, and that the price and other terms of such new issues be consistent with statutory guidelines.

Other aspects of the customer-broker relationship are subject to regulations prescribed by the Board of Governors of the Federal Reserve System (FRS). For example, the Board determines which securities can be purchased on margin and set requirements for brokers extending or arranging credit for customers. It also establishes rules pursuant to which lenders other than members of a national securities exchange or brokers and dealers in securities (e.g., commercial banks) can advance credit to investors.

Registered national securities exchanges regulate, subject to SEC oversight, the trading activities of their members in those instances where transactions are effected on an exchange. These exchanges also set requirements for public disclosures by listed companies.

However, most securities issues are not traded on an exchange. They are bought and sold in the over-the-counter market, sometimes referred to as the *OTC market*. A 1938 amendment to the Securities Exchange Act of 1934 permitted the formation of the NASD, which has assumed considerable responsibility for protecting investors in the vast OTC market. This responsibility includes monitoring trading and sales practices, reviewing underwriting terms and distribution arrangements, administering qualification examinations to those wishing to enter the securities business, and reviewing members' sales materials. The NASD is also charged with examining the books and records of member firms to assure compliance with SEC and FRS regulations and to inform the Securities Investor Protection Corporation (SIPC) of any firms which may be in or approaching financial difficulty. All NASD regulatory activities are subject to SEC oversight. It is within this legal framework that the market operates, and it is within this framework that communications must be directed.

THE SECURITIES AND EXCHANGE COMMISSION

The Securities Act of 1933, or the "truth in securities" law, which created the Securities and Exchange Commission, has two basic objectives: (1) to provide investors with financial and other information concerning securities offered for public sale; and (2) to prohibit misrepresentation, deceit, and other fraudulent acts and practices in the sale of securities generally, whether or not the securities are required to be registered. (See Figures 4–1 and 4–2 for the organization of the SEC.)

Registration of Securities

The first objective applies to securities offered for public sale by an issuing company or by any person in a control relationship to such a company. Before the public offering of such securities, the issuer must file with the SEC a registration statement setting forth the required information. When the statement has become effective, the securities may be sold. The purpose of registration is to provide disclosure of financial and other information on the basis of which investors may appraise the merits of the securities. To that end, investors must be furnished with a prospectus containing the salient data set forth in the registration statement so that they will be able to evaluate the securities and make informed and discriminating investment decisions.

There are, however, certain exemptions from the registration requirement. Among these are private offerings to a limited number of persons or institutions that have access to the kind of information registration would disclose and that do not propose to redistribute the securities, and offerings restricted to the residents of the state in which the issuing company is organized and doing business.

The purpose of registration is to provide disclosure important financial facts so that investors may realistically appraise the merits of the securities offered and thus exercise an informed judgment in determining whether to purchase them. Assuming proper disclosure, the SEC cannot deny registration or otherwise bar the securities from public sale, whether or not the price or other terms of the securities are fair and whether or not the issuing company offers reasonable prospects of success. Moreover, registration does not guarantee the accuracy of the facts represented in the registration statement and the prospectus. The law does, however, prohibit false and misleading statements under penalty of fine or imprisonment, or both.

Figure 4–1
Securities and Exchange Commission

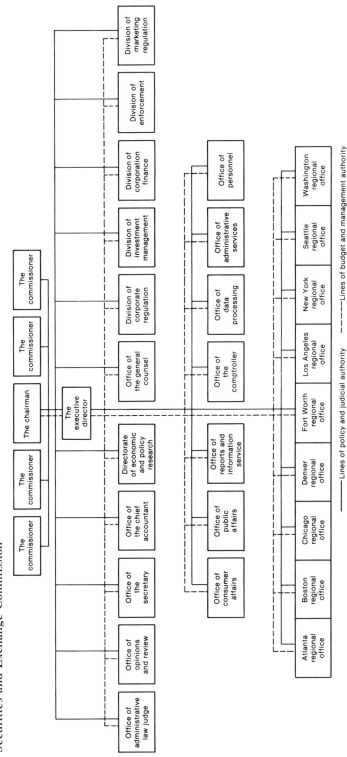

Figure 4-2
Securities and Exchange Commission

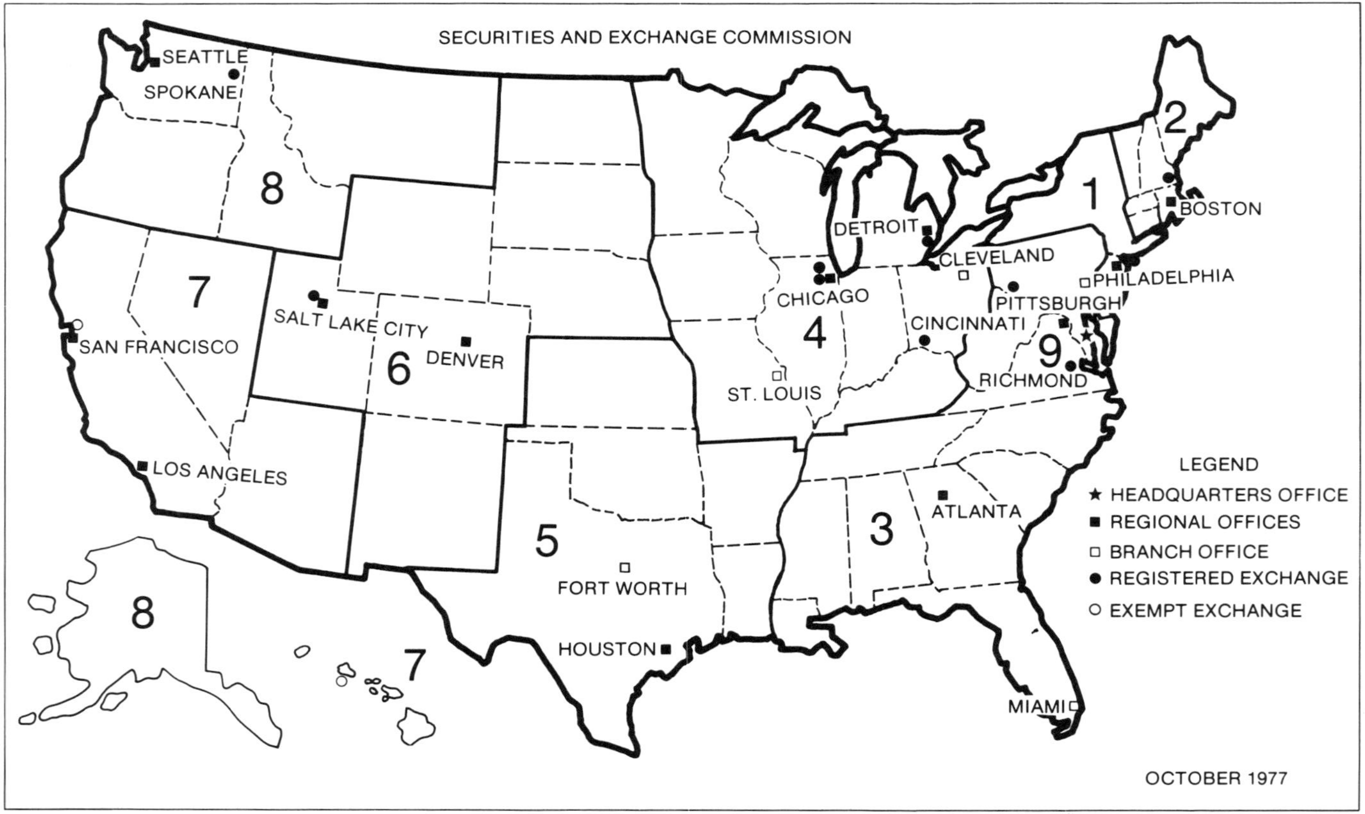

Source: Adapted from a map prepared by the Securities and Exchange Commission.

The Registration Process

To facilitate the registration of securities, the SEC has prepared special registration forms which vary in their disclosure requirements so as to provide disclosure of the essential facts pertinent to a given type of offering while at the same time minimizing the burden and expense of compliance with the law. In general, the registration forms call for a description of the registrant's properties and business, a description of the significant provisions of the security that is to be offered for sale and of its relationship to the registrant's other capital securities, information about the management of the registrant, and financial statements certified by independent public accountants.

Registration statements are examined by the Division of Corporation Finance for compliance with the disclosure requirements. If a statement appears to be materially incomplete or inaccurate, the registrant is usually informed by letter and given an opportunity to file correcting or clarifying amendments. The Commission, however, has authority to refuse or suspend the effectiveness of any registration statement if it finds, after a hearing, that material representations are misleading, inaccurate, or incomplete.

The examination process contributes to the general reliability of the registration disclosures—but it does not give positive assurance that the facts reported are accurate. Even if a verification of the facts reported were possible, the task would involve such a tremendous expenditure of time and money that it would seriously impede the financing of business ventures through the public sale of securities.

Interpretations and Rulemaking

The Division of Corporation Finance also renders administrative interpretations of the law and the regulations to members of the public, prospective registrants, and others so as to help them decide legal questions about the application of the law and the regulations to particular situations and to aid them in complying with the law. This assistance might include an informal expression of opinion about whether the offering of a particular security is subject to the registration requirements of the law and, if so, advice as to compliance with the disclosure requirements of the applicable registration form. Other divisions render similar advice and assistance. The Commission normally gives advance public notice of proposals for the adoption of new or amended rules or registration forms and affords opportunity for comment by interested members of the public.

The fraud prohibitions of the 1933 Securities Act are similar to those contained in the Securities Exchange Act of 1934, under which Congress extended the "disclosure" doctrine of investor protection to securities listed and registered for public trading on national securities exchanges. The Securities Acts Amendments of 1964 applied the disclosure and reporting provisions to the equity securities of companies traded over-the-counter if their assets exceed $1 million and their shareholders number 500 or more.

Since, unlike an offer of securities for sale by the issuing company, trading by and between public investors, whether involving listed or over-the-counter securities, involves transactions between holders of outstanding securities there is no provision for the dissemination of data to investors through the use of a prospectus or a similar medium. However, the reported information is available for public inspection, both at the offices of the SEC and at the exchanges. It is also used extensively by publishers of securities manuals, securities advisory services, investment advisers, trust departments, brokers and dealers in securities, and similar agencies, and thus it obtains widespread dissemination. The law prescribes penalties for filing false statements and reports with the SEC, and it makes provision for recovery by investors who suffer losses in the purchase or sale of registered securities in reliance thereon.

Tender Offer Solicitations

In 1968, Congress amended the Securities Exchange Act to extend its reporting and disclosure provisions to situations where control of a company is sought through a tender offer or other planned stock acquisition of over 10 percent of a company's equity securities. The amount was reduced to 5 percent in 1970. The SEC requires disclosure of pertinent information by a person seeking to acquire over 5 percent of a company's securities by direct purchase or by tender offer and by any persons soliciting shareholders to accept or reject a tender offer. Thus, public investors who hold stock in a corporation may make informed decisions on takeover bids.

Market Surveillance

The Securities Exchange Act also provides a system for regulating securities trading practices in both the exchange markets and the over-the-counter markets. The system seeks to curb misrepresentations and deceit, market manipulation, and other fraudulent acts and practices and to establish and maintain just and equitable principles of trade conducive to the maintenance of open, fair, and orderly markets. The SEC is responsible for promulgating rules and regulations for the implementation of these principles. Thus, the SEC has adopted regulations which, among other things:

1. Define acts or practices which constitute a "manipulative or deceptive device or contrivance" prohibited by the statute.
2. Regulate short selling, stabilizing transactions, and similar matters.
3. Regulate the hypothecation of customers' securities.
4. Provide safeguards with respect to the financial responsibility of brokers and dealers.

Investigation and Enforcement

The investigation and enforcement work of the SEC is the primary responsibility of the Commission's regional offices, subject to review and direction by the Division of Enforcement. Most of the investigations are conducted privately, the facts being developed through informal inquiry, interviewing of witnesses, examination of brokerage records and other documents, reviewing trading data, and similar means. The Commission, however, is empowered to issue subpoenas requiring sworn testimony and the production of books, records, and other documents pertinent to the subject matter under investigation. In the event of refusal to respond to a subpoena, the SEC may apply to a federal court for an order compelling obedience.

The more general types of investigations concern the sale without registration of securities subject to the registration requirement of the Securities Act and the misrepresentation or omission of material facts concerning securities offered for sale, whether or not registration is required. Among the types of inquiries are inquiries regarding the manipulation of the market prices of securities; the misappropriation or unlawful hypothecation of customers' funds or securities; the conduct of a securities business while insolvent; the purchase or sale of securities by a broker-dealer, from or to his customers, at prices not reasonably related to the current market prices therefor; and violation by the broker-dealer of his responsibility to treat his customers fairly.

Assuming that the facts show possible fraud or other violations of the law, there are several courses of action or remedies which the SEC may pursue:

1. *Civil injunction.* The Commission may apply to an appropriate U.S. district court for an order enjoining those acts or practices alleged to violate the law or Commission rules.

2. *Criminal prosecution.* If fraud or other willful violation of the law is indicated, the Commission may refer the facts to the Department of Justice with a recommendation for criminal prosecution of the offending persons. That department, through its local U.S. attorneys (who are frequently assisted by Commission attorneys), may present the evidence to a federal grand jury and seek an indictment.

3. *Administrative remedy.* The Commission may, after a hearing, issue orders suspending or expelling members from exchanges or the

over-the-counter dealers association; denying, suspending, or revoking the registrations of broker-dealers; or censuring individuals for misconduct or barring them (temporarily or permanently) from employment with a registered firm.

Public Utility Holding Company Act of 1935

This act was enacted by Congress to correct the many abuses which congressional inquiries had disclosed in the financing and operation of electric and gas public utility holding company systems. When the act became law in 1935, some 15 holding company systems controlled 80 percent of all electric energy generation, 98.5 percent of all electric energy transmission across state lines, and 80 percent of all natural gas pipeline mileage in the United States. Many of the huge utility empires then in existence controlled subsidiaries which operated in many widely separated states and had no economic or functional relationship to one another. Holding companies were pyramided layer upon layer, many of them serving no useful purpose, and many holding company systems had very complicated corporate and capital structures, with control often lodged in junior securities having little or no equity. These conditions ranked high among the abuses which the act was designed to correct.

The most important provisions of the act are its requirements for the physical integration and corporate simplification of the holding company systems. The integration standards of the statute restrict a holding company's operations to an "integrated utility system," which is defined as one capable of economical operation as a single coordinated system confined to a single area or region in one or more states and not so large as to impair the advantages of localized management, efficient operation, and effective local regulation.

The overall effect of the Commission's administration of the integration and simplification provisions of the law has been far-reaching. From 1938 to 1972, about 2,500 companies were subject to the act as registered holding companies or subsidiaries. These included 227 holding companies, 1,046 electric and gas utility companies, and 1,210 other companies engaged in a wide variety of pursuits, such as brickworks, laundries, experimental orchards, motion-picture theaters, and even a baseball club. Today, the picture is strikingly different. Only 17 active holding company systems are now registered. These comprise 13 registered holding companies which function solely as holding companies, 7 holding companies which are also engaged in utility operations, 91 electric and/or gas subsidiary companies, 57 nonutility subsidiaries, and 16 inactive companies, making a total of 184 companies with aggregate assets of $19 billion. Further, these 17 systems now account for only about one fifth of the aggregate assets of the privately owned electric and gas utility and gas pipeline industries of the nation. Most of the electric and gas utility companies which formerly were associated with registered holding companies now operate as independent concerns.

Trust Indenture Act of 1939

This act applies in general to bonds, debentures, notes, and similar debt securities offered for public sale that are issued pursuant to trust indentures under which more than $1 million of securities may be outstanding at any one time. Even though such securities may be registered under the Securities Act, they may not be offered for sale to the public unless the trust indenture conforms to specified statutory standards of this act that are designed to safeguard the rights and interests of the purchasers.

The act was passed after studies by the SEC had revealed the frequency with which trust indentures failed to provide minimum protections for security holders and absolved so-called trustees from minimum obligations in the discharge of their trusts. The act requires that the indenture trustee be free of conflicting interests which might interfere with the faithful exercise of its duties in behalf of the purchasers of the securities, that the trustee be a corporation with minimum combined capital and surplus, and that high standards of conduct and responsibility be imposed on the trustee.

Administrative Proceedings

All formal administrative proceedings of the SEC are conducted in accordance with its Rules of Practice, which conform to the Administrative Procedure Act and are designed to establish procedural, due process safeguards that will protect the rights and interests of the parties to each such proceeding. Among these are requirements for timely notice of the proceeding and for a specification of the issues or charges involved that is sufficient to enable each of the parties to prepare adequately for the case. All parties, including counsel for the interested division or office of the Commission, may appear at the hearing and present evidence and cross-examine witnesses in much the same manner as in the ordinary trial of court actions. In addition, other interested persons may be permitted to intervene or may be given limited rights of participation. In some cases, the relevant facts may be stipulated in lieu of the conduct of an evidentiary hearing.

Hearings are conducted before a hearing officer, who is normally an administrative law judge appointed by the Commission. The hearing officer serves independently of the interested division or office and rules on the admissibility of evidence and on other issues arising during the course of the hearing. At the conclusion of the hearing, the parties and participants may urge, in writing, specific findings of fact and conclusions of law for adoption by the hearing officer. The hearing officer prepares and files an initial decision (unless this is waived) that sets forth conclusions as to the facts established by the evidence and includes an order disposing of the issue involved in the proceeding. Copies of the initial decision are served on the parties and participants, who may seek SEC review. If review is not sought and the SEC does not order review on its own motion, the initial decision becomes final and the hearing officer's order becomes effective.

A TOUCH OF HISTORY

True or false?
First Philadelphia and later Washington, D.C., were the political centers of the United States.

Wall Street was once the political capital of the United States, just as it is the financial center of the world today. Here the New York Chamber of Commerce, established April 5, 1768, pressed the fight on the Stamp Act and the tax on tea. Here George Washington took the first presidential oath of office; here the first Congress gathered; here the first executive departments of the U.S. government were organized; and here the immortal Bill of Rights was adopted.

It was on Wall Street that the 1789–90 Congress authorized an issue of $80 million in stock to help pay for the costs of the Revolutionary War. There was a scattered market for this government stock as well as for the shares of the banks and insurance companies that were then springing up. Trading was carried on in various coffeehouses, auction rooms, and offices, but it was mostly unorganized, and people were reluctant to invest because they had no assurance that they could sell their securities when they wanted to do so.

The New York Stock Exchange

On May 17, 1792, 141 years before the passage of the first Securities Act, 24 merchants and auctioneers met to resolve this situation. They decided to meet daily at regular hours to buy and sell securities under an old buttonwood tree on Wall Street, only a few blocks from the present site of the New York Stock Exchange.

These men were the original members of the Exchange. They handled the public's buy and sell orders in the new government stock, as well as in shares of insurance companies, Alexander Hamilton's first U.S. Bank, the Bank of North America, and the Bank of New York. In 1793, the Tontine Coffee House was completed at the northwestern corner of Wall and William streets and the brokers moved indoors.

Private financial activity was checked for a time by the War of 1812, but peace brought the formation of new enterprises. New York State bonds, issued to pay for the Erie Canal, joined the issues traded on the new Exchange. Private businesses also expanded. The cotton industry, which boasted only a few mills in 1804, was operating half a million spindles by 1815. The tempo of business quickened as the country headed into a postwar boom.

By 1827, the stocks of 12 banks and 19 marine and fire insurance companies, the Delaware & Hudson Canal Company, the Merchants' Exchange, and the New York Gas Light Company—the nation's first public utility—were traded on the Exchange. Ten years later, the list included eight railroad securities. As other new enterprises developed, their securities came to the Exchange. The builders of our country's pioneer companies had discovered that investors placed marketability high among the requirements for a desirable investment.

Soon after the turn of the century, it became apparent that the Tontine Coffee House was too small to accommodate the volume of trading in securities and the stockbrokers moved to a meeting room in what is now 40 Wall Street. Greater activity brought the need for a more formal organization, so on March 8, 1817, the first formal constitution of the New York Stock and Exchange Board, as it was then known, was adopted.

The constitution provided, among other things, that the president was to call out the names of stocks, fix commissions, and set fines—6 to 25 cents—for violation of procedure or nonattendance at sessions "unless when sick or out of the city." Each trading session consisted of a morning call, at 11:30, of all stocks on the list. As the name of each stock was called, the brokers made their bids and offers.

From 1817 to 1827, the board met in various offices. After that, it moved a dozen times before settling, in 1863, upon the site of the present Broad Street Building, erected in 1903, which contains most of today's trading floor. The adjoining office building at the corner of Broad and Wall streets was erected in 1922. An extension of the trading floor completed in 1969 and known as the Blue Room, the bond trading room, and the public Exhibit Hall of industry and investment are housed in a newer building at 20 Broad Street.

Other historic dates are: 1863, when the name New York Stock Exchange (NYSE) was adopted; 1867, when the first stock tickers were installed; 1871, when the call market gave way to a continuous market; 1886, the first year in which a day's volume topped 1 million shares; 1910, when the Exchange discontinued unlisted trading (previously an unlisted stock could be traded, but the company had no responsibility to comply with Exchange standards); 1915, when the basis of quoting and trading in stocks changed from percent of par value to dollars; 1922, when the questionnaire system for periodic examination of the financial condition of member firms was inaugurated; 1933, when independent audits of financial statements were required of listed companies; 1938, when a sweeping reorganization of the Exchange called for its first paid president; and 1972, when a new board was established, with 10 directors representing the securities industry, 10 directors representing the public, and a full-time paid chairman of the board who was also the Exchange's chief executive officer. (A complete list of significant historic Exchange dates appears in Figure 4-3.)

Figure 4-3
Significant dates in NYSE history

May	17, 1792	Original brokers' agreement subscribed to by 24 brokers.
Mar.	8, 1817	Constitution and the name New York Stock & Exchange Board adopted.
Mar.	16, 1830	Dullest day in history of Exchange—31 shares traded.
Jan.	29, 1863	Name changed to New York Stock Exchange.
Nov.	15, 1867	Stock tickers first introduced.
Oct.	23, 1868	Membership made salable.
Sept.	24, 1869	Gold speculation resulted in Black Friday.
Sept.	1871	Continuous markets in stocks established.
Sept.	18, 1873	NYSE closed through September 29; failure of Jay Cooke & Co., others.
Dec.	1, 1873	Trading hours set at 10 A.M. to 3 P.M.; Saturdays, 10 A.M. to noon.
Nov.	13, 1878	First telephones introduced in the Exchange.
Jan.	29, 1881	Annunciator board installed for paging members.
Mar.	25, 1885	Unlisted Securities Department set up; abolished March 1910.
Dec.	15, 1886	First million-share day—1,200,000 shares.
July	31, 1914	Exchange closed through December 11—World War I.
Oct.	13, 1915	Stock prices quoted in dollars as against percent of par value.
Jan.	2, 1919	Separate ticker system for bonds installed.
Apr.	26, 1920	Stock Clearing Corporation established.
Jan.	3, 1927	Start of 10-share unit of trading for inactive stocks.
Oct.	29, 1929	Stock market crash; 16,410,000 shares traded.
Sept.	2, 1930	Faster ticker—500 characters a minute—installed.
Mar.	4, 1933	Exchange closed to March 14 for bank holiday.
June	6, 1934	Enactment of Securities Exchange Act of 1934.
June	30, 1938	First salaried president elected—William McChesney Martin, Jr.
Sept.	29, 1952	Trading hours changed. Weekdays, 10 A.M.–3:30 P.M. No Saturdays.
June	4, 1953	First member corporation—Woodcock, Hess & Co.
Dec.	1, 1964	New ticker—900 characters a minute—put into service.
July	14, 1966	New NYSE Stock Price Index inaugurated.

Figure 4–3 (*concluded*)

Dec. 28, 1967	First woman member admitted—Muriel F. Siebert.
Mar. 26, 1970	Public ownership of member firms approved.
Dec. 30, 1970	Securities Investor Protection Corporation Act signed.
July 27, 1971	First member organization listed—Merrill Lynch.
Jan. 20, 1972	NYSE reorganization, based on Martin Report, approved.
July 13, 1972	Board of directors, with 10 public members, replaced board of governors.
July 17, 1972	Securities Industry Automation Corporation established.
Aug. 28, 1972	First salaried chairman took office—James J. Needham.
May 11, 1973	Depository Trust Company succeeded Central Certificate Service.
Oct. 1, 1974	Trading hours extended to 4 P.M.
Oct. 18, 1974	Consolidated tape begun; 15 stocks reported.
Apr. 30, 1975	Fixed-commission system abolished.
June 16, 1975	Full consolidated tape begun.
Jan. 19, 1976	New data line handling 36,000 characters a minute.
Mar. 1, 1976	Designated Order Turnaround (DOT) System begun.
May 24, 1976	Specialists began handling odd lots in their stocks.
Jan. 6, 1977	Independent audit committee on listed companies' boards required.
Feb. 3, 1977	Foreign broker-dealers permitted to obtain membership.
July 27, 1977	Full Automated Bond System in effect.
Apr. 17, 1978	Intermarket Trading System (ITS) begun.
May 2, 1978	Registered Competitive Market-Maker category for members approved.
Aug. 3, 1978	First 65-million-share day in history (66,370,000 shares).
Aug. 7, 1980	New York Futures Exchange started trading.
Jan. 7, 1981	First 90-million-share day in history (92,881,000 shares).

Source: *New York Stock Exchange Fact Book, 1981,* p. 62.

The American Stock Exchange

In 1849, as the NYSE was turning a mature age 57, gold was discovered in California. As settlers opened new markets in the vast territories of the West, the young and growing nation needed more and more goods—everything from nails to shovels to steamships. But companies needed capital to make these products. To raise money, many firms sold shares in their businesses to wealthy individuals.

A small group of these investors gathered daily in the streets of downtown New York and began to trade their shares of stocks and bonds among themselves. Like all good businessmen, they hoped to buy low and sell high, and thus to profit from their investments. In time their number grew, and the men found themselves acting as brokers on behalf of an increasing number of public customers. These brokers traded in specific issues at various street landmarks—lampposts, mailboxes, fire hydrants.

As the market, called the *Outdoor Curb Market,* gradually took shape, a more formal organization was established. Brokers were registered, trading regulations enacted, and a constitution adopted.

Nothing stopped these outdoor brokers. Even in the snow and rain, they gathered to put up lists of stocks for sale. By 1900, millions of dollars worth of securities were being traded in mines, farm machinery, life insurance, printing, textiles, and railroads—right out on the street. Some investors even bought stocks in such daring new inventions as the horseless carriage and pictures that moved.

The streets got so crowded that some brokers moved their clerks to windows above the street. The clerks would take customers' orders by telephone, then call them down to their brokers. But this only added to the noise. One day someone got a bright idea—hand signals! These worked just fine in all that noise. Soon everyone began using them. Then, so their clerks could find them more easily in the crowd, brokers began to wear brightly colored hats and jackets. In those days, the Outdoor Curb Market was one of the most exciting and colorful spots in all of America. In 1921, it finally moved indoors to its present site on Trinity Place. But it continued to be known as the Curb until 1953, when its name was changed to the American Stock Exchange (Amex) to signify its national character.

With the growth and sophistication of the exchanges, there was a demand for disseminating information on trading across America. The first stock ticker developed to report transactions on the NYSE went into service in 1867.

The glass bubble ticker, familiarized by movies and cartoons, was an invention of Thomas A. Edison and became standard equipment in 1883. By 1930, a printer was developed to transmit stock transactions at the rate of 500 characters per minute. This device, rapid as it was, could not keep up with the increasing volume of trades and would run behind actual trading.

Both exchanges are now covered by the 900 ticker, which operates at the rate of 900 characters per minute—as fast as the eye can read. Because of the new speed and changes in ticker printing procedures, huge share days have been handled with tape delays of no more than two to three minutes. The ticker is only one of many steps taken by the exchanges to provide investors with a faster, more reliable transaction reporting technique and an expanded, more comprehensive source of market information.

The ticker system at the NYSE is linked to the Market Data System. Thirty-three optical "card readers," strategically located at every post on the trading floor, provide fully automated reporting of stock transactions to the computer. Instantaneously, the stock symbol, number of shares, and price are transmitted to thousands of stock tickers and other display devices in brokers' offices throughout the world. These devices include "moving news bulletin signs" and cathode-ray tube (CRT) units, which resemble television sets.

The Market Data System reduces to seconds the interval between the reporting of a trade and its appearance on the ticker tape. It also enables brokers to serve their customers better through instantaneous access to a variety of statistical and historical data relating to any listed stock or overall market trends.

Modernization continues at the NYSE:

In 1972, the Odd-Lot Automation System was introduced to permit computerized switching of orders of less than 100 shares for automatic execution.

In 1973, the Market Data System was upgraded and improved as MDS II to provide greater flexibility in accommodating additional services as the need arises.

In 1975, the Consolidated Tap began reporting transactions in listed stocks on regional exchanges and the *third market* (the popular term for over-the-counter dealers in listed stocks) as well as on the NYSE, where some 85 percent of such transactions occur.

The NYSE ticker is also seen through commercial and cable television networks. However, all data supplied to the networks are delayed for 15 minutes since the timely information is restricted to the primary subscribers within the industry for their own use and the use of their customers.

All of the NYSE's communications systems are operated and maintained by the Securities Industry Automation Corporation (SIAC), which is responsible for the sales processing and ticker generating equipment and the continuing development and implementation of projects to keep the Exchange in the technological forefront.

Practically every city in the United States is linked with the nation's marketplace. (Although not members of the Exchange, most banks have contacts with one or more member firms.) About 500,000 miles of teletype and telephone wires connect the Exchange with members' offices and many of those offices with nonmember correspondents.

Member firms have offices in all 50 states and about 1,000 U.S. cities, as well as Puerto Rico, the Virgin Islands, the District of Columbia, Argentina, Austria, the Bahamas, Belgium, Canada, England, France, Germany, Greece, Israel, Italy, Japan, Lebanon, Monaco, the Netherlands, Panama, the Philippines, Spain, Switzerland, Uruguay, Venezuela, and Hong Kong.

The 18,000-mile ticker network of Amex covers 871 cities in the

84

United States and Canada. Amex data are also available on a worldwide basis to more than 60 cities overseas through facilities of international communications companies offering global ticker service.

DOING BUSINESS WITH THE NYSE

The NYSE views its most important function as that of allowing the individual to put capital to work whenever he or she so chooses. In a free society, capital must be free to move from one enterprise to another—entitled to the profits when the venture succeeds, ready to stand the losses if it fails.

Membership in the Exchange totals 1,366 individuals. A member may be a general partner or a holder of voting stock in one of the brokerage concerns which, by virtue of NYSE membership, is known as a member firm or a member corporation. There are some 500 such member organizations—about one half are partnerships, and about one half are corporations.

In 1970, the NYSE authorized public ownership for member corporations, and 17 have offered their stock to investors. Seven of these corporations are listed on the Exchange directly or indirectly through a parent company.

About one half of the Exchange members are partners or officers in member organizations doing business with the public—so-called commission houses. These members execute customers' orders to buy and sell on the Exchange, and their firms receive the commissions on those transactions. Many firms have more than one member (see Table 4–1).

About one fourth of all members of the NYSE are specialists—so called because they specialize in *making a market* for one or more stocks. (See Glossary at the end of the chapter for this and other definitions.) To carry out the function of maintaining a fair and orderly market, insofar as reasonably practicable, in the stocks in which he specializes, the specialist often risks his own capital by buying at a higher price or selling at a lower price than the public may be willing to pay or accept at the moment. For instance, let's say that the last sale in XYZ stock was at $35 a share, that the lowest offer to sell is $35 a share, and that $34 is the highest bid. Depending on conditions in the market, the specialist might bid $34⅝ in order to narrow the temporary spread between supply and demand. Conversely, in a rising market the specialist frequently sells stocks for his own account at a lower price than that at which the public will sell.

The Exchange sets specific requirements for specialists, such as market experience, dealer function, and the amount of capital they must have. The specialist's business is concentrated in a particular

Table 4-1
NYSE member firm offices and registered representatives

Location	Sales offices		Full-time producing registered representatives	
	December 31, 1978	December 31, 1977	December, 31 1978	1977
Alabama	29	24	247	232
Alaska	8	8	55	51
Arizona	48	42	478	419
Arkansas	26	20	158	105
California	406	375	5,677	5,437
Colorado	66	61	652	584
Connecticut	72	67	783	690
Delaware	10	10	84	80
District of Columbia	29	28	521	504
Florida	249	214	2,604	2,502
Georgia	60	57	837	767
Hawaii	16	14	196	191
Idaho	19	18	65	50
Illinois	181	171	2,305	2,108
Indiana	65	59	384	346
Iowa	67	57	276	278
Kansas	43	37	158	142
Kentucky	24	28	229	239
Louisiana	37	34	342	312
Maine	14	14	85	91
Maryland	44	41	507	448
Massachusetts	95	91	1,457	1,381
Michigan	124	116	1,076	1,010
Minnesota	46	46	622	625
Mississippi	22	21	88	63
Missouri	102	90	983	880
Montana	12	10	50	34
Nebraska	43	40	265	219
Nevada	12	10	99	87
New Hampshire	13	10	55	41
New Jersey	113	99	1,243	1,116
New Mexico	19	18	124	105
New York	464	462	8,232	7,656
North Carolina	89	82	571	554
North Dakota	8	6	30	21
Ohio	145	142	1,292	1,171
Oklahoma	35	33	326	304
Oregon	41	35	371	332
Pennsylvania	187	185	1,863	1,756
Rhode Island	11	8	137	110

Table 4–1 (concluded)

Location	Sales offices		Full-time producing registered representatives	
	December 31, 1978	December 31, 1977	December, 31 1978	1977
South Carolina	43	37	231	196
South Dakota	10	10	44	34
Tennessee	45	38	468	426
Texas	206	200	2,302	2,103
Utah	18	15	173	159
Vermont	6	7	45	36
Virginia	86	76	581	506
Washington	55	45	662	586
West Virginia	19	18	101	98
Wisconsin	87	81	525	503
Wyoming	10	9	28	32
Total United States	3,679	3,419	40,687	37,720
Foreign countries and U.S. possessions and territories	224	214	1,369	1,314
Total United States and Foreign	3,903	3,633	42,056	39,034

Note: Full-time producing registered representatives include all registered personnel in sales offices who devote at least three fourths of their time to selling, exclusive of partners, officers, and branch managers. The 1977 data have been revised slightly.
Source: New York Stock Exchange Fact Book, 1981, p. 56.

group of stocks at one trading post. Thus, he can act for other brokers who cannot remain at one post until the prices specified by their customers' buy and sell orders—either purchases below or sales above the prevailing prices—are reached. The specialist must assume responsibility for the execution of orders turned over to him. Part of the commission that the customer pays his own broker goes to the specialist when the specialist's services are used. Most of the specialist's earnings come from commissions on orders he executes for other brokers.

The specialist must subordinate his personal interests in the market to the public's. For example, he cannot buy in the NYSE market at any price for his own account until he has executed all public buy orders held by him at that price. The same principle applies to sales.

The function of floor brokers is to assist the commission house brokers. Floor brokers are popularly known as $2 brokers, since $2 used to be the standard commission they received for executing a 100-share order.

Registered traders, some 100 in number, trade for their own accounts while on the floor. Their transactions, which must meet NYSE requirements, contribute to the liquidity of the markets in the stocks in which they trade. Registered traders may be asked to help expedite the handling of blocks of stock bid for or offered on the Exchange.

All members, whatever their function, must own a *seat*. The term traces back to early years when the brokers remained seated while the president called the list of securities. There is nothing sedentary about an Exchange member's day now.

One of the most interesting sights for the hundreds of thousands of NYSE visitors is the constant movement of the people on the floor. At first glance, that movement seems aimless. But after a guide has explained exactly what happens on the floor, the visitor soon realizes that each step is taken for a particular reason. Each broker on the floor executes his customer's orders as rapidly and efficiently as he can— and, in the process, wears out a lot of shoe leather.

The price of a NYSE membership is determined by how much a candidate will pay and by the amount that the owner of the membership will accept. The board of directors maintains complete control over the admission of new members. The price of memberships since 1950 has ranged from $38,000 to $515,000. The initiation fee is $7,500; the dues are $1,500 annually.

In addition to the Exchange members, there are allied members, who are usually either partners in member firms or directors of member corporations. Although allied members may not do business on the trading floor, they are subject to most of the strict rules and regulations that apply to members.

Board of Directors

Rules and regulations governing the conduct of members and allied members are set by the board of directors, which is elected by the members. The board exercises broad policymaking and disciplinary powers that have been designed to represent the security industry, listed companies, and the investing public. Member organizations choose 10 directors, and 10 are chosen from outside the industry. The chairman of the board, selected by the board of directors, brings the board's membership to 21.

The administration of policies made by the board rests in the hands of the staff, headed by the chairman, who also serves as chief executive officer. The NYSE has some 1,600 employees, of whom 600 work on the trading floor.

Organization of the New York Stock Exchange is centered in four major groups. The Regulation and Surveillance Group is responsible for all surveillance activities related to members, the office of the chief examiner, registration and rule administration, enforcement, and member firms compliance. The Market Operations and Membership Services Group is responsible for the listed companies, floor operations, and membership services, including the Stock Clearing Corporation. The Public Relations Division is responsible for educational and informational programs and publications, media relations, investor and corporate communications, the visitors gallery, and the Investors Service Bureau. The Administration Group is responsible for financial services, personnel, and facilities management.

There are subsidiary companies such as the Depository Trust Company, which confirm and balance transactions made on the trading floor and expedite the delivery of securities and the related cash settlements between clearing firms. Often the delivery of shares between clearing firms is accomplished through computerized bookkeeping entries to eliminate the physical handling and delivery of certificates, in much the same way as a checking account reduces the physical transfer of cash.

The Securities Industry Automation Corporation (SIAC) coordinates communications systems, programming, and data processing technology for all NYSE and Amex operations involving computers and is owned jointly by the two exchanges.

NYSE revenues come mainly from members in dues and charges for services and facilities, and from fees paid by corporations whose securities are listed.

The NYSE is a rather unusual form of enterprise because it does not seek to make a profit and it isn't a charitable organization. It is an incorporated association of brokers.

Of all corporations in business in the United States today, less than 1 percent are listed on the Exchange, but those listed represent most of the largest and most profitable corporations.

Almost 80 percent of the companies listed now pay cash dividends, and some 700 have paid dividends every single quarter for 20 to more than 100 years. The listed companies provide jobs for about one fifth of the U.S. labor force, producing practically all of the automobiles and trucks made in this country and more than 90 percent of all the aluminum, copper, and cement made, and operating 97 percent of the telephones in service. In a recent year, these companies paid over $18 billion in federal, state, and foreign income taxes.

Up until 1869, admission of a company's securities to the NYSE list was a highly informal action. All that was necessary was for a member to propose that a certain issue be traded. If a majority of the members consented, the stock or bond was eligible for trading.

But expanding business brought new needs for self-regulation, and over 100 years ago the Exchange laid down its first requirement for listing—that it be notified of all stock issued and valid for trading.

In the years that followed, the Exchange added more requirements, including earnings reports, disclosure of substantial changes in property or business, and maintenance of securities transfer offices.

The philosophy behind the listing requirements is simply this: The investor or trader who owns, buys, or plans to purchase listed securities is entitled to information about the corporation that will help him to make the investment decisions intelligently.

Corporate management has derived many more concrete benefits from having its securities listed on the Exchange than the benefits of having a greater number of shareowners and of having the company's name appear in the financial pages and the stock tables of the nation's press. For example, listed companies enjoy a substantial cost advantage in raising new capital.

Assets and Earning Power

At the time that a company qualifies for original listing on the Exchange, it must be a going concern with substantial assets and demonstrated earning power. The NYSE places emphasis on such considerations as the degree of national interest in the company, the character of the market for the company's product, the company's relative stability, and the company's position in its industry. The stock should have a sufficiently wide distribution to offer reasonable assurance that an adequate auction market in its securities will exist. Normally, the company should have earning power, under competitive conditions, of over $2.5 million annually before taxes. It should have a minimum of 1 million publicly held common shares, with not less than 2,000 round lot shareholders and a minimum aggregate market value of $16 million.

If a company wants to list a new issue or additional shares of an already listed issue, it must get NYSE authorization and, in some cases, stockholder approval. All approved listing applications are made public promptly.

Financial Statements

Some 99 percent of the companies now listed on the NYSE publish earnings statements every three months, and about 1 percent publish earnings statements every six months. The few companies that report earnings only once a year are dependent upon long-term contracts or upon the growth and sale of a crop in an annual cycle.

The standard agreement calls for the distribution to shareholders of the listed company's annual report, with financial statements certified by independent accountants, at least 15 days before the annual shareholders' meeting and not later than three months after the close of the fiscal year. These are important deadlines for the communicator.

The listed company must also agree to have a transfer agent and registrar in New York City, although under certain criteria a non-New York City transfer agent may act in lieu of a New York City agent. A transfer agent records the name and address of each registered shareholder, along with the number of shares owned, and makes sure that certificates presented to him for transfer are properly endorsed. The registrar agrees that no additional shares will be registered without authorization by the Exchange, and the company must agree that no additional shares will be issued without application to the Exchange. To help safeguard investors against spurious stock certificates, the NYSE even requires that the engravings meet specific standards.

The Right to Vote

The Exchange feels so strongly that the right to vote is fundamental to corporate democracy that it has refused, since 1926, to list nonvoting common stock. Moreover, it will consider delisting the common voting shares of a company which creates a nonvoting common stock. The Exchange expects, too, that the owner of common stock in a listed company will have the right to vote in reasonable proportion to the ownership interest represented by his or her stock.

The solicitation of proxies is a requirement for listing the common stock of operating companies. Proxies are an essential element in facilitating the voting right, for they enable shareowners to register their votes freely and conveniently—without having to personally attend annual or other meetings that have been called to consider matters of importance.

Suspension or Delisting

A primary objective of the Exchange is to maintain an auction market for listed securities. The factors involved in continued listing are not measured mathematically; the board may act to suspend or delist a security in any situation where it feels that the security is not suitable for retention. In considering a specific case, the board will give weight to all the factors affecting the security and the company.

For example, suspension of trading or delisting will normally be considered when round lot shareowners total less than 1,200, when the number of publicly held shares falls to less than 600,000 or their market value falls to less than $5 million, or when for other reasons further dealings in the security are not advisable.

Other examples include situations where the size of the company has fallen below $8 million in net tangible assets or in the aggregate market value of its common stock and average net earnings after taxes have been below $600,000 for the last three years, or where liquidation of the company has begun or substantially all of the company's assets have been sold. Delisting of a common stock will also be considered if the issuing company has violated its agreements with the Exchange.

The delisting of preferred stocks will normally be considered when the aggregate market value of publicly held shares is less than $2 million or when there are fewer than 100,000 publicly held shares and, in the case of bonds and debentures, when the aggregate market value or the principle amount outstanding is less than $1 million.

Controls—from Within

Over the years, the Exchange, largely through experience, has evolved a complex system of rules for self-control. But the underlying principle has remained the same: Securities may be bought and sold only at prices that have been arrived at openly and fairly.

The regulations for floor trading repeatedly stress the importance of the open market. Bids and offers are made in multiples of the unit of trading (ordinarily 100 shares), and the highest bid and the lowest offer have precedence. Bids and offers must be called out loud. Transactions are reported promptly over the nationwide ticker system. No floor trades are allowed before or after trading hours.

To understand the controls, it might be well to cite a portion of Article I of the NYSE constitution: "Its objects shall be . . . to maintain high standards of commercial honor and integrity among its members, allied members, member firms and member corporations; and to promote and inculcate just and equitable principles of trade and business."

There is a strict code of conduct, and the relations of member organizations with their clients are subject to a set of requirements prescribed by the NYSE. All member organizations doing business with the public carry some fidelity insurance as protection against possible loss due to fraud or dishonest acts on the part of their employees, general partners, or officers.

Financial Reports for Customers

All customers of a member firm must be offered or furnished a copy of the firm's financial statement once a year. NYSE rules provide that member firms carrying accounts for customers must have a prescribed amount of capital and must file annually a financial questionnaire based on an audit by the firm's independent public accountants. Each member firm must file monthly a Joint Regulatory Report of Broker/Dealer's Financial and Operational Conditions.

Member firms are expected to adhere to the principles of good business practice. A member or allied member found guilty of conduct or proceedings inconsistent with just and equitable principles of trade may be suspended or expelled.

There are also rules and regulations which apply to member firm employees who do business with the public. All applications for employment of these personnel, who are known as registered representatives and who together number more than 30,000, are passed on and registered by the Exchange. The Exchange regularly reviews its rules and regulations in the context of existing market conditions. Among the significant measures stemming from this self-appraisal have been strengthened training standards for registered representatives of member organizations, new qualifying examinations for new members and allied members, and a new inspection program for checking the performance of member organizations' office management and sales activities.

Every day, hundreds of newspapers across the country publish a price record of stocks listed on the NYSE or tell about the market's action in a news column. Many papers do both. Most of the popular averages or indexes are based on a limited number of issues—for instance, the well-known Dow Jones Industrial Average is based on only 30 stocks. Hence, the average does not tell the whole story of the market by any means.

The Dow Jones Industrial Average is compiled by adding the prices of the 30 stocks. This total is divided by a divisor which compensates for past stock splits and stock dividends. The answer is expressed in points, not dollars. The Dow might decline 10 points without any of the 30 individual issues declining as much as $1 a share. The main value of an average is as a gauge of the market's course over a period of time rather than as a measure of daily fluctuations of individual issues.

A new way of looking at the market, the New York Stock Exchange Common Stock Index, was introduced in mid-1966. This index covers every common stock listed on the Exchange. It is considered the most comprehensive and the most accurate indicator of market trends. The index is calculated continuously during the trading day by the Exchange's Market Data System, and it is sent over the international ticker network every half hour.

No aggregate measure, of course, shows how a particular issue acted in the market. The NYSE Index is, however, a practical tool for enabling investors to follow general stock market trends.

THE AMERICAN STOCK EXCHANGE

The American Stock Exchange classifies itself as a leading market for the securities of young and growing companies in the United States. It also lists the shares (or their American equivalents) of more foreign corporations than are listed by any other stock exchange in the country. Options to buy or sell the stock of a number of leading corporations are now traded on the Amex, as are units of U.S. government obligations, such as Treasury notes and bonds. In providing a fair and orderly marketplace for the millions of investors who buy and sell these issues continuously throughout the trading day, the Amex functions as a vital nerve center of the nation's economy.

Trading Floor at a Glance

The trading floor of the Amex covers 20,650 square feet, or an area the size of the main arena of the new Madison Square Garden in New York City. It has 11 circular posts—of which 10 are 20 feet in diameter and the 11th is 15 feet across. Pigeonholes on the outside of each post provide convenient storage space for buy and sell orders in each security traded by the specialist. Bids are filed in descending order by price, and offers are filed in ascending order.

The inside of the post provides a suitable area for the reporting and recording of sales traded at the post. There, specialist clerks use photocopy equipment to document reports of an order's execution. An automated display board located directly above each post indicates the last sale and the "tick" (whether up or down from the previous sales price) for each stock traded at the post, thus providing up-to-date information for brokers in the trading crowd.

More than 1,000 people work on the floor—as commission brokers, specialists, Amex employees, and member firm employees. About 500 telephone and teletype booths are manned by member firm clerks. A clerk receives an order to buy or sell from his brokerage house and relays it to the floor broker. Annunciator boards on the floor may be used to page the broker. Ticker screens (Amex above and NYSE below) are located on four walls above the floor.

Man in the Middle

Regular members, who have been registered as specialists and who work in units, perform an important function for investors. They help to provide continuous markets where an investor can buy or sell stock with minimum price changes between transactions.

The specialist is expected to buy securities in declining markets and to sell stock in rising markets. He buys and sells for his own account in this way, so that prices move in an orderly manner, usually within a narrow range. Thus, he is called *the man in the middle*.

If a broker on the floor receives an order to buy or sell a security at a price *away* (different) from the last sale, he leaves that order with the specialist, who assumes responsibility for it. When the market in that security reaches the point (either up or down) that permits execution of the order left with him, the specialist, as a broker, will execute it.

When a specialist enters the market, he does so under stringent rules imposed by the Amex and the SEC, which keep a constant check on his performance in maintaining markets in assigned securities with reasonable depth and price continuity.

Company List

More than 1,250 corporations are represented on the Amex trading floor. Together, they offer the investing public a list of over 1,500 securities, including stocks, rights, warrants, and bonds.

To qualify for listing and trading, a company must meet certain requirements. Its size, its current earnings, and the market value of its securities are important considerations, as are the number of shareholders and the number of shares publicly held. The Amex also considers other factors, such as a company's pattern of growth, the reputation of its management, and its financial outlook.

Although many new companies are listed each year, others are delisted—for failure to maintain requirements for continued listing or because of merger, liquidation, or other reasons. The net list, however, reflects the pattern of growth that has characterized Amex history.

Public Information

The Amex Communications Center generates coverage in hundreds of newspapers and on thousands of radio and television stations throughout the United States, Canada, and other nations. Up-to-the-minute market lead stories are transmitted directly to 265 major financial and general news services and newspapers three times daily. AP–Dow Jones and Reuters disseminate Amex news and market reports via their overseas facilities throughout Canada, Europe, Central and South America, Africa, and the Far East. The flow of information to the media stimulates stories on Amex and its member organizations and listed companies, and results in daily publication of Amex stock quotation tables in more than 360 newspapers from coast to coast and in many newspapers abroad.

The Communications Center generates approximately 86,000 broadcasts on more than 5,000 radio stations each week. In addition, major television stations bring market news summaries provided by the center to millions of persons daily. Amex also publishes booklets and other literature to help investors, students, and the general public better understand securities and securities markets. Films and the visitors gallery overlooking the trading floor provide further insight into the role and operations of this exciting marketplace.

Private Eye in the Public Interest

Amex rules govern all transactions on the trading floor as well as the relationship of members to their customers. Self-regulation in the public interest is a pervasive concern and is continuously reflected in the activity of Amex members and the Amex administrative staff.

Supervision of the Amex market and the business practices of its members is carried on primarily by 28 floor officials and by the Market Operations and Membership Compliance divisions. The floor officials are regular members who have been vested with supervisory responsibility. They are empowered to act decisively and in the public interest to resolve questions that arise under the rules and policies covering transactions.

The efforts of the Amex staff include monitoring market activity and staying abreast of developments outside the market that might explain or affect market activity. Other functions include processing inquiries from member organizations and the public, auditing the financial condition of members and member organizations, and disseminating trading statistics to member organizations and the public.

THE OTHER EXCHANGES

Those companies not meeting the criteria of the New York and American Stock exchanges have available to them listings on the Boston, Philadelphia, Midwest, Cincinnati, and Pacific exchanges. Except for the Cincinnati exchange, these exchanges are linked to the Intermarket Trading System (ITS). This is an electronic communications network that enables brokers representing public customers, as well as specialists and market makers trading for their own accounts on the floor of one exchange, to reach out electronically to another exchange to obtain a better price.

To execute an ITS transaction, a specialist/market maker or broker in one exchange, seeing a better price on another exchange, sends the other exchange a commitment to buy or sell through ITS. If the bid or offer still stands when the commitment arrives at the other market center, it will be accepted, and the originating specialist/market maker or broker will be advised that the trade has taken place.

ITS was inaugurated on a pilot basis on April 17, 1978, with the New York and Philadelphia exchanges trading 11 stocks. On June 26, the Pacific Stock Exchange joined ITS. The Boston and Midwest Stock Exchanges became ITS participants in July. The American Stock Exchange commenced trading through ITS on August 7.

By the end of 1978, 300 issues were being traded over ITS. Of these stocks, 295 are listed on the NYSE and 7 on Amex, including 2 issues dually listed on the New York and American Exchanges.

As exchanges joined ITS and eligible issues were added, ITS trading rose rapidly. Within nine months of operation, ITS volume approached over half a million shares and nearly 900 trades a day.

THE OTC REGULATORY FRAMEWORK

In 1938, U.S. Senator Francis T. Maloney of Connecticut (author of the Maloney Act) noted, "There can be no large group of people engaged in any industry enjoying potentialities for profit which does not attract the careless and greedy few who bring discredit upon the entire group unless prevented by regulation from doing so." The firms and individuals that engage in unfair or unethical practices constitute a very small percentage of those involved in the securities business. The weeding out of such persons and firms from the securities industry is an important part of the work that NASD does in the public interest and for the protection of investors.

The Maloney Act amended the Securities Exchange Act of 1934 to permit the formation of self-regulatory associations of dealers and brokers that would register with the SEC. Such associations were authorized to establish, with the SEC, rules of proper business conduct for their members and to enforce those rules so as to protect investors from unfair practices and ensure the integrity of the over-the-counter market.

The board of governors is the controlling body of the National Association of Securities Dealers and determines its policy on a national scale.

For administrative purposes, the NASD membership has been divided into 13 districts, with representation on the board based roughly on the numbers of members in each district (see Figure 4–4).

The board of governors has 27 members, 21 of whom are elected by the NASD membership. Five governors-at-large are elected by the board, including two governors who represent investment company underwriters and insurance company members, respectively. The president serves as a continuing member of the board. With the exception of the president, all members of the board serve without compensation.

OTC Market Making

On an exchange, a single *specialist firm* is designated as that exchange's sole market maker in a given security. As such, the specialist firm is responsible for matching buy and sell orders and for maintaining an orderly market by buying or selling from its own inventory as circumstances dictate. By contrast, trading in the over-the-counter market is characterized by competition among a number of broker

Figure 4–4
The 13 districts of the National Association of Securities Dealers

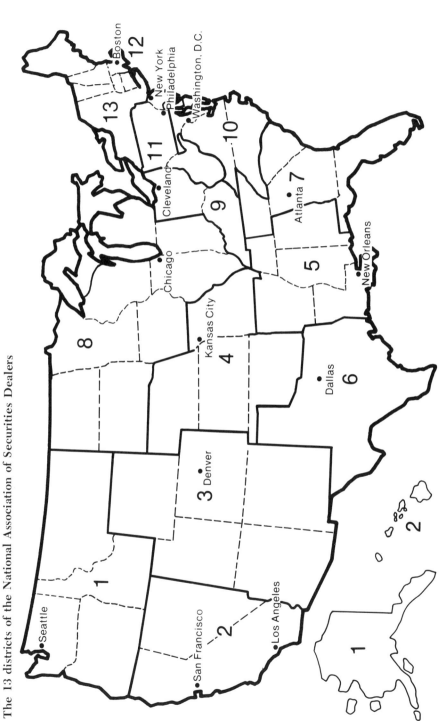

Source: National Association of Securities Dealers, Inc.

dealers who make a market in a particular security. Any number of OTC firms may make a market in a given security, in competition with other firms, by entering bid and asked quotations that indicate their willingness to buy and sell that security.

These procedural differences aside, business conduct in both the exchange and the over-the-counter markets is carefully monitored and is subject to exchange or NASD regulation, as well as regulations of the SEC, the Federal Reserve Board, the Municipal Securities Rulemaking Board, and state securities commissions. However, the NASD has the major responsibility for monitoring business conduct and trading activity in the over-the-counter market.

Although the NASD devotes a significant amount of its time to regulatory matters, its overall programs are much more encompassing. Their underlying purpose is to improve and strengthen financial markets. In recent years, many significant programs launched by the NASD have come to fruition. An over-the-counter quotations system (NASDAQ) and over-the-counter clearing facilities are two examples of the tangible benefits that have resulted from NASD programs. These services have reshaped the manner in which members now conduct their over-the-counter business, and they have done so in a very cost-effective fashion. Other member services now being developed, including automated order routing and a computer-assisted execution system, will further improve the functioning of the OTC market.

The NASDAQ System

NASDAQ is a computerized communications system which stores up-to-the-second price quotations from a nationwide network of dealers for over 2,700 over-the-counter securities. Through NASDAQ, professional traders and investors as well as broker-dealers who retail over-the-counter securities to the public have immediate access to the quotations of all dealers making markets in securities displayed on the NASDAQ system.

Until 1971, over-the-counter quotations were disseminated by telephones, private wires, and printed quotation sheets. Published quotations were generally stale by the time they were disseminated. Locating the best market was, at a minimum, cumbersome and expensive. Important data such as volume and price indexes were unavailable.

With the advent of NASDAQ, the situation changed dramatically. Share volume for the companies quoted on the NASDAQ system has exceeded 3.5 billion shares. NASDAQ has achieved an unprecedented upgrading of the over-the-counter market. OTC share volume has consistently exceeded that of all stock exchanges combined except the NYSE, and the NASDAQ Industrial and Composite Price indexes have outperformed nearly all of the major stock averages.

Advances in Clearing

Crucial to the increased investor participation in the NASDAQ system has been the provision of clearance and settlement facilities for over-the-counter transactions. In the late 1960s, the lack of such facilities in the over-the-counter market was a major cause of the industry's paperwork logjam. Now, through the National Securities Clearing Corporation, the regional exchanges, and the Depository Trust Company and other depositories, over-the-counter transactions are cleared through the same facilities, in the same manner, and at the same cost as transactions that take place on stock exchanges.

Glossary

Amex   Short version of American Stock Exchange.

At The Market   A customer's order instructing his broker to buy or sell a security at the best possible price when the order reaches the trading floor.

Bid and Asked   Also called *Quote* and *Quotation*. *Bid* is the highest price anyone will pay for a security at a certain time; *asked* is the lowest price anyone will take for a security at a certain time.

Bonds and Debentures   A bond is basically an IOU, or promissory note. Bonds are usually issued in multiples of $1,000, although $100 and $500 denominations are sometimes used. A bond is evidence of a debt which the issuer promises to repay on the expiration date and on which the issuer usually promises to pay a specific amount of interest for a specific length of time. The bondholder is a creditor of the corporation and not a part owner, as is the shareowner. So long as the company meets its obligations, such as paying the bondholder interest when due at the rate called for and paying off the bond at maturity, the bondholder has no voice in the business.

A debenture is a form of bond which is backed solely by the general credit of a company and is not secured by a mortgage or lien on any specific property. A debenture may or may not be convertible into common stock.

Bonds, like stocks, are an investment. Shareowners and creditors alike are interested in the welfare of a particular business in very much the same way that a person's family and the bank which lends that person money are both interested in his or her financial well-being.

Broker   An agent who buys and sells securities on behalf of others. The person in a brokerage house who accepts buy and sell orders from customers is known as a *registered representative*. The person on the exchange trading floor who executes that order is known as a *floor broker*.

Commission   The fee that a broker charges a customer for buying and selling securities for the customer.

Common Stock   Some companies list only one issue, usually common stock. The common shareholder of a company is its owner in a broad sense of the word and almost always has the right to vote for its directors. The directors, in turn, select the management such as the president, vice presidents, and treasurer.

If the majority, or even a well-organized minority, of a company's common shareowners become dissatisfied with its administration, they may successfully demand broader representation on the board or effect significant changes in company policy. Any common shareholder may suggest changes in corporate policy or practice that management may act upon or that may require a vote of shareholders.

The number of common shares in a listed company ranges from the minimum requirement of 1 million up to American Telephone & Telegraph's 550 million.

Dividend A payment that is made to shareholders if and as the payment is voted by a company's board of directors. Dividends may be paid in cash or stock, or both, and are distributed to shareholders according to the number of shares they hold in the company.

GTC Orders If you want an order to hold good indefinitely, you give the broker a *good-till-canceled order*. This type of order is carried as an open order—until the broker is able to execute it or until you cancel it.

Investor A person who holds securities in the hope of making a profit, either by selling the securities at a price higher than he or she paid for them or by accumulating dividends and interest.

Limit Orders If a round lot order is entered to buy a stock at $35, it cannot be executed at a price higher than $35, it can be executed below that price. In all cases, though, the broker will try to get the best price available to him on the floor.

Listed Company A company whose securities are listed on an organized exchange and are traded on the floor of that exchange.

Margin Anyone who purchases a listed stock can pay the full amount involved, thereby buying the stock outright; or the purchaser can make partial payment and have the balance advanced by his or her broker, thus buying the stock on *margin*.

Since the Federal Reserve Board first set margin requirements late in 1934, the margin which purchasers of listed stocks have been required to put up has ranged from 40 to 100 percent of the purchase price. Today, the margin rate is 50 percent.

Requirements for the maintenance of margins are set by the exchanges. Generally speaking, a customer's equity in an account may at no time be less than 25 percent of the market value of the securities carried. Frequently, individual member firms set higher requirements for their customers.

NYSE Short version of New York Stock Exchange.

Odd Lot An amount of stock, generally less than 100 shares.

Over-the-Counter Generally, the use of the term *over-the-counter* in connection with securities transactions refers to all such transactions that do not take place on a securities exchange. The term apparently originated during the early years of securities trading in the United States, when investors usually bought and sold securities through private banking houses. These institutions had counters over which stocks and bonds were bought, sold, and delivered.

The over-the-counter market encompasses not only transactions in outstanding securities (those already held by shareholders) but also transactions resulting from the initial distribution of new securities, including stocks, mutual funds, and bonds issued by corporations and by municipalities and other governmental units. Frequently, individuals, institutions, and trusts trade exchange-listed issues in the over-the-counter market, particularly when unusually large blocks of securities are involved.

About 3,400 securities are listed on the stock exchanges. In comparison, quotations on some 30,000 over-the-counter securities are published during the course of a year. Though most of these over-the-counter securities are not actively traded, the dollar volume of transactions in over-the-counter securities greatly exceeds the dollar volume executed on all the stock exchanges combined.

Preferred Stock Such stock is given certain preferential treatment over the common stock. This preferential treatment usually includes:

1. The right to receive a fixed dividend before the common receives any dividends.
2. A prior claim against the assets of the company in the event of liquidation.

Because of these advantages, the participation of preferred shareholders in company affairs is usually limited. Such shareholders generally have no voting privileges, except when a specified number of preferred dividends are defaulted, and they usually cannot expect more than their stipulated dividend no matter how prosperous the company may be. If the company runs into hard times, the preferred dividend may be reduced or omitted. If the preferred dividend is cumulative, an omitted dividend usually must be paid before the company may pay any dividend on the common stock. But if it is noncumulative, any unpaid dividend may be lost.

Round Lot An amount of stock, generally 100 shares.

Seat A term used to describe membership in an organized stock exchange.

SEC Short version of Securities and Exchange Commission.

Securities Evidence of ownership of a business, property, or goods or of a debt owed to the securities holder. Stocks and bonds are two kinds of securities.

Securities Investor Protection Corporation (SIPC) This organization provides funds to customers whose cash and securities are on deposit with an SIPC member firm in the event that the firm fails and is liquidated under the provisions of the SIPC Act. Protection is limited to $50,000 per customer account of which no more than $20,000 may be used for cash claims. The SIPC is not a government agency. It is a nonprofit membership corporation that has been created by an act of Congress.

Short Selling This, basically, is selling shares of a stock you do not own and borrowing the same number of shares in order to make delivery to the purchaser. When you buy the stock later so that you can return it to the lender, you hope to do so at a lower price, thus making a profit. Short selling may not be used to depress security prices artificially, and there are rules to enforce this prohibition. No short sale of a stock is permitted except on a rising price. For instance, there may have been six separate transactions in a given stock at a price of $45 per share, but no stock can be sold short at $45 unless the price before those six transactions was $44⅞ or less. Essentially, short selling is a normal business transaction.

Specialist An exchange member who helps provide a continuous market in issues assigned to him by buying when others want to sell and selling when others want to buy. The specialist also fills orders given to him by floor brokers who are *away from the market*—that is, above or below the current market price. When the price of a security rises or drops to a level which permits such an order to be filled, the specialist does so. For that reason, he is also called a *broker's broker.*

Stock Watch An exchange group which carefully examines each day's trading.

Stop Orders These may be used in order to protect a paper profit or to limit a possible loss to a certain amount. For example, if you bought a stock at $35 a share, you could enter an order to sell the stock at *30 stop.* If the stock declines to $30 or less, your order automatically becomes a market order and is then executed at the best price available to your broker on the floor—which could be $30, or below or above $30, depending upon the market in the stock at that time.

When you give your broker a limit order or a stop order, you can specify that the order is to be good for only one day. This is known as a day order. You can also give a week order or a month order. If the order is not executed during the period you designate, it automatically expires.

Trading Floor The trading area of an exchange where securities are bought and sold.

Trading Post A location on an exchange trading floor at which securities assigned to that location may be bought and sold.

Warrants Options to buy a given amount of stock at a specified price, usually over a specified time period. The life of warrants may be perpetual. However, many warrants have expiration dates after which they are worthless. When a warrant is issued, its exercise price is usually above the market price. Warrants are sometimes attached to bonds or other securities to make them more attractive. Warrants distributed in this manner can usually be detached and traded separately.

CHAPTER FIVE

Behind the Signature

BEHIND THE SIGNATURE AND OVER YOUR SHOULDER

The signature of an accounting firm in an annual report is like a grain of sand in the desert compared to the work that the firm does before signing the report. The accounting firm comes to know your company so well that it even learns how the company dots its *i*s and crosses its *t*s.

Another group which wants to know your company that well is the credit rating agency. It needs complete financial data so that it can publicly publish a rating of your company's financial condition.

Corporate executives have varying levels of involvement with these two groups. In a communications role, top management, accounting, the legal department, and the communicator will be involved in the development of financial statements and disclosure.

While the communicator may encounter the accounting firm primarily at annual and quarterly report time, other managers will interface with it frequently because the firm's accounting team is constantly poring over the financial records of the company and all its divisions. An annual fee in excess of $1 million is not unusual for a medium-sized company.

If your company is a frequent borrower of large sums of cash, financial executives and communicators will have ample opportunities to interface with the rating agencies. Such interfacing may also occur if substantial positive or negative changes in your business prompt the rating agencies to review its financial position.

This chapter contains information that will give you a better understanding of the two groups that are involved with for accounting practices and credit ratings and of the bases for their operations.

THE BIG EIGHT

The odds that your account, if you are a Fortune 1,000 company, will be handled by one of the Big Eight accounting firms are overwhelming. This is not surprising since the skills and resources of large

Figure 5–1

Auditors' Report

To the Stockholders of Trans Union Corporation:

We have examined the consolidated balance sheet of Trans Union Corporation (a Delaware corporation) and subsidiaries as of December 31, 1979, and 1978, and the consolidated statements of income, retained earnings, additional capital and source and use of funds for each of the five years in the period ended December 31, 1979. Our examinations were made in accordance with generally accepted auditing standards and, accordingly, included such tests of the accounting records and such other auditing procedures as we considered necessary in the circumstances.

In our opinion, the financial statements referred to above present fairly the financial position of Trans Union Corporation and subsidiaries as of December 31, 1979, and 1978, and the results of their operations and the changes in their financial position for each of the five years in the period ended December 31, 1979, in conformity with generally accepted accounting principles applied on a consistent basis.

Arthur Andersen & Co.

Chicago, Illinois,
January 31, 1980.

accounting firms are necessary to complete the audit function for major corporations.

Who are the Big Eight? Alphabetically, they are:

>Arthur Andersen & Co.
>Arthur Young & Co.
>Coopers & Lybrand
>Deloitte Haskins & Sells
>Ernst & Whinney
>Peat, Marwick, Mitchell & Co.
>Price Waterhouse & Co.
>Touche Ross & Co.

The ranking of the Big Eight is another matter. Despite the lifting of a ban on advertising by the accountants' professional organization in 1978, little is known publicly about the exact ratings of the firms. There appears to be ethical shadow boxing in which firms use statistics to make claims about their relative importance. For example, one of the Big Eight may claim the largest number of Fortune 500 companies, while another may claim the largest total number of clients. One firm may claim the largest number of professionals worldwide, while another may claim the largest number in the United States.

In general, the Big Eight have from 16,000 to 23,000 employees and 300 to 350 offices located in 70 to 90 countries. These statistics separate the Big Eight from Alexander Grant & Co., which is generally believed to rank ninth, with 2,600 employees in 58 cities.

In a 1973 study, Allen Schiff, assistant professor, Fordham University, and H. Dov Fried, a doctoral candidate, New York University, attempted to determine the relative size and stability of the leading public accounting firms.[1] Their measure was the economic characteristics of the firms' clientele. Included in the measure were the Fortune 500 industrials and the top 50 merchandising, transportation, and utility companies—650 companies in all.

The dominance of the Big Eight public accounting firms, they found, was clearly reflected in the fact that 91.6 percent of the companies included, whose revenues represented 95.5 percent of the total operating revenues, were audited by the eight largest CPA firms (see Table 5–1).

This dominance by the Big Eight extended in similar degrees in the industrial area (92.6 percent of the companies—96.1 percent of the sales), merchandising (92 percent of the companies—94.7 percent of the sales, transportation (84 percent of the companies—87.5 percent of the sales), and utilities (94 percent of the companies—94.6 percent of the sales).

---

[1] Allen Schiff and H. Dov Fried, "Large Companies and the Big Eight," *Abacus* 12, no. 2 (1973):116–23.

Table 5–1
Industrials, merchandising, transportation, and utilities, 1973

Firm	No. of companies	Percent	Sales or operating revenues ($ million) Absolute	Percent	Assets ($ million) Absolute	Percent	Income ($ million) Absolute	Percent
*AA	108	16.60	118,414	13.87	136,801	16.50	7,676	15.70
AY	47	7.20	65,768	7.70	53,529	6.46	3,223	6.59
CL	58	8.90	106,550	12.48	143,093	17.26	7,290	14.91
EE	69	10.60	64,002	7.50	49,534	5.97	2,969	6.08
HS	76	11.60	119,807	14.03	155,205	13.89	6,916	14.14
PMM	87	13.30	91,366	10.70	67,366	8.12	3,937	8.05
PW	115	17.60	183,654	21.51	181,901	21.94	12,565	25.70
TR	38	5.80	65,873	7.71	41,893	5.05	2,502	5.12
O	40	5.40	29,341	3.45	29,899	3.61	1,492	3.05
N.a.	12	1.80	9,032	1.06	9,935	1.20	330	0.67
Total	650	100.00	853,897	100.00	829,157	100.00	48,899	100.00

* These abbreviations are also used in Tables 5–2, 5–3, and 5–5.

AA	Arthur Andersen & Co.	PMM Peat, Marwick, Mitchell & Co.
AY	Arthur Young & Co.	PW Price Waterhouse & Co.
CL	Coopers & Lybrand	TR Touche Ross & Co.
EE	Ernst & Ernst	O Other
HS	Haskins & Sells	n.a. Not available

The names given are those which were used when the study was conducted.
Source: Allen Schiff and H. Dov Fried, "Large Companies and the Big Eight," *Abacus* 12, no. 2 (1973):117.

Schiff and Fried then analyzed a disaggregation of the companies on the *Fortune* list into 34 different industry classifications. It is important to note that any attempt at classifying large companies by industry poses some problems. The classifications that Schiff and Fried used were taken from several sources and may be viewed as "noncompelling" in several cases. Tables 5–2 and 5–3 separate CPA clientele by industry using two measures: number of companies and volume of sales. In some cases, the two measures give identical results; in other cases, the results are quite different. For example, in industry 5—Autos, AA, CL, EE, and HS each has 17 percent of the total number of companies and TR is dominant, with 33 percent of the companies. However, when sales are used as a criterion, AA has 1 percent; CL, 31 percent; EE, 2 percent; HS, 48 percent; and TR, 18 percent. By contrast, in the case of industry 13—Liquor, the positions of AA, AY, and PW are almost identical using both criteria.

This study enables one to identify the leading CPA firms and their relative strength by industry. It is interesting to note that TR focused on relatively few industries.

In late 1975, the U.S. Senate's Committee On Government Operations through its Subcommittee On Reports, Accounting, and Management began a study of the federal government's role in establishing accounting practices. The major purpose of the study was to provide Congress and the public with an understanding of the private organizations and federal agencies that were involved in establishing and administering accounting practices. The work of the subcommittee was presented in a text of 11 chapters (1,760 pages) that summarized the identities and activities of the organizations comprised by the accounting profession. The study, concluded in December 1976, was aptly called *The Accounting Establishment.*

Two of the chapters dealt with the influence of the Big Eight on the principal private rule-making bodies of the accounting establishment, that is, the AICPA and the FASB. The Big Eight were the center of attention of about one third of the study. Their position and activities in the accounting establishment formed the major premise for the government's conclusion that the accounting profession was dominated by eight giant accounting firms. It was the government's contention that these eight firms were so large and influential in relation to other CPA firms that they were able to control virtually all aspects of accounting and auditing in the United States.

It was apparently not their sheer size that the government saw as their source of influence. It was, rather, the size and influence of their clients that were the source of the tremendous influence wielded by the Big Eight. Through their clients, the Big Eight were able to exercise substantial influence on auditing and accounting matters, and therefore on the economy and society in general.

Table 5–2
Percentage of companies audited—number of companies as the criterion, 1973*

	AA	AY	CL	EE	HS	PMM	PW	TR	O	N.a.	Total companies
1. Aerospace	13	20	7	20	7	7	7	13	7	0	15
2. Air transport	19	6	6	19	19	19	6	0	6	0	16
3. Amusements	25	17	0	8	8	25	17	0	0	0	12
4. Auto parts	5	10	0	33	14	24	10	5	0	0	21
5. Autos	17	0	17	17	17	0	0	33	0	0	6
6. Building	30	5	15	10	10	5	10	10	5	0	40
7. Chemicals	11	9	9	2	20	20	18	2	7	0	44
8. Containers	7	7	7	0	20	0	47	7	7	0	15
9. Drugs	17	4	8	13	4	17	25	0	13	0	24
10. Electronics	16	11	11	16	3	11	14	8	11	0	37
11. Home furnishings	0	0	50	0	0	50	0	0	0	0	2
12. Leather and shoes	25	0	0	25	0	50	0	0	0	0	4
13. Liquor	17	17	0	0	0	0	67	0	0	0	6
14. Machinery	28	0	8	15	8	13	18	5	5	0	39
15. Metals—aluminum, copper, fabricating	13	7	40	7	7	13	13	0	0	0	15

16.	Metals—lead, zinc, gold	0	0	17	0	33	17	17	0	17	0	6
17.	Office equipment	9	0	18	0	9	18	45	0	0	0	11
18.	Oil	20	17	10	13	3	13	17	7	0	0	30
19.	Paper	17	0	8	0	25	8	25	8	8	0	12
20.	Communications	8	15	8	15	15	23	8	0	8	0	13
21.	Railroad equipment	20	20	0	20	0	0	40	0	0	22	5
22.	Railroads	0	0	0	0	28	17	33	0	0	4	18
23.	Retail trade—I	11	5	11	7	7	29	7	14	7	0	28
24.	Retail trade—II	20	0	5	10	5	15	15	25	5	0	20
25.	Rubber fabricating	0	0	17	33	17	0	33	0	0	0	6
26.	Soft drinks and candy	25	25	0	50	0	0	0	0	0	0	4
27.	Steel	23	0	14	14	5	9	32	5	0	0	22
28.	Telephone	25	25	25	0	0	0	25	5	0	0	4
29.	Textiles—apparel	0	28	0	8	28	13	8	4	25	0	24
30.	Tobacco	0	17	33	17	33	3	0	0	0	0	6
31.	Utilities—electric	22	0	17	0	31	20	22	0	6	0	36
32.	Utilities—gas	50	0	0	0	10	9	10	0	10	0	10
33.	Trucking	18	0	0	18	18	15	0	18	18	0	11
34.	Food	12	9	5	8	6	25	25	8	8	5	65

Table 5–3
Percentage of companies audited—sales volume as the criterion, 1973*

	AA	AY	CL	EE	HS	PMM	PW	TR	O	N.a.	Total companies
1. Aerospace	14	15	1	22	14	1	10	17	5	0	15
2. Air transport	28	12	12	7	21	9	10	0	1	0	16
3. Amusements	12	13	0	4	22	11	38	0	0	0	12
4. Auto parts	2	5	0	36	25	20	10	3	0	0	21
5. Autos	1	0	31	2	48	0	0	18	0	0	6
6. Building	41	6	16	9	7	4	7	7	3	0	40
7. Chemicals	14	5	5	1	26	14	16	10	9	0	44
8. Containers	6	16	19	0	30	0	22	5	2	0	15
9. Drugs	20	2	11	9	3	15	26	0	14	0	24
10. Electronics	21	20	4	7	0	26	12	5	4	0	37
11. Home furnishings	0	0	44	0	0	56	0	0	0	0	2
12. Leather and shoes	15	0	0	24	0	62	0	0	0	0	4
13. Liquor	15	19	0	0	0	0	66	0	0	0	6
14. Machinery	20	0	4	17	10	14	28	2	4	0	39
15. Metals—aluminum, copper, fabricating	6	3	47	11	10	6	18	0	0	0	15

16. Metals—lead, zinc, gold	0	0	32	0	36	16	9	0	8	0	6
17. Office equipment	4	0	10	0	10	16	60	0	0	0	11
18. Oil	17	19	8	5	1	3	47	1	0	0	30
19. Paper	25	0	12	0	27	3	18	11	3	0	12
20. Communications	5	16	21	14	10	21	3	0	9	0	13
21. Railroad equipment	14	38	0	16	0	0	31	0	0	21	5
22. Railroads	0	0	0	0	42	11	26	0	0	4	18
23. Retail trade—I	6	1	13	3	17	0	7	12	6	0	28
24. Retail trade—II	14	0	2	6	5	16	18	37	2	0	20
25. Rubber fabricating	0	0	24	16	16	0	45	0	0	0	6
26. Soft drinks and candy	10	37	0	53	0	0	0	0	0	0	4
27. Steel	7	0	3	16	9	4	58	2	0	0	22
28. Telephone	2	3	93	0	0	0	2	0	0	0	4
29. Textiles—apparel	0	14	0	6	17	28	6	2	26	0	24
30. Tobacco	0	7	47	31	15	0	0	0	0	0	6
31. Utilities—electric	26	0	14	0	27	2	22	0	9	0	36
32. Utilities—gas	49	0	0	0	11	18	9	0	13	0	10
33. Trucking	27	0	0	18	15	4	0	28	9	0	11
34. Food	15	10	3	4	5	13	29	10	6	3	65

* Some minor errors appear due to rounding.
Source: Allen Schiff and H. Dov Fried, "Large Companies and the Big Eight," *Abacus* 12, no. 2 (1973):122.

112

A research report prepared by the Congressional Research Service (CRS) confirmed the extent of Big Eight concentration. The CRS used the corporations listed on the NYSE and Amex as its data base. It selected average annual sales data for the years 1974 and 1975 as the measurement yardstick for determining the extent of concentration. It used five dependent variables: (1) sales received, (2) profits earned, (3) income taxes paid, (4) people employed, and (5) assets owned. In addition, it studied the concentration of particular firms in 10 selected industries.

The results show that for the NYSE and Amex significant percentages of the respective data categories were associated with Big Eight firms (see Table 5–4). In all cases, on the NYSE the Big Eight represented at least 89.9 percent of the total for each of the five variables. Further, Big Eight clients represented one third of the nation's 62.5 million employees in nonagricultural and nongovernmental establishments and one half of the $2,552 billion in sales for the manufacturing, trade, and retail sectors. The statistics show that there are actually three tiers within the Big Eight. Price Waterhouse is "king of the mountain." The second tier comprises four firms led by Arthur Andersen. The third tier is made up of three firms of about equal size. Based

Table 5–4
Percentage of all corporations listed on the exchanges for which a "Big Eight" firm acts as independent auditor

	New York Stock Exchange	American Stock Exchange
Sales		
Price Waterhouse & Co.	23.8	15.7
Arthur Andersen & Co.	14.6	8.6
Coopers & Lybrand	11.7	6.3
Haskins & Sells	12.5	5.5
Peat, Marwick, Mitchell & Co.	11.5	8.4
Arthur Young & Co.	6.9	8.2
Ernst & Ernst	6.9	8.8
Touche Ross & Co.	5.8	5.4
Total	93.7	66.9
Net income		
Price Waterhouse & Co.	28.1	19.3
Arthur Andersen & Co.	15.6	11.2
Coopers & Lybrand	13.4	5.7
Haskins & Sells	12.7	7.0
Peat, Marwick, Mitchell & Co.	9.6	5.5
Arthur Young & Co.	5.8	7.8
Ernst & Ernst	6.3	5.4
Touche Ross & Co.	2.6	4.8
Total	94.1	66.7

Table 5-4 (concluded)

Income taxes	New York Stock Exchange	American Stock Exchange
Price Waterhouse & Co.	36.0	19.1
Arthur Andersen & Co.	13.1	10.4
Coopers & Lybrand	10.1	7.9
Haskins & Sells	8.7	5.0
Peat, Marwick, Mitchell & Co.	7.0	5.6
Arthur Young & Co.	8.2	6.0
Ernst & Ernst	4.8	6.6
Touche Ross & Co.	2.0	4.4
Total	89.9	65.0
Employees		
Price Waterhouse & Co.	19.6	13.5
Arthur Andersen & Co.	14.8	9.3
Coopers & Lybrand	10.0	4.4
Haskins & Sells	14.8	5.4
Peat, Marwick, Mitchell & Co.	14.0	6.6
Arthur Young & Co.	5.6	9.4
Ernst & Ernst	7.2	8.3
Touche Ross & Co.	8.1	4.3
Total	94.1	61.2
Assets		
Price Waterhouse & Co.	20.3	13.8
Arthur Andersen & Co.	13.9	12.5
Coopers & Lybrand	13.1	6.8
Haskins & Sells	13.8	8.5
Peat, Marwick, Mitchell & Co.	16.6	10.1
Arthur Young & Co.	4.6	9.5
Ernst & Ernst	7.7	6.6
Touche Ross & Co.	3.7	5.0
Total	93.7	72.8

Source: U.S. Congressional Study, *The Accounting Establishment.*

on this evidence, the government concluded that the Big Eight had individual influence as well as a combined clout.

The concentration of particular accounting firms within particular industries is illustrated by Table 5-5. The CRS selected six major industries and the auditors of the 10 leading corporations in each. In the oil sector, Price Waterhouse audited six of the corporations. In the government's opinion, this analysis complemented the stock exchange statistics on Big Eight domination.

The government appears to have made a strong case against the Big Eight of the accounting profession. Whether the evidence collected is of sufficient competence to support the conclusions of concentration

Table 5–5
The Big Eight accounting firms and the top 10
companies in selected industries, 1974–1975

	Accounting firm
Natural resources (fuel)	
Exxon	PW
Royal Dutch Petroleum	PW
Standard Oil—California	PW
Gulf Oil Corp.	PW
Standard Oil—Indiana	PW
Shell Oil	PW
Mobil Oil	AY
Continental Oil Co.	AY
Texaco, Inc.	AA
Atlantic Richfield	CL
Banks and Bank Holding Companies	
Citicorp.	PMM
Chase Manhattan	PMM
Wells Fargo	PMM
Manufacturers Hanover	HS
J. P. Morgan	HS
Chemical New York Corp.	PW
Bankers Trust	PW
Continental Illinois	EE
Western Bankcorporation	EE
First Chicago	AA
Chemicals	
Du Pont	PW
Allied Chemical	PW
W. R. Grace & Co.	PW
FMC Corp.	PMM
Celanese Corp.	PMM
American Cyanamid	PMM
Dow Chemical	HS
Monsanto Co.	HS
Hercules, Inc.	CL
Union Carbide	Other
Drugs and Pharmaceuticals	
American Home Products	AA
Merck & Co.	AA
Abbott Laboratories	AA
Bristol-Myers	PW
Sterling Drugs	PW
Warner-Lambert	PW
Squibb Corp.	PMM
Eli Lilly & Co.	EE
Upjohn Co.	CL
Pfizer, Inc.	Other

Source: U.S. Congressional Study, *The Accounting Establishment.*

and power is still open to question. For example, using the stock exchanges as the sole data base gives results of the "to be expected" variety. In order to enhance their acquisition of capital from the equity markets, only large corporations list their shares on the national exchanges. These corporations need a large CPA firm to audit their activities because only a Big Eight firm can provide the required expertise and staff. In addition, access to the equity market is certainly affected by the ability of an underwriter to distribute a corporation's shares. The corporation's use of Big Eight firm is prima facie evidence of credibility. Only after considerably more research has been completed may one seriously consider the possibility of anticompetitiveness and lack of independence.

Accounting Rules

A substantial change is occurring in the way in which accounting rules are being formulated and in which the accounting environment is affecting companies. During the 1950s and the 1960s, the accounting environment practically stood still. The accounting rule-making bodies did almost nothing. Throughout that period, accounting technology was aimed at balance sheets. This was because in the late 1930s and the 1940s, when the rules were being written, they were rules on balance sheets. Accounting technology was a balance sheet technology when World War II ended. So accountants went through the 1950s and 1960s with insufficient technology for dealing with new types of companies, such as franchisors, lessors, and educational and real estate companies, which became quite optimistic when they recognized profits. There was an enormous amount of front-ending of earnings that became even worse because of another phenomenon—namely, the popularity of *per share* income as a profit measure. The term *earnings per share* was not defined in accounting literature until APB-15 became effective, in 1969. Put all these things together, and you have high-flying companies, ignorant investors, and a measurement called earnings per share which concealed most of the improper accounting practices that were being used in the 50s and 60s.

During this entire period of change, accountants did nothing but make money. The major accounting firms would have been superinvestments. Their real rates were between 10 and 15 percent per year. They did sensationally.

Although many companies became manipulative or highly creative in their accounting procedures during the 50s and 60s, at that time accountants did nothing to develop appropriate accounting rules. Then came the reaction. The excesses of the 1960s spawned a new breed of accountant who found that it was easy to uncover manipulative accounting by utilizing some of the disclosure documents. It was certainly easy to write about it. It became like shooting ducks in a

116

pond. This gave rise to the Monday Morning *Barron's* Syndrome. Someone would come into the office Monday morning after reading a front-page article in *Barron's* that attacked the so-and-so company. He would pick up the telephone, call his broker, and say, "Sell my shares." The broker would reply, "Sorry, the stock did not open."

A variation on the Monday Morning Syndrome was the Friday Night Syndrome. Here the investor would stay awake all night Friday, Saturday, and Sunday wondering whether the stock would open Monday morning after everyone else had had a chance to examine the *Barron's* article. These syndromes led to other reactions. Companies were not terribly happy; auditors were not very happy; and a number of companies got shot so far down that they went into receivership.

When these companies went bankrupt, people began to sue. There was not much point to filing a lawsuit against management. It had no money. So people began to sue the big accounting firms operating as partnerships, whose 500–1,000 partners had homes in ethnically pure suburbs, available for attachment in lawsuits.

All of these factors came together, and a massive number of accounting changes finally took place, including the firing of the old APB and the establishing of the new FASB. In addition, more accounting pronouncements were written in the 1970s than in the entire prior history of accounting.

At present, two problems are occupying the attention of the accounting profession:

1. Accounting issues.
2. Advertising.

With respect to the first problem, many of the accounting issues are really variations on a single theme: Should companies and their accountants deal exclusively with the past? Or should they take a crystal ball in hand and attempt to forecast with future-oriented information?

Forbes likens the action to a battleground.[2] On one side of the battleground stand most of the corporations, extraordinarily reluctant to release to the public the forecasting figures that they produce internally. After all, such disclosure subjects a company to two great fears: the forecasts could be high and wrong—or low and right. Either way, the corporation is in trouble. On the other side stands the SEC, which decided in 1978 to encourage forecasting. And in the middle, manning the mortars, are the Big Eight. The positions of the Big Eight range from Peat, Marwick, Mitchell's interest in trying to Arthur Andersen & Co.'s steaming opposition to the whole SEC forecasting idea.

Rising above the battle, like Greek gods peering down at the Trojan War, are two of the statesmen of accounting. They are John C. (Sandy)

[2] "Relativity Comes to Accounting," *Forbes*, June 23, 1980, pp. 113–14. Copyright © 1980, Forbes, Inc.

Burton, former chief accountant for the SEC and now head of the Columbia Business School's accounting department, and Oscar Gellein, a onetime member of the FASB and retired from Deloitte Haskins & Sells. They have come down on opposite sides of the issue.

Sandy Burton supports future-oriented information on pragmatic grounds. His position is that when the FASB says that the primary objective of financial reporting is to enable investors to predict the amount, timing, and uncertainty of future cash flows, accountants can't reject out of hand the possibility that a forecast might be the most useful information.

Disagreeing, Oscar Gellein insists that the accountant's traditional distinction between the past and the future must be preserved. For him, it gets down to this: Can accountants measure the future with enough reliability for people to believe their reports? He believes that if you tried to mix in everybody's future perceptions, pretty soon you'd have a state of accounting that nobody has confidence in. It's not unreliability that bothers him so much as crossing the traditional borderline from past to future too quickly, because a forecast is not a financial statement. There is a big difference between the two. He questions whether the public would be better served if accounting reports focused on forecasts than it would be if we developed the maximum usefulness of the statements we've got and assumed that sophisticated users should make their own forecasts.

The Big Eight and Advertising

The Wall Street Journal reports that with the ban on advertising lifted, fierce competition has forced auditing firms to enter the alien world of marketing. It gave the following account of the Big Eight:

> The "Big Eight" once considered marketing unnecessary, inappropriate and beneath their dignity. No more. Accounting firms are becoming 20th Century marketers, and as such are doing a lot of the things that Procter & Gamble does—segmenting and studying markets, developing new products for them and marketing them, says Harold Wolfson, a New York public-relations consultant who has Ernst & Whinney as a client.
>
> Accountants aren't about to hustle their wares the way P&G sells soap. "But," says Gary Mozenter, national director of planning and marketing (a new position) at Coopers & Lybrand, "There's no question that we are taking a fundamental and in-depth approach to marketing."
>
> There now is a fiercely aggressive environment, a good deal less gentlemanly than the country-club level of competition a decade ago, asserts Lee J. Seidler, Price Waterhouse & Co. professor of accounting at New York University. Mr. Seidler cites direct solicitation of prospective clients as a practice that's gaining popularity.[3]

---

[3] "Fierce Competition Forces Auditing Firms to Enter the Alien World of Marketing," *The Wall Street Journal*, March 18, 1981, p. 29. Copyright © 1981, Dow Jones & Co., Inc.

118

The Wall Street Journal adds:

> Deloitte Haskins & Sells has been touting its expertise in such publications as *The Wall Street Journal* and *Inc.*, a magazine for small business. Others, such as Peat, Marwick, Mitchell & Co., Ernst & Whinney, and Coopers & Lybrand, have been promoting specific services in publications including *Business Week, Forbes* and trade journals. Price Waterhouse & Co. is advertising a computer-based program to help oil and gas companies do windfall-profits tax returns.
>
> Ernst & Whinney's prime advertised offering has been its software packages, designed to drum up management-consulting and other business to complement the traditional accounting and auditing functions.[4]

Service Expansion

While their focus is on accounting, the Big Eight perform a host of services for clients. Following is a list of Big Eight specialties:

Firm	Specialties
Arthur Andersen & Co.	Management information systems
Peat, Marwick, Mitchell & Co.	Accounting, taxation, and management consulting services
Ernst & Whinney	Banks, S&Ls, insurance, health care, small business, government, manufacturing, executive search, consulting on controls, data systems, human resources, tax planning
Price Waterhouse & Co.	Manufacturing, health care, state and local government, transportation
Arthur Young & Co.	Agribusiness, food service, manufacturing, real estate, law firms, government, utilities, health care, pension funds, associations
Coopers & Lybrand	Not available
Touche Ross & Co.	Manufacturing, distribution, health care, financial institutions, retailing
Deloitte Haskins & Sells	Manufacturing, financial institutions, utilities, transportation

In addition, the Big Eight, scrambling to find new growth areas to compensate for a drought in public offerings, are flexing their competitive muscles by opening separate small-business divisions to pursue aggressively the traditional bread-and-butter business of local accounting firms.

The trend isn't new. Arthur Andersen & Co. has operated a Small Business Department since 1943, and Price Waterhouse & Co.'s Met-

[4] Ibid.

ropolitan Group is more than 20 years old. But unlike the early days, when small-business groups provided basic audit and tax work, the new effort means selling entrepreneurial services in addition to traditional accounting services. "We take the place of the financial vice president or the chief executive officer," claims Ira Edelson, head of the Small and Growing Businesses Group for the Chicago office of Deloitte Haskins & Sells.

Moreover, several of the Big Eight are stepping up suburban expansion plans so that they can compete more aggressively for small, young businesses outside the cities. In the Chicago area, Arthur Andersen has opened four suburban satellites, in Oak Brook, Rolling Meadows, Northbrook, and Olympia Fields. It's too early to know how successful the big firms will ultimately be. But the years of successful, hands-on experience and the loyalty of small companies give medium-size accounting firms an important advantage, if it isn't squandered by indifference to the competition.

Thus, internally, accounting firms have communications and business problems, issues, and opportunities, just as you have in your own business. The preceding inside views should enrich your perspective on these firms. Externally, accounting firms play an important role in the communications process. Their knowledge and data base enable them to estimate the effects of the proposed changes in disclosure and reporting, and thus to provide valuable information to those charged with making changes in accounting standards, such as the FASB.

THE RATING AGENCY

Although of secondary importance to the financial communicator, an audience of importance to a corporation—normally to the treasurer's department—is the rating agency. However, while it is the corporation's financial arm that interfaces with the rating agencies, the communicator can be a valuable resource in the preparation of the company's formal presentations to these agencies. In addition, many portfolio managers rely on rating agency examinations.

The concept of a rating is simple. What is the probability of timely payment of interest and repayment of principal? It's in the implementation of the concept that things get complicated, primarily because of the number, diversity, and complexity of the variables involved. The rating agency's role is to study and evaluate those variables.

The Agency as an Information Source

Opinion Research Corporation (ORC) reports that only one fourth of portfolio managers say that a rating agency's assignment of a company's debt is extremely important in their evaluation of a company's

120

Table 5–6
Weight placed on rating agency assignment
of a company's debt

Rely more on own examination
 of company's situation 51%
Rely more on rating agency
 assignment 19
Rely on both about equally 29

Source: Eugene E. Heaton, Jr., "Current Practices and Attitudes in the Investor Relations Field," *Investor and Financial Relations, 1980 State of the Art Report* (New York: Opinion Research Corporation, December 3, 1979), p. 87. Copyright © 1979, Opinion Research Corporation.

credit (see Table 5–6). Furthermore, when asked specifically about the relative weight they place on the rating agency assignment, one half of the portfolio managers in all institutions (and 8 out of 10 portfolio managers in the largest institutions) say that they rely more on their own evaluations of a company's situation than on the rating agency assignment. However, 2 portfolio managers in 10 (and nearly one half of the portfolio managers in the smaller institutions) say that they rely more on the rating agency assignment, with the balance relying about equally on both the rating agency assignment and their own examination.

Figure 5–2
Standard & Poor's organization chart

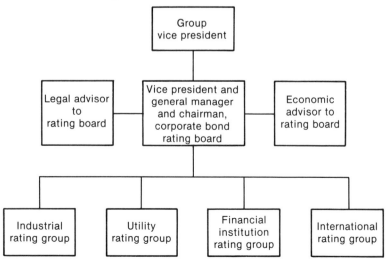

Portfolio Managers Rate the Raters

ORC asked portfolio managers to evaluate the three bond rating services (see Table 5-7). Over one half of portfolio managers say they assess Standard & Poor's most favorably, while just under one half say

Table 5-7
Evaluation of the three leading bond rating services

	Evaluate most favorably	Evaluate least favorably
Standard & Poor's	58%	3%
Moody's	47	6
Fitch	1	74
All about the same	4	2
No opinion	8	16

Source: Eugene E. Heaton, Jr., "Current Practices and Attitudes in the Investor Relations Field," *Investor and Financial Relations, 1980 State of the Art Report* (New York: Opinion Research Corporation, December 3, 1979), p. 89. Copyright © 1979, Opinion Research Corporation.

they rate Moody's most favorably. (Interestingly, the smaller institutions seem more favorable toward Moody's, while the larger institutions are somewhat inclined to favor Standard & Poor's.) Fitch is clearly an also-ran in this three-way evaluation.

In response to a specific question, a majority of portfolio managers expressed the view that the services were not as strict as they should be in evaluating corporate credit (see Table 5-8).

Standard & Poor's

Standard & Poor's is the oldest of the rating agencies. It has been in business since 1890. It is a major publisher of business and financial

Table 5-8
Are bond rating services as strict as they should be in evaluating corporate debt?

Strict as they should be	34%
Should be stricter	54
Other/no opinion	12

Source: Eugene E. Heaton, Jr., "Current Practices and Attitudes in the Investor Relations Field," *Investor and Financial Relations, 1980 State of the Art Report* (New York: Opinion Research Corporation, December 3, 1979), p. 89. Copyright © 1979, Opinion Research Corporation.

information on publicly held U.S. and foreign corporations and municipalities. It was a publicly held corporation until 1966, when all of its common stock was acquired by McGraw-Hill, a major publishing company. Today, Standard & Poor's operates as a wholly owned subsidiary of McGraw-Hill and is independent of any investment banking firm, bank, or similar institution.

Standard & Poor's has been assigning ratings to corporate bonds since 1923, to municipal bonds since 1940, and to commercial paper since 1969. It has outstanding today approximately 8,000 ratings on state and municipal entities and on issues of over 1,700 corporations. In addition, it has commercial paper ratings outstanding on over 700 corporations. Its ratings are distributed through a variety of news media, including its own publications.

Moody's Investor Services

Moody's has business and financial data on some 34,000 corporations and municipalities. Its information pool includes all corporations listed on any U.S. exchange, most over-the-counter traded corporations, and some privately held companies; the transportation industry; public utility enterprises; banking and other financial institutions; and municipalities and government institutions. Its most widely distributed publication is *Moody's Industrial Manual* and *News Reports,* which covers 2,900 companies. (See Figure 5–3 for highlights of Moody's history.)

The most primary and necessary working tool for anyone involved in stocks—from the individual investor to professional financial people—is Moody's *Handbook of Common Stocks*. The *Handbook* tells the story of over 900 issues—those of high investor interest. It gives the reader a quick way to select well-situated companies—plus valuable information that helps warn the reader away from unwise situations.

The Role of Credit Ratings

Standard & Poor's explains that until fairly recent times the extension of credit was based on the close personal relationship between the borrower and the lender, whether the credit was being extended to an individual, a corporation, or a municipality. However, the sheer size of today's public market for corporate and municipal debt necessitates some sort of impersonal credit judgment. No nation in history has been able to build the huge reservoirs of money available for investment that the United States has built through its insurance companies, savings banks, trusts, mutual funds, profit-sharing plans, and pension plans. AT&T alone is accumulating money in its pension plans at a rate

Figure 5–3
History of Moody's

1900   Founded by John Moody
1900   Published first industrial manual, *Railroads and Public Utilities*
1909   Published manual entitled *The Analysis of Railroads*
1914   Published *Public Utilities: An Industrial Manual*
1918   Published *Municipal and Governments*
1925   Began publication of supplements (*News Reports*)
1928   Went public with first stock offering
1928   Published *Banks & Insurance Companies*
1931   Published *Dividend Record*
1936   Published *Bond Record*
1955   Published *Handbook of Common Stocks*
1962   Acquired by Dun & Bradstreet
1970   Published *Over the Counter Manual*
1970   Began invoicing for rating services
1971   Published *Moody's Municipal Credit Reports*
1978   Published *Fact Sheets*

---

of about $2 billion a year. These funds are invested in a multiplicity of debt and equity instruments, and one of the tools that has assisted in their investment has been the nationally recognized credit ratings of firms, such as those provided by Standard & Poor's.

These credit ratings give investors an easily recognizable, simple tool that couples a possibly unknown issuer with an informative and meaningful symbol of credit quality. The corporate issuers range in nature from such public utilities as Commonwealth Edison, to such conglomerates as Gulf & Western. The municipal issuers range from the states of California and Virginia to the New Jersey Sports and Exposition Authority (the Meadowlands) and the Yazoo Mississippi Delta Housing Corporation. To these ratings of domestic issuers have been added such foreign governments as Japan and Finland and such foreign corporations as Nippon Telephone of Japan and ICI of England. Moreover, many issuers sell bonds with varying security pledges, such as first-mortgage bonds and sinking fund debentures.

Ratings are of value only as long as they are credible. The credibility of ratings arises primarily from the objectivity which results from the rater's independence and disinterestedness with respect to the issuer's business. The investor is willing to accept the rater's judgment only where such credibility exists. When enough investors are willing to accept a particular rater's judgment, that rater is referred to as a rating agency.

Credibility is very fragile. Standard & Poor's operates with no governmental mandate or subpoena powers or any other official authority. It simply has a right, as part of the media, to express its opinions in editorials written in the form of letter symbols.

In order to use the credit rating properly, one should understand what a rating is and is not. A bond rating, for example, is not a recommendation to purchase, sell, or hold a security inasmuch as it does not comment on the bond's market price or on its suitability for a particular investor. Although in the course of the rating process, the rater asks many questions in any number of areas, the rating does not mean that Standard & Poor's, or any other rater, has performed an audit, nor does it attest to the authenticity of the information which the issuer has provided and on which the rating is based. Ratings can be changed, suspended, or withdrawn as a result of changes in, or the unavailability of, information. A rating is not a general-purpose evaluation of an issuer. For example, an issuer with a AA obligation is not necessarily "better than" an issuer with a BBB obligation inasmuch as the AA rating may be based primarily on the specific security underlying the bonds.

Ratings do not create a fiduciary relationship between the rater and any users of the ratings since there is no basis for the existence of such a relationship. Ratings by themselves do not justify purchasing, selling, or holding a particular security. The rating performs the isolated function of credit risk evaluation. Since this is only one element of the entire investment decision-making process, it cannot in and of itself constitute a recommendation inasmuch as it does not take into consideration such other factors as market price and the personal risk preference of investors.

A Role for the Communicator

Rating agencies are great consumers of corporate information, so there is a definite role for the communications department as the rating agencies perform their rating processes. The first thing I have done is to make sure that these agencies have been invited to company field trips and seminars for financial analysts where a considerable amount of operating and financial data is reported. Another interface of the communications department is to aid executives of the treasurer's department in making presentations to rating agencies. Here the communicators' communication experience helps assure a logical, sequential, and credible corporate message, well framed with understandable, well-prepared tables, charts, and financial data. Finally, I have the rating agencies on my financial analysts mailing list so that they receive all important literature and announcements from the company.

CHAPTER SIX

Disclosure

DISCLOSURE, DISCLOSURE, AND THEN SOME

Following the passage of the securities acts in 1933 and 1934, annual reports to shareholders were almost exclusively the product of management for 30 years. Although public corporations had to start filing 10-Ks in 1941, it was not until 1964 that the SEC opened the wedge in the floodgate of regulation governing corporate reports.

Because every word and every number in a 10-K had to be cleared by lawyers and accountants, the documents were more reliable than annual reports, whose financial statements were audited but whose other features, such as the chief executive's letter, were included at the corporation's discretion. Some companies were actually telling the SEC one thing in the 10-K, and shareholders quite another in the annual report. This could be done legally by using different data bases for their accounting. For example, a company called Atlantic Research Corporation reported a profit of $1,473,192, 77 cents a share, in its 1961 annual report. The company based its results only on figures for the parent company. But in its 10-K form that same year, Atlantic Research used consolidated figures of the parent and its subsidiaries and reported a loss of $1,066,015, equal to 55 cents a share. (The present Atlantic Research Corporation is a new company with entirely different ownership and management.)

Annual Report versus Form 10-K

To protect shareholders from this kind of double-dealing, the SEC took steps to make the annual report a better yardstick of management's performance. Thus, in 1964, the agency laid down a rule requiring corporations to tell shareholders in what parts of their annual reports the accounting practices used differed from the accounting practices used in their 10-Ks.

Until the early 1970s, annual report financial statements were governed by generally accepted accounting principles (GAAP). SEC actions in the activist 1970s, however, added significantly to shareholder

125

report content by requiring such disclosures as a five-year summary of earnings and a management discussion and analysis. Financial statements were expanded to include such additional information as quarterly operating and compensating balance data.

Even so, the shareholder report and the Form 10-K were marked as much by differences as by similarities. The fact that these differences were expanding necessitated an evaluation of over 40 years of rule making. So, in 1974, the SEC started issuing a stream of amended rules forcing specific pieces of information into annual reports. The agency insisted that annual reports include financial statements for the prior two years "in roman type at least as large and as legible as ten-point modern type," a summary of operations, line-of-business information, the identity of all directors, and high/low prices of the company's stock for the previous two years. In 1976, the SEC required corporations to show quarterly stock prices and also to mention in the annual report that shareholders would find replacement cost data in the 10-K. In 1977, the SEC set down the requirement that corporations must put in their annual reports the same "segment" information (breakouts of numbers by categories such as divisions and product lines) that is contained in their 10-Ks.

10-K as a Benchmark

In effect, the SEC decided that it liked the 10-K more than it liked the annual report to shareholders. So it began to use the 10-K as a benchmark and to pull up the annual report to the level of the 10-K. The 10-K, for instance, includes the compensation of executives and directors, the options granted to management to purchase securities, replacement cost data, and extensive analyses of pending legal proceedings, general business operations, and "forward-looking" data.

The first suggestion that the two documents should eventually be merged came in 1977 as a recommendation by an SEC-appointed Advisory Committee on Corporate Disclosure. Headed by A. A. Sommer, Jr., a former SEC commissioner, the committee described its recommendation as an attempt to shift the emphasis of SEC-mandated disclosures from a dialogue between reporting companies and the SEC to one between companies and the public. What the committee was saying was that investors who relied on annual reports rather than on 10-Ks were being shortchanged. One solution was to force the 10-K data into the annual report. The SEC endorsed this approach by issuing a "guideline" encouraging corporations to publish annual reports that would meet the 10-K standard, and even to file the annual report in lieu of a separate 10-K.

Harold M. Williams, the SEC chairman, holds a fairly low opinion of most annual reports and isn't likely to let up in the long campaign to re-tailor them. He thinks that annual reports often reflect the results of a conflict between the desire to create a promotional document and the need to provide full and fair disclosure—a conflict in which meaningful disclosure frequently loses. In that sense, the attractive but somewhat vacuous shareholders' report is the other end of the continuum which begins with the 10-K. Sommer believes, however, that the threshold of fear among executives is very low for the annual report—and very high for the 10-K.

The SEC's push to make annual reports as revealing as 10-Ks and eventually to merge the two documents raised several important questions: Can a lengthy, complicated annual report filled with technical information still reflect a corporation's "personality"? Exactly how would shareholders benefit from such a report? Should control over the contents and format of annual reports rest with the SEC or with the directors and officers of the corporations?

There was a mixed reaction among corporate executives on the merging of the annual report and the 10-K, according to *Fortune*.[1]

It quoted A. William Capone, Koppers Company senior vice president for finance, as saying: "In our judgment, any investor who puts his money in Koppers is entitled to the same information as the professionals are getting." But executives at some other companies argued that merging the two documents was a bad idea. "I think we're already putting too much 10-K information into our annual report," said GM's Roger Smith. "It gets discouraging for a shareholder to have to read it all." Archie R. McCardell, president and chief executive of International Harvester Company, couldn't agree more. "The legal requirements of today's annual reports are ridiculous," he fumed. "They don't do the average investor a bit of good. All he's interested in is the price of the stock and the company's sales and profits. And he can get that from the newspapers." McCardell said that he had never read an annual report cover to cover—including those of companies where he had worked.

As for expanding the report to accommodate all the 10-K data, McCardell thought that would be not only useless but a waste of money as well. The number of shareholders who request a 10-K is "infinitesimally small," he said. So why spend the extra money to distribute the 10-K to all shareholders as part of the annual report? "I've got a lot better uses for $150,000 around here," McCardell added.

The problem of information overload is one that also bothers the august American Institute of Certified Public Accountants, which con-

---

[1] Herb Myer, "Annual Report Gets an Editor in Washington," *Fortune*, May 7, 1979, pp. 210–22. Copyright © 1979, Time, Inc.

cedes that people have trouble understanding annual reports. The reason for this—according to certified public accountants who audit financial statements—is that people try to read the reports. The institute urges shareholders to treat annual reports as reference documents, not as highly readable magazines. But this is precisely what most executives are trying to avoid. Understandably, they want shareholders to go through their annual reports—to absorb the message, whatever it may be.

The new integrated disclosure rules attempt to minimize the differences between the 10-K and the annual report by achieving an interrelationship among public financial reports. The rules also aim to improve the clarity of disclosure to investors and other users of financial statements and to facilitate the use of the shareholder report in meeting SEC reporting requirements.

Conforming SEC rules to the private sector's GAAP is one thing; conforming GAAP to SEC rules is something else. There is uneasiness that financial statements in shareholder reports are subject to the provisions of the SEC's Regulation S-X in addition to GAAP. This has two undesirable consequences. First, revised SEC-style financial statements will, in many cases, add considerable volume and detail. Second, the prior distinction between GAAP and S-X compliance disclosures has been thoroughly submerged. Historically, GAAP has been conceptually oriented. The SEC has often used GAAP concepts as a springboard to specific S-X disclosures by applying rigid materiality criteria. Most of these criteria have been retained under the new rules. Furthermore, any audited financial statement disclosure appearing only in an SEC filing was, in years past, presumably an S-X compliance disclosure and *not* a GAAP requirement. That distinction has disappeared under the new rules.

The Basic Information Package

The nucleus of the new integrated disclosure rules is the basic information package. The basic information package consists of selected financial data for five years, audited uniform financial statements, and management's discussion and analysis of financial condition and results of operations. The content of this package must be the same in shareholder reports and SEC filings requiring annual financial statements. The package is designed to capture the key financial attributes of each registrant. As a result, it should probably be approached as a single unit rather than as separate items.

Selected financial data for five years. The selected financial data replace the five-year summary of earnings mandated in previous years. The new summary's minimum disclosures include:

Net sales or operating revenues.

Income from continuing operations.

Earnings per share from continuing operations.

Dividends per share.

Total assets.

Long-term obligations and redeemable preferred stock.

Registrants should also disclose any other data needed to highlight trends. For larger companies, GAAP requires disclosure of data concerning the effects of inflation. Such data can be included where applicable in the package.

Audited uniform financial statements. A comparison of the previous and new requirements for financial statements reveals what may be sweeping changes for some companies (see Table 6-1.) The re-

Table 6-1
Comparison of requirements for financial statements

	Old	*New*
Balance sheets	Two years	Two years
Statements of income	Two years	Three years
Statements of changes in financial position	Two years	Three years
Standards, procedures, and regulations governing auditor report and form and content of financial statements and notes	GAAP and generally accepted accounting standards (GAAS) for shareholder report; GAAP, GAAS, and Regulation S-X for Form 10-K	GAAP, GAAS, and Regulation S-X for all public documents

quirement that the statements of income and changes in financial position include an additional preceding year is based on the SEC view that sufficient detail should be available to permit investors to analyze and understand the registrant's operations for the two most recent years; therefore, three years must be shown. The related footnotes must also conform to this requirement.

An analysis of common stock and other shareholders' equity is required, either in a footnote or in a separate statement, for each period for which an income statement must be filed. As noted, Regulation S-X now governs the form and content of financial statements in shareholder reports as well as SEC filings. Newly mandated S-X compliance information includes the following.

1. *Income taxes.* The revised rules retain prior S-X disclosure requirements and add a requirement to segregate pretax book income between domestic and foreign.

2. *Redeemable preferred stock.* The revised rules have the effect of applying the full burden of existing S-X disclosure to the annual report financial statements.

3. *Related party transactions.* Current professional standards require disclosure in broad and aggregate terms, but the revised S-X requires substantial explicit disclosure in each of the primary financial statements, including footnotes. This requirement is also applicable to other financial statements contained in the shareholder report or filed only in SEC documents. Where related party relationships and transactions are numerous, the new rule could result in substantially increased detail.

4. *Restrictions on intercompany dividends.* Disclosure of the most significant restrictions on the payment of cash dividends by subsidiaries to the registrant must now be included. This requirement encompasses situations where the viability of an entity is threatened because of restrictions on the intracompany flow of funds. Similar disclosure must accompany the five-year selected financial data and the management discussion and analysis.

5. *Materiality tests.* S-X rules require disclosures that are not mentioned explicitly in the professional literature. In addition, a greater number of materiality tests for individual amounts or account balances in financial statements for SEC filings must now be applied in determining amounts or accounts to be set out separately in the annual report financial statements. However, registrants have the flexibility to make most disclosures either on the face of the balance sheet or in appropriate footnotes.

6. *Oil- and gas-producing activities.* The SEC's reserve recognition accounting data, previously limited to SEC filings, must now be in the shareholder report. This requirement is not the result of the new rules; rather, it results from the timing of machinery independent of the new rules. These data can, but need not be, an unaudited supplement to the three-year financial statements.

Management's discussion and analysis (MDA). For a number of years, the SEC has required registrants to provide a discussion and analysis of their summary of operations. For the most part, the registrants' response has focused on period-to-period fluctuations in line items—information that certain parties concluded did not give readers much insight into the business. Needless to say, the SEC has been disappointed with the results. Under the new rules, the SEC clearly signals its intention to significantly increase its expectations for the MDA. If compliance falls short of SEC expectations, we can expect the kind of haggling that took place when segment disclosure was required.

The new rules expand the MDA to include a discussion and analysis of the *full* financial statements (including relevant statistical data and segment information), changes in financial condition, and results of operations for the three-year period covered by the financial statements. The discussion must provide information concerning liquidity, capital resources, and results of operations by identifying such indicators as needs, trends, uncertainties, material changes, and the effects of inflation. The SEC encourages registrants to focus specifically on events and uncertainties that they know would keep reported financial information from being indicative of future financial conditions.

Registrants are also encouraged, but not required, to supply forward-looking information. Such information is distinguished from known data that will impact future operating results, such as known future increases in costs of labor or materials. Any forward-looking information supplied is expressly covered by the untested safe harbor rule for projections.

The liquidity discussion, designed to assess the registrant's ability to generate adequate cash to meet its requirements, should include, where applicable and of importance, the following matters:

1. Known trends, demands, commitments, events, or uncertainties that are likely to materially affect liquidity.
2. Courses of action that will be taken to remedy any apparent cash deficiency.
3. Internal and external sources of liquidity.
4. Material unused sources of liquid assets.
5. Future cash outlays for taxes that exceed current tax expense.

The discussion of capital resources should include:

1. Material commitments for capital expenditures as of the end of the current year.
2. The general purpose of the commitments and anticipated source of funds to fulfill such commitments.
3. Known material trends in capital resources.
4. Expected material changes in the capital resources mix.
5. The relative cost of capital resources.
6. Any changes in equity, debt, and off–balance sheet financing arrangements.

The disclosures related to the results of operations should encompass:

1. Unusual or infrequent events and transactions or significant economic changes.
2. Known trends or events likely to affect revenues, the cost/revenue relationship (gross margin), or net income.
3. Reasons for material increases in revenues or expenses (that is, volume related, price related, new products, and so on).
4. The impact of inflation and changing prices on net sales, revenue, and income from continuing operations for years beginning after December 25, 1979 (that is, the effective date of SFAS 33).

The SEC has characterized the statement "a meaningful description of the registrant's business and financial condition" as being a key component of its basic information package. It is also evident from other such statements that the SEC considers MDA to be an important part of its integrated disclosure system. The SEC has underscored MDA's significance by stating that management is in the best position to know what information about its company is important to the users of its reports and that management need not await the development of specific disclosure requirements by the Commission.

An unfortunate result of the SEC's approach is that specific advice as to how to meet the new MDA requirements cannot be offered in checklist fashion. The SEC's background comments on MDA, its MDA instructions, and the preceding quotation demonstrate that the SEC expects each registrant to tailor its MDA to its own specific circumstances. In the SEC's view, the MDA is the registrant's means to tell its own story, a story that only the registrant's management is in a position to tell. Not until registrants have worked with the subjective provisions of the MDA will a discernible pattern of disclosure begin to emerge.

What one can see is the manifest absence of a coherent, widely shared disclosure policy. This ideological void was gleefully highlighted by Roberta Karmel, a former SEC commissioner, before her resignation in 1980. Karmel made a point of dissenting from most SEC actions and of speaking out on the inconsistencies and inadequacies of new SEC rules and proposals. Her words found more than a few receptive ears.

The SEC, however, has not cornered the "illogic" market. The two-step requirement by the Financial Accounting Standards Board (FASB) on disclosure of the impact of inflation is a good example of a problem in search of a solution. The prevailing regulatory attitude is: Do something, even though it may not be the right thing.

Hence, the new rules result in two additional pages in most annual reports and the kind of cranky, self-canceling language that IBM used in its 1979 report. After telling shareholders that the figures didn't measure current values, that the Consumer Price Index didn't measure the real world, and other things that a shareholder should not assume, IBM said, "Accordingly, management believes that the restatement of IBM earnings prepared under the Constant Dollar Method does not properly reflect the effects of inflation on the company." And if you didn't catch its drift the first time, it went on to say, "The methods promulgated to quantify these effects are still experimental in nature, and will need refinements over time. A great deal of education and understanding will be required by preparers and users before gaining acceptance for purposes of measuring the effects of inflation on corporate financial results."

IBM is in the mainstream. It seems likely that most companies will do everything short of stamping a "Don't Read This" in red across the new pages to avoid the possible misunderstandings that these imperfect rules could generate.

What of the ideological grails of yore? What, for example, of corporate governance? The idea is still around, and it actually generated some liberalizing of the proxy rules. But in the trendy world of disclosure, it is not at the moment a hot topic, other than in the context of the independent director's role.

A number of external forces are at work to dampen enthusiasm for more, or more innovative, disclosure. There has been a major exodus of talent from the SEC to beat government rules that would make it inconvenient for a former SEC lawyer to join a law firm to help corporate clients evade the snares of the very SEC he or she left behind.

There is continuing, and now more effective, complaint about the cost of all types of government regulation, which makes the whole idea of new areas of disclosure politically and popularly unappealing. There is a small but growing attack on certain SEC personnel who, it is felt by some, may be kicking companies around far more than Congress intended. And there are serious questions about the quality of some of the SEC's legal work.

REPORTING REQUIREMENTS

Numerous other reporting requirements are mandated by the SEC, the New York Stock Exchange, and the American Stock Exchange. Communicators, lawyers, and accountants should know them. These requirements are listed under the following headings, the SEC requirements being listed just under each heading.

Annual Report to Shareholders: Contents

Certified financial statements for last two years. Explain any difference between financial statements in annual report and statements filed with the SEC. Summary of operations for last five years and accompanying management analysis. Identify directors' principal occupations. Stock market and dividend information for prior two years. Notice of Form 10-K availability. Brief description of business and line-of-business breakout similar to description in 10-K. Summary of quarterly results in footnote. Supplementary inflation accounting. NYSE and Amex—requirements fulfilled.

Annual Report: Form 10-K

Required by Section 13 or 15(d) of Securities Exchange Act of 1934 on Form 10-K. Three complete copies and five copies without exhibits to be filed with SEC and one copy to be filed with exchanges where listed no later than 90 days after close of fiscal year. Companies which file pursuant to Section 15(d) must submit four copies of printed annual report with 10-K. NYSE and Amex—file three copies.

Annual Report to Shareholders: Distribution

Annual report to shareholders must precede or accompany delivery of proxy material. Seven copies to SEC with preliminary proxy material or when annual report is given to shareholders, whichever is later. NYSE—published and submitted to shareholders at least 15 days before annual meeting but no later than three months after close of fiscal year; three copies to NYSE. Amex—published and submitted to shareholders at least 10 days before meeting but no later than four months after close of fiscal year; 10 copies to Amex.

Accounting: Change in Auditors

8-K. Include information on disputes over past two years and on whether opinions in last two years were adverse or qualified. Former accountant files letter as exhibit commenting on company explanation. Impact of any changes made by new firm. In proxy statement, give name of current accountant and of accountant of the previous year, if changed, along with details of disagreements. NYSE and Amex—prompt notice when 8-K is filed.

Accounting: Change in Method

10-Q. Independent public accountant must file letter indicating whether he or she approves of "improved method of measuring business operations." NYSE—prompt notification required. Amex—notify before change is made, and disclose the impact in succeeding interim and annual reports.

Amendment of Charter or Bylaws

10-Q if matter is subject to shareholders' approval or if change materially modifies rights of holders of any class of registered securities. NYSE—four copies of any material sent to shareholders in respect to proposed changes; certified copy of changes when effective. Amex—10 copies of any material sent to shareholders; 10-Q must be filed with Amex when effective with certified copy of (*a*) charter amendments and (*b*) directors' resolution as to charter or bylaws.

Annual Meeting of Shareholders

10-Q following meeting when shareholders' vote required except as to procedural matters. NYSE—four copies of all proxy material sent to shareholders; notice of calling of meeting; publicity on material actions at meeting; 10 days' advance notice of record date or closing transfer books to NYSE. Amex—same, except 10 copies.

Bankruptcy or Receivership

8-K immediately after appointment of receiver. Identify proceeding, court, date of event, name of receiver, and date of appointment. 10-Q requires description of any bankruptcy, receivership, or similar proceeding. NYSE and Amex—notify immediately.

Contracts

Disclosure of progress on material contracts in such filings as 10-K, 10-Q, and registrations. Disclosure should include earnings losses, anticipated losses, and material cost overruns. NYSE and Amex— immediate publicity when news spreads beyond top management and confidential advisers.

Default upon Senior Securities

10-Q if actual material default in principal, interest, or sinking fund installment or arrearage in dividends for preferred, registered, or ranking securities is not cured within 30 days of any stated grace period and if indebtedness exceeds 5 percent of total assets. NYSE and Amex—immediate publicity and notice to exchange.

Directors or Officers

8-K if change in control of corporation. Report who acquired from whom, terms, terms of any loan involved, and amount and source of consideration used to gain control. 10-Q requires disclosure of newly elected directors and directors still in office unless proxies were solicited, there was no opposition to management's nominees, and all nominees were elected. New directors and officers must personally file Form 3 upon election. NYSE and Amex—prompt written notice of any change; immediate release if change material.

Dividends

Notice of dividend declarations pursuant to Rule 10B-17 required. Over-the-counter companies must provide advance notice of record date for subsequent dissemination to investors. NYSE and Amex— prompt notice and immediate publicity, which means notice and publicity even while directors' meeting is still in progress; 10 days' advance notice of record date.

Earnings

10-Q required for each of first three fiscal quarters (10-K for full year). Include unaudited income statement for current quarter, same quarter prior year, year-to-date data for two years; balance sheet for end of latest and year ago quarter's sources and applications of funds for year to date for two years; management analysis of changes between current and prior quarter, quarter a year ago, and comparison of two years to date. NYSE—publicity required quarterly; shareholder mailing recommended; four to five weeks after close of period considered usual. Amex—should be published quarterly within 45 days after end of fiscal quarter for all four quarters.

Earnings: Forecast or Estimate

SEC guidelines permit inclusion of forecast in filings such as registration statements and prospectuses. Safe harbor rule limits liability for incorrect forecast. NYSE—immediate public disclosure when news goes beyond insiders and confidential advisers. Amex—public disclosure not required unless earnings forecast has been released and later appears to be wrong.

Extraordinary Charge or Credit

SEC expects discussion in management's discussion and analysis. NYSE and Amex—disclosure recommended for material provisions for future losses, discontinued operations, foreign operations, future costs.

Foreign Currency Translation

FASB 8 requires quarterly report of foreign currency translation gains or losses. NYSE and Amex—no requirements.

Form, Nature, Rights, or Privileges of Listed Securities Changed

10-Q if constituent instruments defining rights of shareholders have been materially modified or limited. NYSE and Amex—20 days' prior notice of change in form, nature, or rights of securities or certificates; timely disclosure of all relevant information as soon as those other than insiders are involved in planning discussions.

Inflation

FASB 33. Companies must also include in annual reports current-cost and constant-dollar disclosures. NYSE and Amex—no requirement.

Merger, Acquisition, or Disposition of Assets

8-K if company or majority-owned subsidiary acquires or disposes of significant amount of assets or business other than in course of business (10 percent of total assets). NYSE—8-K if filed; immediate public disclosure; prompt notice with asset disposal. Amex—8-K if filed for acquisition or disposition of assets; immediate public disclosure.

Prospectus

Must be filed as part of registration statement. Copies distributed to underwriters and dealers in securities offerings and to investors. NYSE—seven copies of final prospectus; may be used as part of listing application covering the new securities. Amex—one copy of complete registration filing.

Proxy Material

Five preliminary copies filed at least 10 days prior to shareholder mailing; eight final copies when sent to shareholders. Five preliminary copies of additional soliciting material subsequent to proxy filed two days prior to mailing; eight final copies filed when mailed. NYSE—immediate publicity on controversial issues; four copies of definitive proxy material. Amex—10 copies of all proxy material when sent to shareholders.

Shareholder Proposals

Written notice to management if proponent intends to personally present proposals at a meeting. Proposal must be submitted at least 90 days before annual meeting solicitation. Company must give in proxy materials final date for receipt of shareholder proposal for next annual meeting. NYSE and Amex—no requirement.

Stock Split, Stock Dividend, or Other Change in Capitalization

10-Q required if exceeds 5 percent of amount of securities of the class previously outstanding. NYSE and Amex—immediate public disclosure and exchange notification. Issuance of new shares requires prior listing approval.

Tender Offer

Schedule 14D-1 increases disclosure required of tender offerers, who are required to disclose position and reasons toward tender offer within 10 days of commencement of offer. NYSE and Amex—consult exchange stock list department in advance; immediate publicity and notice to exchange.

FASB Statement No. 33

The extremely complex and most controversial regulation is FASB Statement No. 33, "Financial Reporting and Changing Prices," which requires the nation's largest public companies to report the effects of inflation on their financial statements. Donald J. Kirk, the FASB chairman, describes the statement as meeting an urgent need for information about the effects of changing prices. He cites the following possible consequences of not providing this supplemental information: investors' and creditors' understanding of a company's performance and their ability to assess future cash flows might be severely limited, and government officials might lack necessary information on the implications of their decisions on economic policy.

Disclosures have been effective for the fiscal years ending after December 24, 1979, but only public companies having either $1 billion of assets or $125 million of inventories and gross properties at the beginning of the year are required to present the supplemental information. All enterprises, however, are encouraged to make these disclosures. Many banks, insurance companies, and other large financial institutions which did not have to report under the SEC replacement cost rule are covered by the FASB standard.

The deliberations on the changing prices standard generated a great deal of controversy among preparers, auditors, and users of financial statements over how the FASB should proceed on its inflation-accounting experiment. Realizing that a consensus could not be reached on how to report the effects of inflation on business enterprises, the FASB concluded that companies should report under two fundamentally different measurement approaches—historical-cost/constant-dollar accounting, which deals with general inflation (i.e., changes in the purchasing power of the dollar), and current-cost accounting, which addresses specific price changes.

Early in 1979, the FASB appointed task groups to study the implementation and measurement problems in six specialized industries—banking and thrift institutions, insurance, forest products, oil and gas, mining, and real estate. These task groups issued preliminary reports, conducted public hearings, and published interim reports containing their recommendations to the FASB.

The task groups generally reported that no distinctive problems would be encountered in implementing the proposed historical-cost/constant-dollar disclosures. But a wide range of views was expressed on the current-cost disclosures and on the need to disclose values in lieu of, or in addition to, current-cost disclosures. The FASB considered the views of the task groups when it finalized Statement No. 33 and decided that all six specialized industries would be required to report historical-cost/constant-dollar data.

Although a task group was not established for long-term contractors (e.g., the aerospace and construction industries), Statement No. 33 provides guidance on how to determine the current cost for assets assigned to contracts in process. The FASB decided that items such as materials assigned to partly completed contracts should be measured at their current cost at the date of use on or on commitment to the contracts. Changes in the current cost of such assets will not be recognized after they have been committed to a contract. But in many cases these contracts in process will be monetary assets, as they are effectively receivables, and therefore they should be considered when the gain or loss in purchasing power is computed.

Financial institutions, such as banks and insurance companies, are not given any special guidance in Statement No. 33. At a minimum, the purchasing power gain or loss on net monetary items would have to be presented and some financial institutions would have to report the constant-dollar date (and possibly the current-cost date as well) for their properties because the effect on depreciation expense would be material to income from continuing operations. These entities generally have not had experience in applying inflation accounting since they were not subject to the SEC's replacement cost rules. If they have not previously aged their properties, their first-year implementation efforts could be significant.

140

Realizing that understanding the mass of new disclosures will entail a substantial learning process, the FASB believes that clear narrative explanations and presentations are essential. Therefore, it has organized an advisory task force of senior corporate executives to develop illustrative disclosures on ways to present and explain the inflation-accounting disclosures.

In addition, the FASB intends to assess the usefulness of the experimental changing prices disclosures required by Statement No. 33. This ongoing assessment process is expected to provide a basis for decisions on whether the dual approach should continue and on whether other requirements should be changed. The FASB has also announced plans to "undertake a comprehensive review of this Statement no later than five years after its publication."

FASB Statement No. 14

On the other hand, FASB Statement No. 14, "Financial Reporting for Selected Segments of a Business Enterprise," offers management an ideal opportunity to reexamine its organization structure, management information system, and internal operations. The resulting improvements readily offset the cost of compliance, improve decision making, and bring progress and profit.

For companies reporting on FTC Form LB or public companies registered with the SEC, there are two procedures for selecting segments or lines of a business:

1. The procedures required by Statement No. 14 and also by the SEC. Both requirements are closely related and are selected by management according to stipulated guidelines.

2. The procedure required in reports to such government agencies as the FTC, the Census Bureau, and the IRS. This procedure is based on or modified from the Standard Industrial Classification Manual (SIC). It is used to select lines of a business (often referred to as segments of a business by government agencies).

It should be recognized that segments of a business result from taking the enterprise as a whole and analyzing it, dissecting it, disaggregating it into its several pieces, and then aggregating the results into logical segments according to the guidelines of Statement No. 14. Paragraph 5 of the statement says:

> The purpose of the information required to be reported by this Statement is to assist financial statement users in analyzing and understanding the enterprise's financial statements by permitting better assessment of the enterprise's past performance and future prospects. . . . information prepared in conformity with this Statement may be of limited usefulness for comparing the segment of one enterprise to the similar segment of another enterprise.

Although this refers specifically to the user of financial statements, the segmentation of data by product lines, departments, cost centers, or other organizational units has even greater use and value internally, to management at all levels. Aggregating or disaggregating such units will lead to segments which combine many of the units that make up the business enterprise. Much can be learned about a company by studying the various pieces that make up the whole.

For many years, companies with reasonably sophisticated management information systems have employed segmented reporting of their operations for internal purposes. Management in these companies was motivated by its requirements for the budgeting, reporting, and control of company activities and was not influenced by any external requirements other than such contract responsibilities as royalty payments, bonuses, or rentals that were measured by revenues or activities.

However, prior to the issuance of Statement No. 14, the data aggregated by product lines or profit centers were so limited as to be useless for determining segments. According to Statement No. 14, systems such as the SIC and the Enterprise Standard Industrial Classification (ESIC) are unsuitable for use in determining industry segments. The determination of an enterprise's industry segments must depend to a considerable extent on the judgment of its management.

Three basic steps are suggested by which reportable segments can be determined,

1. Identifying the individual products and services from which the enterprise derives its revenue.
2. Grouping those products and services by industry lines into industry segments.
3. Selecting those industry segments that are significant with respect to the enterprise as a whole.

Statement No. 14 refers to several criteria that must be met in the process of determining segments. These should be considered throughout the three steps.

1. The 10 percent rule requires that each segment represent 10 percent or more of the combined revenues, or 10 percent or more of the operating profit or the operating loss, or 10 percent of the combined identifiable assets. These criteria must be applied separately for each fiscal year, and a segment must satisfy one or more of the criteria.

2. The 75 percent test provides that the combined revenues from sales to the unaffiliated customers of all reportable segments must constitute at least 75 percent of the combined revenues from sales to the unaffiliated customers of all segments.

3. It is suggested that the reportable segments be limited to 10.

4. If an enterprise operates in a single industry or if a dominant portion of an enterprise's operation is in a single industry segment, the segmented reports required by the statement need not be made, but the industry must be identified. An industry segment may be regarded as dominant if its revenue, operating profit or loss, and identifiable assets each constitute more than 90 percent of the related combined totals for all industry segments and no other industry segments meet the 10 percent rules.

The SEC has long been considering the need for segment disclosure to shareholders in the various forms filed with it, and it was the first to issue specific instructions on how to report segments. Initially, registration statements filed on Form S-1 or similar forms required a description of business, including a statement of the principal products made and the principal services rendered and the markets and method of distribution for those products and services. The current SEC requirements are quite similar to those of Statement No. 14. Public companies that comply with the SEC would, in essence, also be complying with Statement No. 14.

Forecasting Gets "No" Vote

In 1975, the SEC issued proposed guidelines regarding the forecasting of sales and earnings by publicly held corporations. Although the guidelines did not require public forecasting, they established a series of requirements which corporate management would have had to follow if it elected to make sales and earnings projections. Essentially, the SEC proposal included the following provisions:

1. A "projection" could cover future revenues, sales, net income, or earnings per share. It could be expressed as a specific amount, a range of amounts, or a percentage variation from previous results. It could also be a company's confirmation of a projection by a noncompany source.

2. The filing of projections on Form 8-K would be required within 10 days after they had been announced publicly. An 8-K filing would also be required when a company believed that a past projection no longer had a reasonable basis or when a company decided to stop issuing projections.

3. The filing of an 8-K would be optional when a company "disassociated itself" from an outside projection. However, a company would not be required to "disassociate itself" from an outside projection.

4. Companies would be required to include, in registration statements and Form 10-K, projections that they had issued for the previous fiscal year, together with comparisons between the projections and the year's actual results.

5. Companies that had been issuing projections would be required to include a new projection for the current fiscal year or the first six months of the year in their annual reports or 10-Ks, or explain why they had stopped issuing projections. Any projections disclosed in Form 10-K would also have to be disclosed in the annual report.

The major public relations firm Burson-Marsteller conducted two surveys to determine the potential impact of implementing the SEC's proposed rules. First, the chief financial officers of the Fortune 1,000 industrial corporations were polled to determine whether they would provide "projections" if these rules were enacted. Of those polled, 325 responded and disclosed that if required to file an 8-K: 93 percent would not be willing to forecast performance to a member of the investment community; 92 percent would not grant a press interview if doing so would prompt a management projection; and 92 percent would not confirm or negate a projection made by another individual.

Four hundred financial analysts at brokerage firms and institutions were polled to determine to what extent they were currently guided by companies in developing their estimates and how this situation could change if the SEC's rules were approved. Of those polled, 83, or 21 percent, responded. The survey disclosed that on average an analyst followed 27 companies. Of these companies, 37 percent gave earnings per share estimates or projected increases/decreases in revenues or earnings last year and 48 percent confirmed or negated the analyst's estimate or indicated that it was a "ball park" figure. Of the analysts who replied, 93 percent contended that the reporting policy proposed by the SEC would restrict the flow of information from corporations concerning future performance potential and 77 percent believed that the SEC's disclosure system would not be in the best interest of the investing public.

In a survey conducted by Newsome & Co., 60 percent of the responding companies submitted to interviews with Dow Jones (*The Wall Street Journal*).[2] During the interviews, management normally discussed the business outlook for the next quarter or for the remainder of the fiscal year. Of these companies, 35 percent reported that they would not continue with the interviews if the SEC proposal were enacted. Several companies commented that they would like to continue with the interviews because these permitted management to gain a broad dissemination of its views on present business conditions. However, they felt that doing so would subject them to the new SEC forecasting requirements. They, therefore, would elect not to participate in the Dow Jones interviews if the SEC proposal were enacted as it then stood.

---

[2]"Proposed Forecasting Rules Get Negative Vote," *Public Relations Journal*, September 1975, pp. 12–14. Copyright © 1975, Public Relations Society of America.

Although the corporate structure is embroiled in arguments with the SEC over certain reporting requirements, many of the SEC regulations offer the communicator opportunities for publicity. In fact, in reviewing the corporate reporting requirement list, it should be noted that publicity is mandated in many instances. Examples include earnings, dividends, contracts, default on senior securities, and changes in directors, officers, or ownership. Other regulations, while they do not mandate publicity, offer the creative company opportunities to get in print. Examples include changes in listed securities, the filing of a prospectus, and annual report mailing.

From this and previous chapters, you now know the breadth and scope of the financial community. You know the major reporting requirements. You know the makeup of the "model" professional. You know the makeup of the "model" individual investor. You know how they think, what turns them "on," and what turns them "off."

You are ready to communicate!

CHAPTER SEVEN

With Pen in Hand

ARE YOU READY TO COMMUNICATE?

Now that you have absorbed the information in the preceding chapters, you may feel that you are ready for communications in your company. But you are *not*. You must first direct a considerable amount of your time and talent, along with some funds, to research and evaluation of that research, program planning, and message positioning in order to develop a program that is flexible, reviewable, and measurable. All of this is necessary before Word No. 1 of a program can be executed successfully.

Your First Steps

Your first step is to evaluate the current situation of your company, such as its strengths and weaknesses. The company's position and image with shareholders, the image and recognition factors of the company in its markets, management philosophy and goals, industry position and characteristics, financial structure and policy, size, earnings record and prospects, geographic profile, shareholder distribution and mix, P/E ratio trading volume, yield, volatility relative to the market, stock price, and stock exchange listings all affect the kind of program that you can design for your company. Some of these factors are strengths inherent to maximum potential, while others may be weaknesses that limit certain types of programs, but they must all be known and understood.

Next, you will want to develop program objectives along with your communications department. What do I want to accomplish? In what kind of time frame? With what kinds of resources? You may need to expand, correct, or even downplay your image; improve your visibility; increase brokerage house and institutional interest and research coverage; revalue the stock price; change your shareholder mix for greater or lesser trading (to reduce volatility); defend against possible tender offers; and improve communications with current shareholders. The key is to establish priorities among objectives, develop strategies,

145

plan your program activities, and decide how you are going to measure the results. You should have your public relations agency at these meetings along with your in-house staff.

Planning begins by assessing the resources of time, budget, internal staff, and outside counsel. You plan by objective, choosing the activities that can contribute to the achievement of your objective. Your starting point is a benchmark study for the communications program. Such a study tells you what your current status is with each of your audiences. You then have your activities monitored as you implement them, so that you know at any given point how the overall program is going.

By periodically measuring and evaluating the results of the program, it is easy to refocus and fine-tune your ongoing program activities to meet your objectives. Some activities may take more time, some less, than you planned. Some may become less important if the current situation of your company changes, so that you can change priorities. Then you start the cycle over again, beginning with your new currently achieved status.

Know Your Audiences

Despite this excellent advice, I have found that many communications professionals will continue to plunge headlong into a program or pieces of programs without planning or without knowing the desires or needs of the audiences for their informational materials. One successful part of a program, for example, can be direct mail—if it is utilized in conjunction with an overall program and if it is very well conceived to provide substantive material, not "blurbs." Otherwise, corporations waste money, often large amounts on investor relations mailings.

Many analysts instruct their secretaries to discard anything with a public relations organization's name on the envelope, as well as mailings from companies outside the industries they follow. A representative of the New York Society of Security Analysts (NYSSA), which sells industry specialists' mailing lists to companies, says that the NYSSA tries to dissuade companies from mass mailings because irate analysts call the association to complain when they receive mail from companies outside their areas of industry specialization.

Furthermore, officers of major national and regional brokerage firms say that they don't encourage registered representatives to recommend issues not approved by their research people. Surveys tend to confirm the existence of policy barriers and, even more discouraging, to cast some doubt on the value of corporate financial mailings, particularly annual and interim reports, to registered representatives.

Other brokers say that they are generally cool to most standard direct mail vehicles with the exception of the annual report. But I have known them to reverse themselves by showing interest in product literature, speech texts, or corporate fact books. Still, time is precious and these types of materials generally take too long to digest. Finally, brokers have told me that a reprint of a brief national business magazine article can be a helpful selling tool, along with continuing contact through financial reports, press releases, and clippings.

Success with direct mail, in my experience, can be achieved by matching the appropriate materials with the appropriate audiences. I have found, for example, that financial analysts and institutional brokers have ferocious appetites for news, despite disclaimers in surveys. Most of my mailings to them have consisted of practically every piece of printed information, ranging from annual reports and corporate brochures to simple new product press releases. The response has been an increase in names on the mailing lists and requests for additional copies of materials for both immediate and research library uses.

Registered representatives, on the other hand, have proven to be highly selective in the materials they desire. For example, they prefer a condensed version of the annual report, highlights of speeches, and flash cards on new developments.

However, obtaining or expanding brokerage firm coverage often requires aggressive activity by the CEO and the investor relations manager. Passively waiting for the stock to be discovered is usually ineffective. The investor relations manager or the CEO should feel free to call on brokerage firms to see whether there is interest in research coverage. Meetings, speeches, and company tours are all important tools in this endeavor.

So, too, with the cultivation of financial analysts because this is fundamental to attracting national brokerage firm analysts. Management need not wait to be asked. It can initiate an appearance at one or more of the 51 societies in the United States and Canada. The NYSSA, with more than 5000 members, is by far the largest. More than ,350 companies appear before the group annually, but very few of them request the appearance. A person speaking for the NYSSA wishes that more companies would initiate such appearances.

The Financial Analysts Federation (FAF) produces industry seminars in major areas, such as energy, retailing, and banking. The programs are arranged by FAF headquarters staff, but analysts recommend the panelists, and typically about one third of attendees are from corporations and about two thirds are from the financial community.

Monitoring for Effectiveness

The effectiveness of communications programs *can* be monitored, even though several key members of the National Investor Relations Institute (NIRI) say that almost no evaluation is being done. If you use as a benchmark the analysis undertaken before your program is initiated, you should be able to establish a checklist for periodic comparison. Depending on your objectives, the checklist may include:

Number and type of requests for business press interviews, especially as an industry representative.

Number of articles published about the company in the business and trade press.

Number and types of requests for annual report, quarterlies, and other financial data.

Annual report reception and awards.

Number of published research reports.

Number of requests for analyst interviews with management.

Number of appearances at professional societies and business seminars.

Analyst attendance at meetings for your company.

P/E and trading volume relative to market and competition.

Stock price movement versus competition and the market.

Stock ownership change, by type of owner and geographic area.

One NYSE-listed corporation monitored the results of its investor relations program two years after its inception. Its analyst mailing list increased by a factor of five; the number of regional and Wall Street analysts who published research on the company increased from 4 to 12 (despite mergers and consolidations on the Street); lengthy analyst telephone calls and visits averaged 12 and 8 per month, respectively; the company made 15 presentations to the investment community in a year; analyst attendance at company-sponsored meetings more than doubled; the company's stock consistently sold at a premium P/E multiple; trading volume in the stock, relative to the market, increased 50 percent; and institutions held 20 percent more of the stock than they did before the company's investor relations program was started. My program has attained similar results, along with a couple of others. Each year for several years our daily trading volume increased, as did requests from business publications for information, particularly views on industry and general business trends.

It Begins with the CEO

For an investor relations program to be effective, it is an absolute necessity to have the commitment of the CEO. Without his presence, any investor relations activity is likely to be ineffective, inconsistent, inaccurate, and frustrating to his staff. It is only the CEO who can objectively evaluate the company and interpret that evaluation for the development of investor relations objectives. He must be involved with determining the corporate profile, or personality, so that strategies can be executed, in large part, by the company's investor relations manager. Without the CEO's personal attention and allocation of the adequate corporate resources of time, money, and staff, the program is likely to be haphazard and to leave the CEO open to criticism.

Agreement of the need for management involvement comes from Richard D. Lewis, chairman of Corpcom Services, Inc. But he says that the first level, the president and the chairman, is usually no trouble. He cites surveys indicating that some chairmen are spending upward of 50 percent of their time on external communication. They understand the need, and they are willing to cooperate.

There is an even more fascinating group of corporate executives in those surveys. They are the men and women who are one level from the top. Usually, they have been operating people all of their lives. Now, suddenly, if they want a shot at the top job, they must change their style and start focusing on the outside world. They must become public people. They must make speeches, testify in Congress, and field questions from financial analysts.

My own experience is the opposite. I find corporate executives aware that they are obligated to the owners of the business to consider legal and ethical measures to reduce the cost of capital, to facilitate expansion, to motivate company officers, to compensate investors for the use of their money, and to tell the financial community about it. I have rehearsed intensely interested executives past midnight before they made speeches so that they could contribute to the credibility of management.

And I have seen, despite the ground swell of advice, some chief executives tend to be reticent, reclusive, and unsure and almost untrusting of either the audience or themselves. Henry Ford reluctantly authorized advertising only because all of his competitors were using it. In the same way, some managements have considered financial public relations nothing more than an unpleasant, defensive necessity. This kind of corporate attitude doesn't work. The practitioner of financial public relations, or investor relations, becomes a functionary; the practice of financial public relations becomes merely a repetition of everybody else's mistakes; and the company suffers.

As more CEOs change their views, financial public relations will get the support it needs in order to function effectively. So, the number one priority for success is that the CEO must understand the marketing of stocks as well as he understands the marketing of products or services.

It is possible for the CEO to assign the program of interfacing with the financial community, but only under highly controlled conditions. First, no matter what the CEO's level of involvement, he must make the initial commitment to communicate. Next, his choice of his per-

150

sonal emissary must be well thought out. Otherwise, the emissary will inject his personality, not that of the CEO.

At Trans Union Corporation, the CEO was able to successfully assign the responsibility to his chief financial officer, basically, because of the attitude and personality of that officer. In this instance, the CFO was knowledgeable and aggressive. He followed three policies that were greatly appreciated by the financial community:

1. Open door.
2. Open telephone.
3. Complete, frank disclosure.

Performance—The First Ingredient

In his book *Management Briefing: Developing a Plan for Marketing Corporate Shares,* Mark J. Appleman agrees that the commitment to an investor relations program must start at the top, but one vital ingredient is required first. It is performance. He states:

> Unless the traditional measures of corporate achievement sales and earnings are translated into dividend payouts and capital appreciation, shareowners are not inclined to be enthusiastic about management claims to performance bonuses. To the owners, after all, higher sales and earnings are not an end in themselves but only a means to an end. Higher profits that remain unreflected in higher share prices are purely academic accomplishments to investors whose test of good management is not an income statement or balance sheet but a dividend check and the latest stock quotation.
>
> The big problem is that in companies approved for purchase by financial institutions, investor relations officers maintain contact with analysts and portfolio managers; and financial public relations officers deal with the financial press, and sometimes send analysts, registered representatives and portfolio managers annual reports and interim reports and other makeshift marketing materials. Often the investor relations and financial public relations officer work out of different departments with different corporate objectives and separate budgets. The company's precious price/earnings multiple is like a pop fly falling between two outfielders—because there is no corporate share marketing plan.[1]

Corporate Share Marketing

One of the first corporate leaders to comprehend the challenge of corporate share marketing was the late Eli Goldston, chairman of Eastern Gas and Fuel Associates. He said that the way to deal with the

---

[1] Mark J. Appleman, *Management Briefing: Developing a Plan for Marketing Corporate Shares* (New York: Corporate Shareholder Press, 1977), p. 4. Copyright © 1977, Corporate Shareholder Press.

crisis in the securities industry was for each company to take steps to market its own shares. To develop a realistic marketing program, Goldston recommended that corporate executives take into consideration five fundamental propositions:

1. Securities are not bought; they're sold.
2. A marketing plan is essential to a successful selling effort.
3. The selling effort for securities must be quite different from the one used for the company's products or services because, for one thing, the sales channel—the stockbroker—and the marketplace are regulated and outside the control of management.
4. The proper marketing approach is to identify the different markets for the company's securities and to develop specific marketing plans for each.
5. Management must take positive steps to make the company's stock stand out from the rest of the market in order to gain the attention of prospective investors.

Sound marketing of a stock, Goldston contended, should begin with management's perception of the company as an investment vehicle. The marketing manager must ask himself these questions: What is my product? How is it perceived? Who are the prospective buyers? What are their investment objectives? How do I persuade them to buy? Finally, what will get their attention and move them to act?

What Goldston was advocating, according to Appleman, was not stock promotion and nothing akin to "touting"—but *marketing*. With marketing, you seek to redistribute the company's shares among investors whose objectives would be compatible with the goals of management and who would therefore be potentially more loyal, long-term holders. Nothing less than a coordinated, adequately budgeted marketing program, Goldston suggested, will enable a CEO to meet his responsibility to shareowners and company management.

Despite the turmoil in the financial community since the early 1970s, many top managements and their professional advisers are still divided about the advisability of corporate share marketing. They feel safe with standard communications techniques. These techniques are largely a vestige of earlier times, when corporate share marketing would never come up in the boardroom. However, marketing can and has been used to describe a variety of activities, including some proscribed by the SEC. For lawyers and accountants alarmed at any departure from the tried and true, the mere hint that a company may market its shares can switch on a red light or at least a caution blinker.

Many CEOs believe it inappropriate for a company to address current and prospective shareowners in a manner that is other than "educational." Their position is to stay with mandatory disclosure data plus background information and timely interpretive comments. Other

CEOs are all for an aggressive corporate program when the stock enjoys favored status among analysts and portfolio managers, but quickly drop to low profile when the bloom is off the rose.

Corporate share marketing is a great deal broader than stock promotion, though. It is also something less—in that it stays within the rules laid down for publicly held companies.

The differences, as developed by Appleman, are these: Stock promotion, or sales promotion of a registered security, is a regulated function of investment professionals and is appropriate only for individuals and firms meeting requirements established by the SEC, the various state securities bodies, the stock exchanges, and the National Association of Security Dealers. Sales promotion of company shares is definitely not worth exploring. Corporate share marketing may be defined as the principles and procedures employed to identify and cultivate investors, both individual and institutional, whose financial goals and investment time frame are consistent with the company's plans and prospects. In short, corporate share marketing is a disciplined approach to constructing a shareholder consitituency.

Should a Company Promote Its Stock?

"Yes, a company should promote its stock" is the answer of Carol J. Loomis, board of editors, *Fortune* magazine. The reasons are so good, she says, that it almost seems strange that the question needs to be asked. The initial problem, she notes, is the unsavory connotation of the word *promote*. "Promote," according to the dictionary, is "to present a product for consumer acceptance," she points out. She defines the word more specifically by saying that to promote your stock is to present it for consumer acceptance fairly and factually, with the goal of securing a price for it that adequately recognizes its underlying value.

Another problem, she points out, is that stock promotion is too often done for the wrong reasons. She adds,

> Stock promotion should always be done in the interest of the company—in the interest of its shareholders—and at least part of the time the preservation of the existing management is not in the company's interest. Managements which only worry about their stock price because they want to fend off raiders are usually foremost among those who do not deserve preservation.
>
> A third problem is that even those managements who do promote their stocks in the interests of their shareholders sometimes do it with a strong sense of embarrassment. A company's executives, after all, are usually among its larger stockholders, and beyond that they typically hold options. Clearly, these executives are going to be among the chief beneficiaries if their company's stock goes up. It is a fact that makes many managers

somewhat self-conscious—a little defensive about any drum beating they
do for their stocks.[2]

Her advice is to stop being self-conscious, to stop being at all defensive about any honest, straightforward, law-abiding steps you may take
to try to improve the public's opinion of your stock. There are just too
many good reasons why you should be doing exactly that.

Among the good reasons is the fact that a company's stock is its
currency. It is currency that can be used in a merger—to buy another
company or a part of another company. And it is currency that can be
used on those occasions when a company makes a public offering of its
stock to buy "cash."

Communicating Performance

A good stock price resulting from corporate performance and communications is beneficial in the sense that such a price is likely to
favorably influence the attitudes of the company's publics. When a
company is well regarded, customers think better of its products;
suppliers are more eager to do business; executives and other employees are easier to hire and keep; and shareholders are more contented.
Also, the higher the degree of acceptance of equity and debt securities,
the easier it is to raise additional funds, make acquisitions, and reward
executives for performance.

Corporations take every conceivable position in calling attention to
their securities. Their activities range from the issuance of the barest
quarterly financial statements to the establishment of elaborate communications departments that are called the keepers of the P/E ratio.
There may be nothing wrong with this. In fact, a great deal of good can
come from a company's active involvement in the dissemination of
information to current and potential shareholders. The prime responsibility for disclosure, after all, is the corporation's. If the corporation
can get the investment community to listen, then it has done itself and
its investors a service. If it can get a potential investor to be interested
and to look at the available factual and analytic information, then it has
also performed a service.

Communications Begins with Disclosure

The pressure is for more disclosure, not less. The SEC has encouraged projections and has encouraged corporations to provide factual

---

[2] Carol J. Loomis, "Should a Company Promote Its Own Stock?" 1973 *Fortune*
Corporate Communications Seminar, pp. 50–51. Copyright © 1973, Time Inc. All rights
reserved.

154

information even during a registration period. It has also encouraged corporations to include more information in the annual report and to present it in a way that can easily be interpreted by the investing public. The regulating agencies are encouraging the corporations to do more, not less, so that individual investors feel that they are in the mainstream of information.

Although the SEC is now working on guidelines to help in the particularly sensitive area of projections, specific answers may not come to all the questions. As a result, chief executives naturally raise the yellow flag of caution on projections.

This really puts a burden on the corporation. The danger is that rather than take any chances, it will cut off the flow of information. If this occurs, there will be an erosion of investor confidence. Corporate disclosure linked with interpretation by investment company research forms the basis for Wall Street customer service. To cut off the corporate information flow would do extensive damage to the system.

However, James W. Davant, chairman of the board of Paine Webber, warns that if business has not deliberately deceived the public, some of its attitudes and practices have had a deceptive effect. He notes,

> In the 60s, we somehow got the cart before the horse. We began to view the purpose of financial public relations as promoting the price of stock. The effectiveness of financial public relations was measured by its success in the games business played with multiples.
>
> The purpose of financial public relations is not to promote stock prices. It is to present the capacities, performance, and prospects of a company clearly, fairly, fully, accurately, and promptly. The work of a company's financial public relations department should no more be measured by the company's multiple than should the activities of the accounting department.
>
> The obsession with multiples was a special aspect of the American corporation's recent regrettable obsession with "image." "Corporate image," a phrase which worked its way into the business vocabulary in the 50s, subtly shifted corporate consciousness toward appearance. It is perfectly obvious that a company should pay some attention to what it looks like. But most of the emphasis must be on the accuracy of that image. Public relations cannot be perceived as an activity—disconnected from reality—which seeks to alter public attitudes by altering appearances.
>
> Image consciousness invites an empty and superficial pretentiousness in corporate communication. And the American people are fed up with pretense—in their political leaders, in most of their institutions, and emphatically in the communications of American companies. Business needs now to begin the painstaking process of winning back the confidence and goodwill of the public. The question is how to go about it.[3]

---

[3] James W. Davant, "Financial Communications," 1975 *Fortune* Corporate Communications Seminar, pp. 47–52, Copyright © 1975, Time Inc. All rights reserved.

There is, of course, no single answer. People form their attitudes about business in many ways, and the corporate response to a crisis in confidence will have to be a broad response. It will involve the way products and services are advertised. It will involve how a corporation performs. It will involve how a company explains and interprets its behavior. It will involve response to community issues. It will involve dealing with employees.

But one aspect of the corporate response—and one which will depend heavily on the effectiveness of financial public relations—is rebuilding the public's direct, individual, independent participation in our capital markets.

One stumbling block, according to Richard E. Cheney, executive vice president of Hill and Knowlton, Inc., is the SEC. It is too much of a negative force in the communications process:

> I think the SEC really should do more to encourage companies to take their story to the investor. Too often, whether it intends to be or not, the SEC is thought of as an inhibiting force. We still find some law firms fearful of SEC reaction to an effort to get companies better known in the investment community. Just how farfetched their caution can become was illustrated recently by one client who was told by his lawyer he couldn't hold meetings with security analysts because he had convertible stock outstanding. Because the price of the underlying common stock was such that conversion looked imminent, the lawyer said our client was in the midst of a security offering, during which talking to security analysts would be a so-called selling effort and hence would violate the securities acts.
>
> Why is this silly? Because communications are constructive if they're responsible, whether a company is about to sell securities or not. In my view, the commission can't emphasize too often—and it's tried to do this in the past—the importance of a company maintaining its communication effort during a registration period. In fact, with the 10-K today, it might be said to be in registration all the time. There's another point which can't be made too often. The commission should make sure that in its zeal for full disclosure, it doesn't cause companies to swamp investors with so much information that they turn away in disgust to real estate or the racetrack.[4]

Management is in the best position to relate, in understandable, readable presentations, what financial data mean in terms of operation, financial condition, and prospects. However, some CEOs fear a loss of credibility if a high profile from communications is followed by disappointing results. While the investment community hates surprises, credibility is not maintained by having a low profile and avoiding surprises. Management's willingness to talk in both good times and bad is cited by financial analysts as an important factor in motivating

---

[4] Richard E. Cheney, "A View of the Securities Market," 1976 *Fortune* Corporate Communications Seminar, pp. 92–97. Copyright © 1976, Time Inc. All rights reserved.

them to follow a company. Understatement is no more effective than overstatement in preserving a company's credibility; and neither passiveness nor aggressiveness offers any kind of insurance.

Statements—the Heart of Disclosure?

Financial statements and related financial information are the heart of disclosure as far as many companies are concerned. The problem is that the development of financial statements having meaning for investors, including financial analysts, has been difficult and, occasionally, tempestuous. A simplistic approach to financial reporting, as advanced by corporate outsiders and by some suspicious and impatient members of Congress, seems to assume that the whole difficulty arises from corporate management's penchant for self-serving deception, the mercenary character of the public accounting profession, and the indecision of the SEC. The problems are far more complex. It would be a better world if all CEOs were guided by a passion to tell their publics the whole truth, if all auditors were entirely free of any selfish instincts, and if the SEC were always fearless in the pursuit of right and good. These changes, however, would not solve many of the problems in this area. The question is whether or not there is meaningful communication.

The accounting profession has never found it easy to achieve a consensus on accounting principles. For years, the Accounting Principles Board of the American Institute of Certified Public Accountants had a hard time getting agreement on anything at all argumentative. The development of accounting principles is now vested in the Financial Accounting Standards Board (FASB), which consists of persons from the profession and from industry who have given up their former careers to serve full time. The best hope for improved financial communication, at least to the extent that it is based on formal financial reporting, lies with the FASB.

Disclosure Is Not Full Communication

Disclosure, however, is not the same as communication. A persistent criticism of the entire disclosure apparatus under the federal securities laws is that it does not actually result in the communication of much useful information to anyone who can understand it. Few investors read prospectuses or 10-Ks. You could count on two hands all of the yearly requests for 10-Ks that I get. Even then, I am not sure whether the reader understands them or whether he asks for them only because they are free. So, does this mean that the whole business is an expensive fantasy for the benefit mainly of auditors, lawyers, financial printers, and the egos of legislators?

The fact that the SEC-required disclosure documents are not read-able by the average person of reasonable intelligence has been de-plored by the SEC itself. SEC chairmen are fond of lecturing on the excessive use of legalisms, so impenetrable by most everyone but law-yers. Disclosure documents filed with the SEC are called liability documents—if you make a mistake, you can be sued. Management must regard itself as accountable to its shareholders with full and truthful reporting of its stewardship on a regular basis in order to maintain its credibility. If this is not done, then the only institution to fill the void must be the government.

Is Your Message Effective?

Corporate communications have come a long way since that time when there were no financial public relations executives on corporate staffs. Annual reports were not as explicit in detail and presentation then as they are today. Meetings for financial analysts were held in dimly lit restaurants offering tacky food. This environment drew few people.

After the expenditure of much effort and money on corporate and financial communications by both industry and the investment com-munity, there are still stocks selling at five, six, and seven times earn-ings. American industry is far more valuable than multiples in recent years would indicate. Does that mean communications have failed? Not necessarily. First, most of the low P/Es are owned by low-profile companies. Second, some companies have tried to communicate with-out performance. Finally, there is value in what corporate officials are seeking to accomplish. Therefore, judging from the dismal P/E statis-tics, it would appear that the communicator has not totally answered the needs of the investor.

Part of the problem, in looking at the advertising part of communica-tions at least, is the problem of deception, according to Lewis A. En-groran, chairman of the Federal Trade Commission (FTC). He says that the individual exaggerations of the advertising industry are not major deceptions, but in the aggregate they lay waste the nation's precious and fragile reserve of public trust. In the end, people are not persuaded that a bowl of breakfast cereal will enable them to pole-vault 15 feet. Nor are they persuaded that by pushing against the doorjamb for three minutes a day, they can look like Charles Atlas.

What they are persuaded of is that they should take what they are told with a grain of salt . . . and then two grains . . . and then three grains . . . until the end result is total suspension of belief. When that happens, all institutions are damaged, Engroran observes. Skepticism is a healthy check on institutions. Reflexive incredulity is not. It is paralytic. We have not yet reached that state, but we are too far down the road not to view with concern the possibility that we will be paralyzed.

So, what should be your message to the investment community? I feel that your message should be whatever resources you have to turn on the investor, the institution, and the brokerage firm analyst. In the silly 60s, the key corporate buzzwords were *growth, synergism, flexibility, opportunistic, young*, and *aggressive*. In today's toned-down environment, the key words are *strong, dominant, conservative, solid, stable, quality*, and *growth*. It is necessary to be sensitive to the investment climate and to create the right image for your company by describing it in terms that are attractive to the investment community at any given time.

Another message which management should get across is that it is maintaining business candor. In this age of skepticism, with financial analysts carefully studying every corporate release, the firm that tells it like it is, brings out the problems, and articulates what management is doing about those problems is going to gain credibility. The company that buries its problems in footnotes at the back of the annual report and talks only about its successes in the past year is going to lose credibility.

I remember one September when my CEO was appearing before the New York Society of Security Analysts. One of our divisions had been expected to have a super fourth quarter, but early warning indications were that it would barely break even. The CEO told that to the audience immediately instead of waiting until fourth-quarter results were announced in January. There wasn't a ripple in the stock, and the CEO got excellent marks for credibility.

The corporation should also clearly discuss its business philosophy, its strengths, where it sees itself going short term, and its overall long-term objectives. In my view, it is very important to leave the financial community with a relatively simple conceptual picture of your company. There are many companies, from Polaroid to Xerox, that, besides being very fine companies, have also projected a clear conceptual framework to the investment community.

The corporate message should emphasize the relevant businesses and opportunities rather than the irrelevant. A discussion of some obscure business that will never have a meaningful impact on the company will turn off the analyst and the investor.

Finally, in communicating with the investing public, management should emphasize the key growth characteristics of the company. We do this by listing five-year tables in our annual report to show how our segments of business has grown relative to the industry in which each does business.

Building a corporate image communications program is difficult, but few things are tougher than changing a corporation's negative image with investors. It can be done, and to prove this, *Institutional Investor* magazine focused on six companies that did it.[5] The publication called them the "Six Secrets for Turning Around an Investor Relations Program." The six proven masters of the art were Westinghouse Electric, Armco, Chase Manhattan, Levi-Strauss, Times-Mirror, and Coca-Cola.

The secrets were:

1. Join a company where the treatment of shareholders has been so bad that any improvement seems to be sent from heaven. In 1974, Coca-Cola, after having done just about everything you could think of to aggravate its investor constituency, announced that its financial statements would henceforth be released only through the news services—financial analysts, money managers, and others need not apply. But in 1975, Coke realized that existing shareholders and their professional surrogates needed attention too. The skimpy annual report has been beefed up, and calls from financial analysts are now taken or returned immediately.

2. Concentrate on those who call most often: the financial analysts. At Armco, investor relations prior to 1978 were carried out on an ad hoc basis by the public relations department and were slanted to shareholders rather than to professional investors. Now the company is focusing principally on professional investors—in recognition of the fact that they have different and more specific needs than those of the general investor.

3. If you're going to concentrate on financially trained professionals, put a finance person in charge of investor relations. Westinghouse said there was a recognition that a financial background is an aid to someone who is given that kind of a job because it may be easier to make a communications person out of a finance person than vice versa.

4. Work for a company where top management for one reason or another shows a sudden renewed interest in investor relations. This can happen for reasons ranging from something as simple as the retirement of a longtime investor relations officer to a change in top management itself. In 1974, Times-Mirror got a new president who was a more communicative person than his predecessor. His feeling was that if the investment community wanted certain kinds of information and providing it didn't pose a business problem, then provide it.

5. Force top management to put its time where its mouth is. That means exposure to investors, and a common tactic for an investor relations turnaround artist is to arrange dialogue between top management and the analysts who cover the company. Westinghouse continually sets up lunches and dinners at which the company's senior managers meet with analysts in major financial centers.

---

[5] "Six Secrets for Turning Around an Investor Relations Program," *Institutional Investor*, May 1980, pp. 191–94. Copyright © 1980, Institutional Investor, Inc.

160

6. It is much easier to persuade management to open up when there is something nice to say. At Armco, the reformed investor relations effort was born when the company finally had some good news: that it had begun to diversify and thus might, to some extent, escape from the malaise affecting the rest of the steel industry. The timing of the invigorated Levi-Strauss investor relations program had a similar origin. Some operating problems in Europe had produced the only quarterly loss that Levi-Strauss had ever sustained. The company spent a lot of time explaining that one—it didn't dodge the issue—but after that there was a feeling that Levi-Strauss needed a few years of improved performance before going out again to tell its story.

These Institutional Investor vignettes emphasized the success of the individuals in charge of communications, but the companies did learn lessons. Among them are: communicate bad news as well as good; never return to a low profile; and be more anxious to talk when there are problems on the horizon than when there are not, particularly when there are unresolved problems.

The central question for the investor relations field: How much were these companies really helped by their investor relations efforts? The stock of some of the companies has doubled in the last few years, but most companies would deny that there is a correlation.

Targeting Your Audiences

In devising the communications plan, it becomes apparent that you must rifle in on targeted audiences to achieve the most message-efficient and cost-effective program. Audience ranking is the most exciting part of the whole strategy development. Audience ranking simply amounts to breaking down, in a detailed fashion, your key audiences, evaluating them, and establishing priorities among them in the order of their importance to your company.

In working on communications strategy, you will often start with perhaps four major communications categories: financial, employee, government and social do-gooder, and customer-supplier. In each of these categories, break down the list into as many as 20 or more specific audiences. For example, under the financial audience, you have, among others:

Individual shareholders—large and small	Bondholders
Potential shareholders—large and small	Directors
	The financial press
Employee shareholders	Advisory services
Retired employee shareholders	Bank loan officers
Bond rating agencies	Acquisition candidates

European investors   Investment counselors
Registered representatives   Holders of other financial
Financial analysts   instruments, such as equipment
Portfolio managers   trust certificates

To go a little deeper, you can buy from mailing houses a list of portfolio managers, broken down into several categories of institutions by several different categories of portfolio size, from $5 billion down to $50 million. You can do much of the spadework in-house. The communications department can work closely with the chief financial officer and the CEO, for example, to develop lists based on telephone calls from the financial community in which interest has been expressed in your company. Also, have the professionals who attend your meetings fill out registration cards, and work with the Financial Analysts Federation to determine which analysts follow your industry.

Once you determine who the really important people are, you can afford to spend quite ample time to focus on them. Start honing in on your important audiences, first, of course. Among the estimated 15,000 analysts, for example, 35 to 40 may be important to you, with 5 or 6 of them following you very closely. Similarly, among the more than 60,000 registered representatives, 2 to 4 percent may be of value. In the extremely broad field of individual investors—30 million plus— 700,000 may be constituents for your company.

You can go for the tops in the field with the aid of *Institutional Investor*, which surveys the financial institutions annually to identify the best analysts in each industry area. It dubbed these experts the All-American Analysts Team. The team has great significance for the corporation that is trying to communicate with the insitutional marketplace. *Institutional Investor* identifies in each industry three or four major analysts who are, in its judgment, the best and who have the most impact on their respective institutional clients.

The All-American Analysts list is a handy tool for any corporation that wants to gain exposure in the institutional marketplace. If the corporation can get its story across to two or three analysts on this list, the chances are that roughly 80 percent of the institutional marketplace will be reached and that the company story will be well presented to that large marketplace. The team differs annually, so contact the magazine for the most current list.

For this varied audience, you can develop separate kinds of corporate literature:

For the shareholder, you have the annual report, the quarterly report, dividend announcements, and dividend reinvestment information.

For the registered representative, you can produce what is called a rep book. This tends to be a small booklet designed (1) to grab the attention of the registered representative and (2) to give him a short sales pitch which he can then repeat on the telephone to his customers. Remember, the registered representative is in a telephone business where the sales message may last less than 30 seconds. The Trans Union rep book was an 8-page condensation of our 64-page annual report.

For the portfolio manager, the most popular approach is to provide summary information that tells the corporate story in a very concise way. Thus, you have a book that is the same as or similar to the one you have for the rep.

Research, of course, must be part of the strategic communications plan. It makes no sense to build a large program and charge forward without having a benchmark survey that will enable you to know from whence you came and how far you have traveled toward your objectives.

Even more important, once you zero in on key audiences, you use research to get inside their collective heads, to find out what they are all about. With this, your communications will be responsive to their real needs.

That's really what strategic communications is all about. Determine your key audiences. Then talk to them so that (1) they hear you and (2) they respond in ways that support corporate objectives.

The Forgotten Financial Audience

Numerous economic, government, and industry surveys focus on the ever-growing shortage of the investment capital needed to fuel the continued growth of our economy. Behind that shortage is the most overlooked audience in the financial community—your friendly banker. "There is a capital shortage in the aggregate, but never for companies that communicate to bank sources," says the treasurer for a large Chicago corporation.

He points out that while loan agreements have disclosure requirements somewhat akin to those of the SEC and the stock exchanges, some companies, including his own, have taken a more aggressive approach to communicating with bankers.

This treasurer controls 700 accounts with 160 banks. Among them are 60 line banks, including 14 of the top 20 banks in the United States and Canada. His company will have $300 million in line credit and $200 million in commercial paper at any given time, and it finances $200 million in long-term debt annually.

When the capital shortage first loomed in the mid-1970s, the company was concerned about having sufficient credit available at reasonable rates. I was called upon to plan and execute a communications program. After evaluating the company's needs and surveying and determining the needs of the audience, I established a mailing list so that bankers would receive important information on the company in addition to 10-Ks, the annual report, and quarterly statements. This information included major press releases, speeches of executives, and new product releases. I developed an annual report for a major finance lease subsidiary that was a large user of cash and relied heavily on banks for financing. Speeches on major company innovations, such as a sophisticated, computer-based cash management system, were directed to bankers, with reprints being distributed to all financial mailing lists.

An annual bankers' conference was also instituted, just like those that many companies sponsor for financial analysts. The top conference drew 110 representatives from 75 banks, including 9 of the top 10 line banks. Each year, the company presents information on how its cash was used during the prior fiscal year and how it is currently being used. The company's perception of its cash needs for the forthcoming two years is provided as well.

Each year, the bankers are polled in advance to determine their desires for program content. As a result, one conference featured presentations by top management, another featured line management, and a third focused on management in the leasing subsidiaries. The complete proceedings of each conference are printed for distribution to the entire banker mailing list and are available to new bank representatives on the account.

"The results have been amazing," says the treasurer. The first major achievement of the communications program was to assure the company of more than sufficient lines of credit to conduct its business. The company was then able to secure funds at rates it believed appropriate. And we even saved a considerable amount of money just on things like having banks move up their month-end closes to match our information systems.

Bank relations are particularly critical for the smaller companies, particularly those whose revenues range from $2.5 million to $100 million. As a group, these firms have major problems where financing is concerned. They are not well known, and they lack Wall Street sponsorship. Because most of them are not actively followed by financial institutions, their securities are undervalued and they have to seek financing in a negative environment.

The most important aspect of such a company's work with bankers is to develop a financial outline that can be left with the investment banker following the initial discussion with a bank. The public relations professional must guide and shape the company's understanding of which banker is most appropriate for the company's requirements. It is obviously easier for an over-the-counter company to deal with a small bank than with a large one.

Another important feature of the small company's financing efforts is to follow up the initial discussion with consistent financial public relations programs that will make investment bankers aware of how the company is operating and how it is progressing. Keep them informed!

CHAPTER EIGHT

Moving the Message

The next breakthrough in corporate communication will be a company with the guts to dramatize its limitations. That communication will indeed have integrity.
ALEXANDER S. KROLL, President, Young & Rubicam, U.S.A.

NOW IS THE TIME TO COMMUNICATE

Kroll's comment was made with tongue in cheek, but there is powerful meaning behind it. Obviously, the communications needs of a company will never be in perfect alignment with the information needs of the professional. But how close, or how far apart, are these two needs?

For the company, the problem in communicating with the financial community is immensely more complex than it was in the halcyon days before Mayday 1975, when fixed commission rates for block transactions were abolished, and before the back-office methods of the early 1970s shoved many competent brokerage firms into marriages with larger or better-run broker-dealer organizations.

It is with good reason that chief executive officers and chief financial officers find that the securities marketplace may undervalue their common stock. There just are not that many people out there paying that much attention to the *average* company with less than $250 million net revenue and with much less than 3 million shares outstanding. This is not to imply that any amount of time and money spent on communicating to the financial community is going to move your stock upward. But it may help.

There are compelling reasons for relating to the financial community. One is the ongoing spate of tender offers, from which not even the largest corporation is immune. (Tender offers are discussed in Chapter 13.) If your stock is flirting near book value and your bottom-line performance is anywhere from excellent to turnaround, it is time to get out there and tell your story.

You know the motivations and needs of the investment professional

165

and the individual shareholder. This chapter will scrutinize how investor relations programs are perceived internally and externally and the communication needs of your audiences and will provide advice on meeting those communication needs.

How Good Is Investor Relations?

To find out how close need and performance are in communications, Robert E. Kennedy, professor of finance, University of Arkansas, Fayetteville, and Mollie H. Wilson, a university graduate and a vice president of Merchants National Bank, Fort Smith, Arkansas, sought out:

1. The goals of corporate investor relations programs.
2. The extent to which those goals are perceived to have been accomplished.
3. The degree of activity of investor relations programs.
4. The effects of those programs on stock price performance.
5. The perceived quality of corporate information.[1]

Questionnaires were sent to investor relations specialists who were members of the National Investor Relations Institute (NIRI) and to sell-side financial analysts who were chartered financial analysts (CFAs).

In setting goals, investor relations specialists focus primarily on providing useful corporate information to investors—in general, the function prescribed by custom, law, and regulation (see Table 8–1). However, they also give high priority to the price performance of their companies' securities, using such expressions as "fair valuation," "fair stock price," and "maximum stock price." Maximizing share price is typically considered an economic objective of the company. Many theorists, however, believe that capital markets are too efficient for prices to be influenced by corporate investor relations programs. In this context, the goal of maximizing share price could be considered grossly misplaced.

CFAs uniformly agree with investor relations specialists on the need for timely, reliable, and useful corporate information. But they don't feel that stock price performance should be a major goal of corporate investor relations programs, even though they view investor relations programs as having a favorable impact on stock price performance. This seemingly contradictory response is not unreasonable when one considers that financial analysts do indeed rely on the information supplied by investor relations programs.

---

[1] Robert E. Kennedy and Mollie H. Wilson, "Are Investor Relations Programs Giving Analysts What They Need?" *Financial Analysts Journal*, March–April 1980, pp. 63–69. Copyright © 1980, Financial Analysts Federation.

Table 8-1
Goals

NIRI: List the principal goals or objectives of your company's investor relations program.

Percent

1. Provide solid understanding of company—fair valuation 57
2. Maintain "fair" stock price 40
3. Increase investment community interest 31
4. Keep investment community informed 29
5. Broaden (diversify) shareholder base 26
6. Increase price-earnings ratio, maximize stock price 16
7. Meet needs of, and provide information to, shareholders 14
8. Improve, maintain liquidity (trading volume) 11

CFA: What do you believe should be the principal goals and objectives of the investor relations programs of those companies you follow on a regular basis?

Percent

1. Disseminate information ("timely," "reliable") 81
2. Make business understandable; provide insight and interpretation, explain corporate philosophy 26
3. Encourage an honest, unbiased, and balanced (both positive and negative) view of company 18
4. Open up "access" to management, insight into management philosophy 14
5. Inform shareholders specifically 8
6. Forewarn financial community of significant new developments, fundamental changes in business 7
7. Provide reliable contact for inquiries 7
8. Cultivate high (also stable) stock prices 5

Source: Robert E. Kennedy and Millie H. Wilson, "Are Investor Relations Programs Giving Analysts What They Need?" *Financial Analysts Journal*, March–April 1980, p. 64. Copyright © 1980 Financial Analysts Federation.

There is a deep-seated conflict between the practicing CFA and the academic investment theorist on the question of price setting. The academic theorist's efficient markets hypothesis states that stock prices, at any given time, are good estimates of fundamental values (i.e., "in equilibrium"), whereas the empirical results obtained by Kennedy and Wilson in another study show that 60 percent of CFAs "disagree" with this statement, 30 percent "agree" with it, and 10 percent are "neutral." Although most CFAs disagree with the academicians on this point, they also do not believe that corporate investor relations programs should concern themselves with security price setting.

Both NIRI members and CFAs are generally satisfied that appropriate goals are being accomplished despite fundamental differences in how these two groups perceive the goals. NIRI members rated their achievement at 74 percent—only slightly higher than the CFAs' 68 percent. Corporation specialists feel that investor relations specialists have done a good job in accomplishing their goals. Analysts generally believe that their information needs are being met.

It is not surprising that investor relations specialists rate themselves highly, because each specialist is rating his own program or his own performance. The resulting bias toward self-serving exoneration is one reason why the CFA responses are important to the assessment of corporate investor relations programs: They act as a check on the goals, accomplishments, and quality of these programs. There was broad agreement by both NIRI members and CFAs on the level of activity of investor relations programs. About 76 percent of both groups rated the programs as active in terms of seeking investor recognition.

The greatest variance between the two groups involved their views on stock price performance. Of the NIRI members, 46 percent rated stock price performance as having "great importance" as a corporate objective, while only 26 percent of the CFAs viewed it as that important. Stock price performance was considered as having only "average importance" by 53 percent of the NIRI responses and 56 percent of the CFA responses, and only one in six CFAs saw it as having "no importance." It is clear, Kennedy and Wilson concluded, that stock price performance has much higher priority with investor relations specialists than with CFAs.

Kennedy and Wilson also determined that 81 percent of the NIRI members saw company programs as having a favorable impact on the corporations' stock prices, compared with only 60 percent of the CFAs. CFAs apparently see investor relations activities as being separate from stock price performance, whereas NIRI members see the two as inextricably mixed. While 74 percent of the investor relations specialists asserted that they did a good job in achieving their investor relations objectives, they felt that they had failed to achieve the corporate objective of bringing their stocks to "full valuation."

Kennedy and Wilson zeroed in on the perceived quality of corporate information by examining how each group perceived the other group's performance of its professional duties. If financial analysts are widely perceived by investor relations specialists as doing an unsatisfactory job of evaluating corporate risks and values, then corporations may choose to ignore analysts in favor of other information conduits in the capital market, such as stockbrokers and portfolio managers. This would be unfortunate, since analysts constitute the principal information processing network in the capital market. Similarly, if analysts perceive investor relations specialists as doing an unsatisfactory job of supplying the kinds of corporate information that facilitate analysis, then analysts may tend more and more to rely on other sources of information—scarcely a happy prospect for investor relations.

Table 8–2 shows that the investor relations specialists and security who were surveyed gave each other relatively high ratings: 79 percent

Table 8–2
Nature of Business

NIRI: How well do the security analysts who follow your company on a regular basis understand the nature of your business?

CFA: How well do the companies you follow on a regular basis supply you information that allows you to understand the nature of their business?

		(1) Very poorly	(2) Below average	(3) Average	(4) Above average	(5) Very well	Totals
NIRI	Frequency......	1	6	31	89	53	180
	Percent.........	0.56	3.33	17.22	49.44	29.44	
CFA	Frequency......	—	6	31	80	30	147
	Percent.........		4.08	21.09	54.42	20.41	

Source: Robert E. Kennedy and Millie H. Wilson, "Are Investor Relations Programs Giving Analysts What They Need?" Financial Analysts Journal, March–April 1980, p. 67. Copyright © 1980 Financial Analysts Federation.

of the NIRI members said that analysts did a good job of understanding the nature of their business, and 75 percent of the CFAs said that corporate investor relations specialists did a good job of supplying the information necessary for such an understanding. Frankly, this result was somewhat surprising, since corporate executives commonly complain that analysts do not really understand their companies and that this surely accounts in considerable part for the low valuation of their common stock.

Table 8–3 shows that only 51 percent of the investor relations specialists believed analysts did a good job of estimating the earnings of their client corporations and that only 33 percent of the CFAs felt the specialists were doing a good job of supplying the information needed for earnings estimates.

On the issue of stock valuation, the results deteriorated further (see Table 8–4). Only 37 percent of the investor relations specialists felt that analysts did a good job of estimating the value of their corporate stocks; 53 percent felt that analysts did only an "average" job of stock valuation. On the other hand, only 20 percent of the analysts thought corporations did a good job of supplying information that assisted them

170

Table 8–3
Earnings potential

NIRI: How well do the security analysts who follow your company on a regular basis estimate your future earnings?

CFA: How well do the companies you follow on a regular basis supply you information that allows you to estimate their future earnings?

		(1) Very poorly	(2) Below average	(3) Average	(4) Above average	(5) Very well	Totals
NIRI	Frequency......	—	16	72	60	32	180
	Percent.........		8.89	40.00	33.33	17.78	
CFA	Frequency......	7	19	69	44	3	142
	Percent.........	4.93	13.38	48.59	30.99	2.11	

Source: Robert E. Kennedy and Millie H. Wilson, "Are Investor Relations Programs Giving Analysts What They Need?" Financial Analysts Journal, March–April 1980, p. 67. Copyright © 1980 Financial Analysts Federation.

Table 8–4
Stock value

NIRI: How well do the security analysts who follow your company on a regular basis estimate the value of your stock?

CFA: How well do the companies you follow on a regular basis supply you information that allows you to estimate the value of their stocks?

		(1) Very poorly	(2) Below average	(3) Average	(4) Above average	(5) Very well	Totals
NIRI	Frequency	1	16	93	47	18	175
	Percent	0.57	9.14	53.14	26.86	10.29	
CFA	Frequency	15	28	67	25	3	138
	Percent	10.87	20.29	48.55	18.12	2.17	

Source: Robert E. Kennedy and Millie H. Wilson, "Are Investor Relations Programs Givin Analysts What They Need?" Financial Analysts Journal, March–April 1980, p. 67. Copyright © 1980 Financial Analysts Federation.

in the valuation process; 49 percent rated the information they received as "average"; and 31 percent gave corporations negative marks.

It is a curious fact that over half of the investor relations specialists surveyed believed that analysts did a good job in projecting earnings, while the analysts, in turn, did not feel that corporations had supplied them with good enough information to make this estimate accurately.

Clearly, the two groups disagree substantially on the type and quality of corporate disclosure that enable analysts to estimate future corporate earnings and investment values.

THE PROFESSIONALS

It must be recognized that financial markets are structured in such a way that the companies concerned with equity and debt financing have relatively little direct interaction with the ultimate buyers—portfolio managers and individual investors. The decision-making and communications channels include intermediaries positioned between the companies and the buyers. For example, on the institutional side are investment committees, while between the firm and the individual investor is the registered representative. As a result, firms rely principally on the "push" theory of selling by marketing equity or debt offerings to intermediaries positioned along the decision-making/communications channels. Thus, information on these offerings is pushed to the marketplace through intermediaries—the professionals.

One way in which a company can bypass intermediaries is by communicating to the ultimate buyers. This is the "pull" concept of bringing in individual investors through communications to either invest directly or be the contact with the professionals.

Tips for communicating with each of these two broad groups follow.

Many companies believe that professional investors require more communication time not because they deserve "advanced" or "special" treatment but because they carry a large dollar responsibility. The analysis done in a major institution controlling a number of large investment pools may result in the formulation of a number of different units of market impression.

An important factor in an analyst's impression of a company is whether the analyst views its projected earnings performance as realistic. This depends on the analyst's perception of management. The analyst tries to judge company management on some key factors:

1. Executive development and motivation.
2. Long-range planning capability.
3. Profit planning and control techniques.
4. Corporate flexibility.
5. Research and product development capability.
6. Marketing skills.
7. Financial structure.

The following steps are logical in approaching the marketplace to ensure that the professional investor has an adequate understanding of the company's management strategy and basic economics:

1. The company must to have its own internal plan for performance.
2. Management must believe in the plan and understand how it compares with representations being made by competitors.
3. Begin to show a quarterly earnings pattern which is consistent with the plan.
4. Develop and maintain a list of the leading security analysts who may be interested in your company.
5. Assign one person the responsibility of actively initiating contacts with professional analysts, but do not allow this to preclude the analysts' contact with other persons.
6. Introduce the key people in making the plan work to those in the marketplace who play an important role in formulating impressions of the company.
7. Help the analyst develop a perception of the company that will enable him to anticipate and understand major changes in its performance. This is best done individually.
8. Remember that the investor is not buying your company. He is considering an investment alternative. He is analyzing (a) the possible total return on an investment and (b) his confidence factor in that return.

Tips on Talking to Analysts—Myth versus Reality

Organizations hostile to the financial community have been known to drive away potential investors, so it should follow that those companies which boast formal investor relations programs are creating a more receptive environment for their stocks. Right?

In fact, conversations with portfolio managers and analysts at brokerage firms and institutions reveal that merely having an investor relations effort does not guarantee happy investors. Many companies, analysts complain, haven't figured out what their audience wants and cling to a host of myths and misconceptions, such as the following.

1. *Something is better than nothing.* Analysts generally agree that poor investor relations is worse than none. They dislike funneling inquiries through an investor relations manager who is unknowledgeable or uncooperative or who doesn't know how to communicate. Such a manager is only a roadblock between the analysts and the senior executives, so nothing meaningful develops from approaching him. Poor-quality analysis and the cultivation of "back-door" contacts result, if the analyst isn't discouraged from even following the stock. Analysts accuse certain companies of deliberately keeping their investor relations people in the dark, excluding them from meetings where policy is set, and giving them low status within the organization. To the frustration of analysts, the investor relations manager in such com-

panies will not return phone calls because he or she has no solid information.

2. *Top management can do the job.* Usually, a company with this attitude will give the responsibility for analyst contact to the chief financial officer. It believes that in this way it is satisfying the need to furnish someone close to the decision making. The chief financial officer may be aware of current developments in the company but is also involved with so many other activities that he cannot give an immediate response to phone inquiries from analysts. Analysts do not have the luxury of playing the waiting game, so they would prefer to deal with a full-time investor relations manager who will give immediate answers than with a decision maker who will respond eventually. To satisfy investors' desire for easy access, some companies will hire an investor relations manager, only to keep that person uninformed or busy on lengthy trips around the country to tell the company story. Analysts want someone home at all times to answer questions.

3. *For good investor relations, hire an investor relations expert.* Analysts prefer to deal with people who have been in the organization for at least 10 years. But they are receptive to an outsider, if the outsider is familiar with the industry and with the company's finances and operations, and has the skills to put it all in perspective and communicate the information. An analyst suggests that a company which lacks such a person should compensate for a while by inviting analysts to meet with senior corporate and/or operating management.

4. *A good investor relations manager eliminates the need to see corporate management.* The presence of a strong investor relations manager reduces the urgency of seeing top management. Members of the financial community appreciate sources who are "data banks" and are close to the people making major policy decisions at their companies. But no matter how well the investor relations manager grasps and interprets corporate policy, he or she does not set it. Well-informed investor relations people are adequate in discussions of day-to-day operations but not in discussions of the company's philosophy, where the company is heading over the next five years, and what strategy management will use to get it there. Analysts also like to meet middle managers to see how they are interpreting and executing corporate strategy on the operating level.

5. *An investor relations expert can overcome poor performance.* Corporate performance is vital. A silver-tongued orator will never overcome poor performance. If anything goes wrong, top management must meet directly with the analysts, first, to explain the problem, but also, and more important, to explain how the problem will be addressed. Afterward, the role of the investor relations person is to keep analysts updated on progress toward the solution.

6. *Big meetings save time for everyone and still get a company's message across.* Group meetings are helpful, and analysts usually flock to such functions for "defensive" reasons. But many confess that they find it difficult to stay awake at most of these mass sessions and that they usually come away with very little, unless a program has been very well conceived and executed. The problem as analysts see it is that company representatives must often water down their remarks so as to appeal to large and diverse audiences. This difficulty can be overcome by addressing key issues, allowing ample time for questions, and setting aside time for informal sessions between analysts and management. At Trans Union, for example, we allotted one half of the speech time to the question-and-answer period. Thus, on a 30-minute speech, we would set aside 15 minutes for questions and answers.

7. *If you can't con analysts, dazzle them.* Elegant meals, multimedia presentations, and three-day boondoggles are widely used techniques to dazzle analysts. Analysts are almost unanimous in panning organizations preoccupied with form rather than substance. But my experience has been that analysts enjoy form—if there is substance too. Dazzle can be dull. Dazzle and substance can bewitch them.

8. *When in doubt, punt.* Some investor relations people refuse to give out critical data, put a wall around top management, and design bland and basic presentations under the guise of inside information. These people suffer from one of two afflictions: uncertainty about their jobs or fear of disclosure. In the first instance, they don't know how to do the job. In the second, they may be reflecting corporate worry that communicating anything not in a press release might get the company into legal hot water or aid the competition. These objections don't sit well with analysts, many of whom call them "a lot of baloney." The analysts get annoyed when conglomerates persist in calling themselves "one-product-line companies" so that they won't have to furnish an adequate breakdown of details, such as operating earnings by business segment or sales and earnings profits on a quarterly basis.

9. *The more numbers the better.* Many companies do an admirable job in providing data at various types of meetings and in fact books and annual reports. But a few firms practice what one analyst has labeled "obfuscation by detail." They give so much information at meetings that it knocks listeners off their feet and, not so coincidentally, discourages questions. One oil analyst told of taking so many notes during a company presentation that he had nothing more to show for it than a broken arm and a sore hand, and three quarters of what was said could have been printed up. Rule 2 is to make sure that voluminous information is printed and that the analysts are so informed. Rule 1, which I follow, is to send the material to analysts two weeks before the meeting. This allows them to become familiar with the information and to hone in on any questions they may have.

10. *Play games with the analysts.* If putting your best foot forward in annual reports, fact books, and meetings doesn't get analysts interested in your stock, resort to other forms of persuasion. Common techniques include giving bearish analysts the cold shoulder or harping on a part of the business that is faring exceptionally well. Some investor relations people go a step farther to coercion. They do this by bragging to one analyst about the great work that another analyst is doing for the company. Such pressures are an intrusion on analytic freedom, and they rarely work. Still, several companies, most notably electric utilities, are said to be flagrant examples of such practices.

The lesson to be learned from these myths is clear. Analysts are not apt to rave about companies that shield valuable information from them. They don't like companies that lie outright, obfuscate, or twist the facts. The companies that analysts find most frustrating are those which assign a low priority to investor relations and put a slow, inexperienced person in the post. How far companies are willing to go to right these wrongs depends on how much they want to woo investors.

Look Inward First

Once what the investment professional thinks of communications and what he needs are known, the actual communications process can begin. However, in order to communicate externally, the financial communicator must first communicate internally. The financial communicator must start by understanding the historic strengths—both operational and financial—of the company. He or she must know where the corporation is going and how it plans to get there. What will be done to expand operations, enlarge market share, strengthen the balance sheet, bring profits to the bottom line on the income statement, and motivate management in the years to come? Once these factors have been determined, the story line begins to emerge.

It is also necessary to know how the corporation is viewed from the outside. Different views are probably held by investment bankers, commercial bankers, rating agencies, and—of particular importance—financial analysts. Thus, a second element of an effective communications program begins to emerge with the understanding of the perceptions held by the financial community.

Another critical element is the process of identifying the audience to whom the emerging story will be told. It is no surprise that very few of the 11,000 traded companies are all things to all people. The individual investor and the institutional portfolio manager rest easy when their holdings consist of blue-chip stocks.

The point is that some companies are not of institutional grade. Time may be wasted in talking about them to anyone but brokerage firm analysts or stockbroker clubs. For the vast majority of companies

176

in the middle, however, gaining access to portfolio managers still holds appeal.

Tips on Talking to the Portfolio Manager

There are companies that can afford a broad national program, taking senior management to the major financial centers for presentations to large and small groups. Some companies can justify strong regional programs aimed at analysts, portfolio managers in smaller institutions, and shareholders. Some have the staffs to arrange one-on-one visits to large and small institutions through a friendly investment banker, a professional financial public relations firm, or corporate contacts. Some companies can even tailor presentations to specific types of portfolio managers.

There are many different types of portfolio managers who work for different types of institutions and run different types of funds for different types of investors. The standard equity funds and bond funds compete with balanced funds, money market funds, aggressive funds, and defensive funds—and there may even be a fund which holds positions only in those corporations that don't threaten the snail darter.

The portfolio manager has strong defenses against the invasion of his consciousness by communications. The portfolio manager's ability to screen out messages of no interest is a major defense of sanity. The credibility of the information provided and the credibility of the source of that information are critical. Making the presentation effective through the use of suitable individuals and attractive media, such as annual reports and audiovisual materials, is of prime importance. Not to be forgotten is timing. While an analyst will dig for details about a company at almost any time, the portfolio manager, influenced to a *much* greater degree than the analyst by macroeconomics and industry-wide factors, will not listen to a company's story if the timing is wrong.

To review: In order to inform and influence portfolio managers, you must:

Gain the interest of your audience.

Provide credible information in a credible manner.

Prepare attractive materials.

Watch your timing.

Money Managers

What money managers rely on most heavily is a corporation's published reports. Money managers claim that they would never start from an ad or a business story in *The Wall Street Journal* and then go out and buy. What really counts are the corporate reports published under SEC and NYSE scrutiny, they say, though they admit that a story in *The Wall Street Journal* may trigger them.

Good money managers keep corporate reports on hand for many years and keep track of what has been said over the years, checking the consistency of the statements. Money managers also pay a great deal of attention to —and not nearly enough companies issue them—statistical booklets.

There are companies that publish booklets on every conceivable ratio. Putting everything about the company on the table, the good news and the bad news, makes a very good impression on an analyst. Most money managers are smart enough to know that not every company is going to have a good year every year. Money managers know you are going to have bad years, and they want to know whether you are facing up to this, so that they can judge how bad the bad years are going to be.

Money managers are swamped with information, so how do you reach them? Since money managers are human, they can be reached by all of the communication techniques that are used to reach other people. Money managers are not a group apart.

In the corporate world, there are middle managers who are assigned to maintain contact with money managers and who deal out information that is quite sterile, devoid of any real insights and of enthusiasm. There are also other corporate managers who are very enthusiastic when not in the presence of investors. These corporate managers don't give inside information, but they do discuss their company and their industry with enthusiasm and with insights that can be especially helpful. Wise money managers will seek out such people because in this way they often get many insights that the normal Wall Street contact feels constrained to keep to himself.

Do not be afraid to tell the whole story. Money managers would rather have the whole story than have part of it held back. If you mislead them, you will pay the penalty for a long, long time to come.

Reaching the Registered Representative

Many investor relations people, discontented with heavy market institutionalization, are rediscovering the use of the registered representative, or retail securities salesperson, as a bridge between the corporation and the individual investor.

This approach was used in the past, but it fell victim to the "institutionalized" market. As individual purchases fell off and brokerage firms cut back rep staffs, corporations turned to institutional analysts and money managers with their messages.

The pendulum has swung the other way, however. In a Conference

Board survey, out of 251 corporate executives representing a broad range of listed companies:

  31 viewed institutional ownership favorably.
  133 viewed institutional ownership unfavorably.
  78 had mixed or indifferent views.
  9 didn't respond.

Also, smaller and medium-sized companies, unable to attract an institutional following, have come to feel left out—excluded from the market and overlooked by financial analysts.

A top-heavy market made it necessary for second-tier companies to find a more realistic market for their securities and for top-tier companies to seek a broader shareholder base. While institutions are still the primary investor relations target, companies of all sizes want to attract the small investors as they come back into the market. The most direct means of communication with this audience, for some companies, is through the registered representative. Two developments have made it easier to reach registered representatives—the advent of the broker mailing list and the advent of parallel broker societies.

The broker list is unprecedented, since it was once difficult for companies to determine how many representatives were working in the field or who they were—a considerable stumbling block to distributing corporate messages widely or effectively.

Some companies find the registered representative invaluable if he or she is approached properly. Communications must be consistent and must contain information that the broker really wants. For other companies, the list has confirmed the lurking suspicion that broker turnover and movement are high. In light of this, they wonder, are the mailings to brokers worth it?

Communicating directly with the registered representative can pay off in two ways. It can attract individual investors, and it can get research department attention for a company. If enough representatives push a company's stock, financial analysts in the research department will almost certainly follow it. The catch is the danger of running afoul of brokerage firm policy. Some broker managements are upset by corporate mailings to their representatives and are wary of legal hassles resulting from the illegal sale of securities.

Companies can avoid antagonizing broker managements by being sure that their stock has the brokerage firm's sanction before going ahead with a mailing to its registered representatives. Most of the larger firms maintain two lists: *recommended*—securities recommended for sale by the research department; and *approved*—securities not specifically recommended, but salable. Companies should determine, firm by firm, whether their stock is on the recommended or approved list before they send communications to securities salespersons.

Research on broker attitudes could be valuable in probing these areas, but very little has been done. One example of such research is a study conducted by Technimetrics, Inc., a New York financial mailing list company, on broker attitudes toward corporate mailings. The results revealed that registered representatives are interested in receiving corporate financial news but receive very little. Representatives are open to corporate mailings and to attending company meetings. Also, representatives do their own research and a representative's recommendation carries a lot of weight with his or her clients.

Tips on Talking to Stockbrokers

Today's retail stockbrokers claim to be far more sophisticated and professional than their predecessors. By communicating with them, you can anticipate productive results from your time and money. That anticipation, it should be noted, is not based on any conclusive research.

Retail stockbrokers claim a very high incidence of recall about companies. Many of them state that the mere listing of a company on an upcoming meetings announcement is enough to spark interest in that company. The theory is that the company will probably have good news to relate and that the attention it generates through such efforts will have a positive effect on the market price.

Your objective in communicating to the retail market is to get stockbrokers to mention your company to their customers at an opportune time and to be sure that they continue to remember you.

Because registered representatives are securities salespeople, they should be approached differently from financial analysts and portfolio managers. It is difficult for a company to know what brokers need and want from its communications. The best approach is the simplest one. Corporate messages should be concise and should present company highlights right at the start. The representative needs a sales pitch, and company communications must help him develop one. The information presented should be straightforward and should tell the broker within the first two paragraphs why the company's securities are a good investment.

An attractive or high-demand product or service should be stressed, regardless of whether it contributes significantly to company earnings. Such products can be great selling tools for the representative, and they have magnetism for the individual investor. Courting the registered representative is popular, but it may not be for every company.

Nevertheless, brokers should be treated with respect because many brokers are as smart as many of the financial analysts. In dealing with them, it is important for your CEO to understand what is happening in the marketplace and that you have his strong backing. A well-coordinated program will use a variety of tactics since no one method can be relied upon to reach the registered representatives.

The one big difference between financial analysts and brokers is time. While the financial analyst wants to explore every facet of a company's operations, the broker does not have time. You must do the work for the broker—prepare a broker booklet and tell the broker how to sell your stock. Advertising alerts the broker, but the attention must be reinforced by the broker booklet, reprints of articles about the company, broker cards, and meetings. Brokers whom I have encountered seem to like to see as well as hear. Therefore, slide, film, and video presentations go over better than just a speech. Some companies have found that working with the National Association of Investment Clubs is a cost-effective method for reaching both investors and brokers. Brokers also appreciate an 800 telephone line so that they can get a quick update on your company. And, of course, you must tell the broker both the good news and the bad news. If you hide when the market is down, the broker remembers you when the market is up.

The Basic Plan for Professionals

Discipline is the primary need, preceded by a need to recognize some major pitfalls.

The pitfalls are:

1. *Starting without a plan.* This is the biggest problem in investor relations, impacting every activity and every dollar spent. Reasonable objectives should be set before the communication elements of a program are determined. The discipline must start at the top of the corporation, and it must include dedication and direction.

2. *Trying to do too much.* If too many tentacles are put out at once, the company may be leaving itself open to unfavorable comparison with companies whose communications and follow-up are more concentrated.

3. *Prepackaged mass programs.* Investor relations is a very personal kind of business. If you try to do it in a prepackaged or mass kind of way, you're only asking for no impact. It is estimated that some 90 percent of corporate investor relations programs are addressed to the largest institutions which follow every industry, but miss the point that each type of institution and each money manager has a different set of attitudes based on different investment needs and philosophies.

So, the following should be included in the basic communications plan:

1. Establish objectives. Decide what you hope to accomplish.
2. Review time. Determine how much time to devote to various elements, such as current shareholders, institutions versus brokers, and prospecting.
3. Review existing programs to see whether they measure up to current objectives—philosophically and budgetwise.
4. Research the investment community. Start with firms that are currently following your company. How is your company perceived? What do sophisticated investors want to hear about your company and its products?

Learning how you are being perceived is an ongoing process requiring constant feedback from various markets. One often overlooked source in the financial community is the enormous computer capability now in place. Quantitative methods are being used increasingly by brokerage houses.

Separate research departments are being formed to provide buy-side clients with computer screening services in selecting smaller companies. The data bases come from a variety of sources, such as Value Line and Compustat, which track upward of 3,500 companies from their 10-Ks and other published materials. In addition to serving the buy side, Shearson Hayden Stone and other firms are inviting investor relations people to come in and learn how their companies stack up against the competition and are actually helping to prepare numbers and ratios needed by the buy side.

Most institutions and money managers use sell-side screens for input on smaller companies. Those with their own terminals usually plug into a service bureau and don't need tailor-made programs. But some buy-side firms are starting to tailor-make their own programs and are offering them to investor relations practitioners—the very people who are trying to reach them. Firms offering quantitative research capabilities include Kidder, Peabody; Donaldson, Lufkin & Henrette; Goldman, Sachs; First Boston; and Merrill Lynch.

You can obtain the results of general surveys showing the attitudes and needs of investment groups, such as retail brokers, from established research organizations, if you feel that you cannot afford your own personalized survey. The major advantage of a personalized survey is that you can use it to sample analysts immediately after a corporate presentation to learn what impact, if any, was made and how follow-up contact work or future presentations might be improved.

Such surveys may also determine:

Whether a money management firm is on the ascendancy or whether it is cleaning house and reducing portfolios. If the latter, you're wasting your time, no matter how large the firm is.

Who is making the investment decisions. At many of the large institutions, the portfolio manager *does not make them*. It is done by members of the investment committee.

Whether your industry is viewed as in a favorable or an unfavorable position by a particular institution. If the latter, stay away from the institution. No amount of talking on your part is going to sway it.

If there is a single conclusion, it is this: Communicating with today's investment decision makers requires a rifle approach. While shotgun methods or sitting back and waiting for targets of opportunity to pop up may still serve on occasion, a passive approach is not likely to compete successfully for favorable attention among a diminishing sell side and a growing, widely scattered buy side with a variety of investment objectives.

Management must be prepared to think selectively about prospective investors; to identify the most likely targets; and to use ammunition of the highest quality and consistency, with emphasis on future-oriented information.

Effective marketing of corporate securities requires discipline. The place to begin is with a thorough analysis of costs and programs. Realistic budgets should be set to carry out goals. At the same time, any tendency to overlook existing constituencies must be curbed. The very core of a successful corporate share marketing effort is sophisticated planning to retain and strengthen the more "loyal" elements of the shareholder base.

WOOING THE INDIVIDUAL

Predicting the future used to be a simple matter for the witch doctor, who tossed dried bones and examined the pattern in which they fell; or for the Delphic oracle, which was consulted on important occasions by the ancient Greeks; or for the gypsy fortune-teller, who professed to see visions in crystal balls.

We know that those foretellers of the future enjoyed a high degree of credibility. It would be interesting to speculate how they would have fared if they had been regulated by some ancient SEC, with detailed prescribed rules. Many companies feel that predicting the future today is a hazardous undertaking similar to Russian roulette. The information that the investor wants most is information the company cannot provide.

If you were to ask the question "Are we adequately communicating with the investor?" You could get widely different responses, depending on who is answering it. The individual investor may say no because he doesn't read everything you send in the mail and because he isn't sure what else he wants. The investment analyst or professional investor may say no even though he does read what you give him. He always thinks there is something else he would like to know. He probably reads financial reports with a suspicion that something important is being hidden behind complicated accounting gimmicks or self-serving language.

So, the basis of the problem in communicating with the investor is the nature of expectation. There is no well-defined criteria as to what constitutes "adequate information" to the investor. Even financial statements are prepared without any defined objectives as to their purpose because they are prompted by legal requirements, not by the desire to communicate. Thus, companies pour out great volumes of data, frequently couched in legalistic terms to comply with SEC dicta, with the hope that the reader can sort out what he or she needs.

The one thing that interests the investor is the future. In more precise terms, he wants to know when and by how much the market price of your stock is going to go up or down. But the future is getting harder and harder to predict, so the investor is in a state of panic. Corporations try to ease that anxiety by shoveling out complicated data which are frequently more confusing than helpful.

The typical investor rightly believes that future stock prices are largely a factor of future earnings. Consequently, he spends a lot of time and effort trying to predict what those future earnings will be. He pores over the record of the past to detect trends and patterns that he can extrapolate into the future. Presumably, historical income statements help him make this extrapolation. They should present as clearly and objectively as possible the economic results of the company's activities in producing and selling its products and services.

Of all the business enterprises in the world that rely on public capital markets, corporations in the United States provide shareholders with the most reliable and informative financial statements in annual reports. Even here, however, the income statements provided to the investor often fail as reliable measures of earning power.

The knowledgeable and persistent investor who is truly interested in what a company's resources and obligations are can piece that information together if he is a good appraiser, a good accountant, and an avid reader of footnotes. But, if a company has a problem communicating through its annual report, how can its communication with the rest of its investor relations program draw investors in the first place? A couple of effective tools are financial publicity and advertising, which can evoke buyer awareness of and interest in a company as an investment opportunity. The problem is to determine the themes or concepts that will trigger awareness and interest. This can be done through research. Two considerations affecting the design of the research are worth noting. First, while such basic themes as financial history, diversification, and management competence are effective in attracting the attention and interest of buyers, it is naive to apply these themes indiscriminately.

Corporate financial communications, like any communications, is a two-way street. Investors will react to corporate messages according to their familiarity with a company, their perceptions (correct or incorrect) of the company, and their financial orientation. Thus, a communications strategy aimed at individual investors which is appropriate to a highly visible, well-known company may not be the most effective strategy for another company. Similarly, the strategy of a multiproduct company may be inappropriate for a single-product company. Further, the reputational strengths and weaknesses of a company as perceived by investors are critical in determining what will evoke their interest as investors. In short, corporate financial publicity, publishing, and advertising aimed at investors must start with an understanding of how a company is currently perceived.

A clear distinction should be made between a corporate theme and its execution. While a particular theme may be effective in achieving desired communications goals, the execution magnifies or attenuates its impact. I have used the following research plan to assess the themes that will best serve my company, not the specific execution embodied in an advertisement or a publicity placement. The research program is not intended to make people experts on communications.

The Research Plan

The research plan has two objectives:

1. To position the awareness and perception of your company by investors.
2. In the context of investors' awareness and perceptions, to determine what corporate messages or themes will evoke interest in your company as an investment opportunity.

The approach, as described below, is a form of communications concept testing. As such, there is less value in exposing large samples to highly structured questionnaires than in submitting smaller samples of investors to an intensive probe on the subject. The research is qualitative rather than quantitative. From it, a company can obtain a sense of the appropriateness of its specific corporate financial communication themes against the background of investors' knowledge and perceptions of the company. You will also investigate the type of information investors desire so that they can judge the company as an investment possibility.

You begin with focus groups; four of them are needed. Two groups consist of individual investors with minimum securities portfolios of

$40,000, and two consist of portfolio managers. Each group consists of 10–12 people who are invited to attend the session and are paid for their cooperation. The sessions should be directed by a trained moderator. The moderator works from a Topic Outline Guide to direct the flow of the discussion. All sessions are tape-recorded to permit detailed content analysis of the discussions.

The scenario of the focus group sessions follows a predesignated plot, such as this:

1. Participants fill out a questionnaire measuring familiarity with your company and perceptions of its reputation. Participants also indicate the type of information that would evoke their interest in the company as an investment.

2. Moderator leads discussion with group based on their answers in 1. The purpose is to explain why the participants selected the information they did in the context of their knowledge of the company.

3. Participants are exposed to a variety of corporate themes either in written statements or as mock-up ads. Mock-ups are recommended over final versions to minimize the effects of format, color, or other elements of the presentation on the participants' responses. Moderator leads discussion dealing with the fit of the theme with the participants' perceptions of the company and with the information the participants desire about the company.

4. Participants fill out a second questionnaire assessing the effectiveness of the theme in matching their information needs vis-à-vis the company as an investment prospect. They discuss their attitude toward the theme and ways in which the theme would be made more appealing to them.

In order to "mask" the interest in a particular company, the scenario is applied to one and possibly two other companies per session.

Familiarity with your company and the other companies will be measured by using a five-point rating scale—"know very well," "know fair amount," "know just a little," "heard of, know almost nothing about," and "never heard of."

Reputation will be measured by choosing from a number of statements which are thought to apply to the companies concerned. Examples of such statements are:

A diversified company.

Makes high-quality products.

Has a very competent management.

A dynamic company.

Other.

Investment information sought will be measured by having the participant rank subjects in importance as advertising themes.

Financial information
Price-earnings ratio
Dividend history

Company strength information
Competence of management
Company size

Futures information
Backlog of orders
Involved in growth industry/products
Other

In order to focus responses, participants will rank the investment information sought according to what they know or do not know about the companies. This approach has several advantages, including the quick generation of reasonably accurate answers. All comments and analysis usually can be completed within a month. In addition, this can be done at low cost, either in-house or by the company's communications counsel.

It is important for a company to understand the investment criteria as viewed by the individual investor because a careful identification of earnings growth has been the key to above-average equity investment performance 90 percent of the time. This will undoubtedly continue to be the case, but the time has come to analyze price as well as the outlook for earnings and to try to identify the factors which may be supporting high price-earnings levels.

The market price of a stock inherently implies that a given rate of earnings growth is worth a certain P/E multiple. Among the points that individual investors often cite in support of a given price-earnings ratio are the following:

1. The quality of a company's name, its reputation among consumers and in its markets, and the franchise or product patents that it holds.
2. The depth of earnings or the degree of confidence that an analyst can have in earnings growth. This also includes the degree of management's control over earnings levels.
3. The maturity of an industry or of individual products. Some companies which were considered growth companies in the 1950s are not considered growth companies today because product growth has waned.
4. Supply and demand for the security itself, which is sometimes determined more by fads than by fundamentals.

The most practical way to get more individuals to own stocks is to establish close relations with those who already do, but most corporations are not moving in this direction, says Georgeson & Co., the nation's largest stockholder proxy solicitation firm and one of the largest practitioners of financial public relations. Georgeson believes that:

"Overdisclosure" in annual reports and other financial communications is alienating small investors—just the opposite of what corporate officers think.

Companies must stop relying on the press to get news to their shareholders and must start mailing bulletins to them directly, expensive as this may be.

"Something dramatic" is required to "recapture the confidence" of shareholders—possibly an "Individual Investor Day" each year, special representation of small investors on boards of directors, or a limitation on the percentage of a corporation's stock which institutions can hold.

Corporations seem reluctant to mobilize shareholders to support business in its battles with government—perhaps because they are afraid that, once organized, the shareowners will "become a new monster to be fed."

Georgeson has expressed these views in a brochure entitled "The Reluctant Marriage," which it published in 1978 in conjunction with Lind Brothers, Inc., designers and printers of financial materials. Surveys that the two companies conducted among individual stockholders and corporate secretaries provided background for some of the opinions in the brochure.

Here are some excerpts:

The "tenuous relationship" between the individual investor and corporate management is "in trouble," and "the reason is simply—they are not communicating."

Most investors want to increase their participation in the market, assuming that the investment climate improves, but they are disheartened and puzzled, and this could presage the doom of shareowner democracy.

Many individual investors feel that:

They are handicapped by lack of access to timely investment information.

Institutional investors are a disruptive influence in the market.

Corporations favor the institutions and give them preferential treatment.

The financial community receives inside information and acts in its own interests before passing the data on to individual investors.

The individual investor and the corporate officer speak two different languages, according to Georgeson.

Corporate officers tend to produce financial communications which reflect their own needs and reading habits, as well as noncommunication criteria such as accountability and potential legal liability.

The result is that individuals, rather than admit ignorance, assume that the corporations are trying to pull a fast one or that the report is intended for institutional investors rather than for them.

Georgeson suggests some ways to establish person-to-person contact with investors:

Hold more regional shareholder meetings to supplement annuals.

Answer all shareholders' inquiries by telephone. Shareholders are usually overwhelmed and extremely pleased when this is done.

Provide a WATS line to permit shareholders to call with questions or hear the latest corporate information. Advertise the service in the annual and interim reports.

Provide space on the proxy form for shareholder questions.

List in the annual report the name, address, and telephone number of the person responsible for investor relations.

Form an advisory committee to the board of directors composed of three to five randomly selected investors with fewer than 1,000 shares, or let one small investor actually serve on the board each year.

Include shareholder relations experts on boards of directors.

But for some chief executives, the very idea of trying to cultivate shareholders is repugnant, if not actually threatening. Many corporate officers—and the attitude increases with length of service—are accustomed to thinking of management as *the company* and of shareowners as a legal euphemism for speculators. It is not uncommon to hear corporate executives say that the investor may construe any attention above mandatory requirements as an invitation to tell management how to run the business. After all, management is already burdened by the government telling it how to run things.

Profitable companies with confidence in the future are in a position to help themselves gain goodwill with the investment community. For thriving corporations, there are shareholders who, if encouraged, wish the company well, buy its products or services, and even express support for a common interest. Unless investors are encouraged to feel that they are in a kind of partnership with management, there can be no shareholder constituency.

CHAPTER NINE

The Annual Report

One thing you can't make twice is a good first impression.
WILL ROGERS

Today, the overwhelming choice of investor-owned companies as a means to make a good first impression is the annual report. This was not always true. History records times when managements were furtive and arrogant toward the owners of the company, namely the shareholders. But the annual report has become the single most visible and important document of the investor-owned company. In this chapter, therefore, I will concentrate on the growth and development of the annual report from the perspective of history, the early influences, and the modern trend setters. This will be followed by a discussion of what the annual report is in the minds of many managements, whether the annual report is worth all of the effort from a readership viewpoint, and how to build extra value into the annual report. Then, a brief look will be taken at the other financial reports issued by corporations and non-profit organizations. Finally, there will be a challenge to overcome problems with annual reports.

Closed lips hurt no one; speaking may.
CATO

THE HISTORY OF ANNUAL REPORTS

In 1973, a manufacturer of business forms printed its annual report cover over in red ink and told its shareholders: "The cover means what you think it means. . . . it was a bum year, and we have too much respect for our stockholders to try to sugarcoat it. Now we're bounding back. But maybe you won't believe that."

The corporate communications executive works hard to fill the an-

189

190

nual report with pertinent facts. And it might bring a smile to the lips
when he or she learns that the emergence of double-entry bookkeeping in medieval Renaissance Venice made it all possible.

The Early Days

Venetian businessmen built their shops as literal forts. This protected these businessmen from pillage and guarded their new bookkeeping entries against theft by a competitor. Centuries later, as stock
markets began to develop, the public began to thirst for corporate
information in the form in which it is available today. Eager people
watched the stock markets emerge from the back alleys and cof-
feehouses of London and New York. But in the 19th century, there
were still very few businessmen who would admit even to their wives
that they were putting together corporate financial statements.

One commentator of that day remarked, perhaps half-humorously,
that "nearly cooked reports and captivating prospectuses were the
main machinery of speculation." Shocked that even the press was
bribed by the gifts of options in shares which were sold at a premium,
the *London Morning Chronicle* published a mea culpa: "We blush to
say few editors in the metropolis are not to be found in the list of those
benefited."

A good deal of information going to shareholders of companies in
that period was produced by the secret counsels of the Rings and
Cliques, an association of railway, steamship, and telegraph directors,
presidents, and heavy shareholders who found it consonant with their
consciences and their purses to water stock and to pay dividends out of
capital, thus inventing that anomalous feature in finance known as
capitalized earnings.

As the 19th century wore on, more annual reports were issued, but
only at irregular intervals and with a minimum of financial information.
Yet, the 1836 report of the Baltimore and Ohio Railroad, issued nearly a
century before the SEC, was embarrassingly honest, admitting "that
the foregoing statement is an approximate estimate of the present situation of the company and may not be strictly accurate, but it certainly
comes within two or three thousand dollars."

Those who manned the rolltop desks of Wall Street may not have
gotten much information, but they probably got a few chuckles from
the statements of the day. The 1866 report of the St. Joseph Lead
Company, for example, contained no balance sheet or capitalization
data. But it did itemize the company's capital equipment and supplies,
including "23 comfortable dwelling houses for miners . . . one frame
ready for a store; one stable with cows, hogs, etc., and wood enough for
one year's supply." The Western Railroad report, directed to the Massachusetts legislature in 1837, remarked that its progress was "not

local in its character; not local in its benefits; but made, like the dews of Heaven, to fertilize every portion of our territory."

At that time, corporate communicators weren't very long on information. In 1866, the treasurer of the Delaware, Lackawanna and Western Railroad Company, responding to an urgent request for information from the NYSE, replied that his company made no reports and published no statements. Also around that time, a congressional committee threw up its hands in frustration, disclosing that "such active stocks as those of Amalgamated Copper and the American Sugar Refining Companies were dealt in on the exchange for many years without the public having any information regarding their affairs."

In 1892, the Pennsylvania Railroad Company issued a 197-page report, complete with index, to its shareholders, a volume that resembled an almanac. In 1903, U.S. Steel published a 60-page annual report filled with facts and statistics and liberally illustrated with photos of smoke-belching steel mills. Bethlehem Steel and General Motors followed with long annual reports, attractive by the standards of the day.

The clamor for better, not more, corporate information intensified because of substantial gaps in reports. Balance sheets were sometimes published in detail. But the reports provided only the barest income statement, showing sales, a few major expense items, and current profits. Often there were no comparisons with previous years and no per share data. One consumer products company rejected shareholder requests to issue an annual report as late as 1932. One insurance company's annual report in the late 30s contained only four pages, consisting simply of a sketchy balance sheet and a list of directors.

Such brevity might have been dictated by the times. By and large, the printing style of those days made most annual reports look like restaurant menus or programs for society benefits. Shareholders, generally disillusioned by the lean stock market of the 30s, weren't as tuned in to reading annual reports. And the news from the corporate suite was hardly uplifting. For instance, the annual report of Royal Typewriter Company noted that "the government prohibited the sale of typewriters to the general public . . . and on October 31, 1942, Royal is scheduled to stop all manufacture of typewriters for the duration of the war."

"V for Victory" was the favored theme in the majority of the annual reports during World War II, with red, white, and blue being the most popular color motif. Few corporations failed to display Army-Navy E pennants in their 1943 reports, and a large number reproduced citations and letters of commendation from military and other government agencies. The most popular illustrations were facsimiles of service flags, and practically every report paid a fitting tribute to employees in the armed forces, many by means of honor rolls listing such employees by name.

After World War II, the door to corporate communications opened wider. As shareholders' interest grew, there was heightened awareness of the importance of the annual report. The use of per share data became more widespread. The need for comparative data was recognized. Longtime periods were included in financial comparisons. The effectiveness of comparative data was increased with the use of percentage increases or decreases for the years covered.

The annual reports began to include details that allowed shareholders to compute important indexes of efficiency, such as the operating ratio, the turnover of total capital, and the turnover of inventories. Corporate executives were alerted to the fact that windfall gains and nonrecurring sources of income should be disclosed and explained adequately. Management became more receptive to suggestions that annual reports include an outlook for the industry and the company.

Companies began to use the modern annual report not only to tell a story to shareholders but also to rap with employees, customers, potential investors, and community leaders. With the expanded audience, the annual report was made more aesthetically pleasing. The use of color photographs increased sharply in the 1960s. Modern design and typography techniques were directed at helping the readers— investors, analysts, suppliers, customers, and employees—understand the financial facts and figures in the shortest possible time.

The mid- to late-1960s found many corporations experimenting in their annual reports and rearranging the conventional location of the annual report features. For instance, financial figures began to be moved toward the front. Annual reports came in odd sizes and shapes so that they would be singled out. The chief executive officer's message to shareholders attempted to indicate more about plans and expectations for the future.

For all of its thinness or thickness, lack of numbers or preponderance of numbers, confusion or clarity, the annual report, for more than a century, was a year-end statement on the financial condition of a business. Change was occurring, but at a pace so slow that a snail would have become impatient.

Then, as business conditions worsened with the dawning of the 1970s, corporations were challenged to explain declining sales and earnings trends in their annual reports. New ways were found to make the reports more readable and more candid, such as the question-and-answer technique utilizing an interview with a top corporate executive.

Suddenly, change was to hit like a bolt of lightning. Booming in the thunderclouds were:

1. Pressures for corporate responsibility which led many organizations to rely on the annual report as a means of gaining public

confidence in management and in the integrity of products and services.

2. A huge governmental lunge in the regulatory arena on social responsibility and rights for workers, investors, and consumerists—a lunge hastened by the push for equality of minorities.

3. The formation in 1972 of the Financial Accounting Standards Board (FASB), the designated organization in the private sector for establishing standards of financial accounting and reporting. For all the positive contributions that the FASB has made to the preparation of financial reports, it has erased one item from them forever—brief footnotes with the financial statements.

4. The SEC's list of commandments, first issued in 1974 and updated and expanded annually since then.

The Early Influentials

The demand for more complete information from U.S. corporations actually began as the 19th century came to a close.

NYSE. In 1899, the NYSE set down a rule that each listed company must publish at least once a year a properly detailed statement of its income and expenditures—and also a balance sheet giving a detailed and accurate statement of the company's condition at the close of its last fiscal year.

The IBA. By the 1920s, the desire for more and better corporate information had risen to a clamor. The Investment Bankers Association (IBA) issued repeated calls for financial disclosure that included an "adequate" and "understandable" balance sheet with at least some comments on such items as inventory, working capital, and depreciation policy as well as earnings presentations and comparisons. The IBA demanded, among other things, more information from holding companies, particularly details about their subsidiaries.

Criticizing corporate indifference to the investing public, the IBA said that some of the best companies objected to furnishing full information that would go beyond the eyes of their investment bankers.

The SEC. After the stock market crash of 1929, the U.S. government made its first entry into the financial accounting and reporting field with the securities exchange acts of 1933 and 1934. Although the SEC had statutory authority to establish accounting and reporting standards, it had a laundry list of items which were optional for several years before they became mandatory for all companies in 1977. The initial standards were minimal, however, such as the requirement that Roman type at least as large as eight point (one ninth of an inch) be used. After companies had used large and more legible typefaces for several years, the SEC changed the rule to require that Roman type at least as large and legible as 10-point Modern be used; that financial statements, but not notes, be in Roman type at least as large and legible as 8-point Modern; and that all type be leaded two points. Furthermore, throughout the SEC's early history, its policy was to rely on the private sector to set standards in fulfillment of their responsibility to serve the public interest.

Financial World. It took another cataclysmic year—1941—to bring the next wave of change. The stock market was plummeting, and NYSE volume was running under a million shares a day. Added to those problems was the national focus on the impending war. In that year, *Financial World*, an investor-oriented magazine, conducted a formal survey of the corporate annual reports available to American investors. The survey of 250 reports was meager by today's standards (*Financial World* now receives more than 11,000 entries in its competition), but it reflected a broad representation of the disclosure to investors at that time.

Of the 250 reports examined, only 25, or 10 percent, could be classified as meeting the "modern" disclosure standards of the time. Moreover, the survey showed that only 45, or 18 percent, of the companies had even attempted to upgrade their standards during the 30s, despite the obvious lessons of the 1929 crash, when investors could not judge companies on the basis of the information that companies provided to them.

There were no really outstanding winners in that competition— merely the disclosure that only 16 of the 25 annual reports were considered to be adequate for shareholders. But that first survey helped lay the foundation for important corporate reform. For one thing, independent and objective scrutiny of annual reports and the nation's corporate disclosure system had begun—something that was in the wind but had been discussed only in theory since the SEC was established. For the first time, corporations had an arena for comparing the quality of their annual statements and an incentive to improve their annual reports through public competition.

In 1942, *Financial World* introduced a competitive system awarding two different citations to the presidents of corporations with annual reports that reflected "certain degrees of excellence" in the magazine's view. One citation was the Highest Merit Award for distinguished achievement in annual reporting as compared with that of a decade earlier. Each company's annual report was judged on the basis of text and illustrations, typography, format, and public relations and was compared directly with the same company's report 10 years earlier.

At the same time, *Financial World* told the corporate community that it would look primarily for continual improvement in annual reports rather than an arbitrary standard of excellence. Thus, the competition took on the spirit of encouragement rather than criticism for mistakes.

The change wrought by competition was evident even in a year's time. Companies embraced the competition, with entries tripling to 766 annual reports in 1942. Of these, 21 percent were classified as meeting modern standards and 37 percent as showing improvement; the number of reports that hadn't changed their standards in over a decade had dropped to 42 percent of the total. In 1943, *Financial World* surveyed 1,000 annual statements and found that 25 percent could be classified as modern. Although only 36 percent were regarded as improved, the proportion that showed change from the 30s had increased to 61 percent.

The competition served to foster the spirit of increased corporate candor even in those early years. *Financial World* reported in 1944 that there was evidence that more and more managements were pursuing the policy of taking the shareholders into their confidence by supplying all essential information, and in a form that could be quickly and easily understood.

In 1944, too, the magazine announced that the competition from then on would be judged by an independent board to ensure objectivity in selecting winners. The five-member board was chaired by Dr. Lewis Haney, professor of economics at New York University School of Finance, who wrote a syndicated business column for the Hearst newspapers and was the author of a number of books on economic history and business forecasting. The other members were C. Norman Stabler, the financial editor of the *New York Herald Tribune* and an influential member of the New York Financial Writers Association; Raymond C. Mayer, a public relations expert and president of the National Association of Public Relations Counsel; Glen Griswold, who had been one of the earlier publishers of *Business Week;* and Norman Bel Geddes, an industrial designer and artist who, among other things, had designed the first streamlined ocean liner. Thus, the board was a group with a keen understanding of financial reporting. The board's philosophy in picking winners played an important role in the evolution of today's annual-reporting standards. It believed that companies should break information down to a per share basis so that the shareholder could see more definitely what the data meant and that pictures of plant additions and important new products should be included.

The first gold trophy award for the best annual report was presented in 1945 to Caterpillar Tractor Company at a banquet that featured Robert A. Taft, U.S. Senator from Ohio, as its principal speaker. The awards banquet has become an annual tradition.

By the early 1950s, standards for writing the annual report had been set that are still valid. One of the best enunciations of these standards appeared in 1949, when *Financial World* listed the requirements needed to qualify for a Merit Award in the contest:

1. *Cover design.* A dramatic photograph or other illustrations appropriate to the corporation or industry represented—one that will attract attention or arouse curiosity to look inside the annual report.

2. *Highlights page.* A panel of essential operating and financial statistics presented in comparison with those of the previous year to show the immediate trend. Many figures can be shown on a per share or per employee basis.

3. *Table of contents.* A listing by page numbers of all editorial and financial material, as well as significant charts, maps, tabulations, and other illustrations. An alphabetical index of editorial and statistical features should be added to annual reports running 24 pages or more.

4. *Management.* Clarification of the duties of each officer of the corporation when not indicated by his title. Identification of each member of the board of directors who is not an executive of the company.

5. *President's letter.* A crisp and readable message, preferably one page in length and no more than two pages, explaining and interpreting data of vital interest to investors, plus an appraisal (not a forecast) of prospects.

6. *The narratives.* The reviews of the progress and developments of the past year, offered in paragraphs suitably subheaded to indicate the contents of each discussion. Here charts, photographs, and other illustrations can be used to emphasize the editorial contents of each page.

7. *Income-outgo chart.* A pie chart or other graph device to show at a glance the relative sources of revenue and how the income dollar is distributed.

8. *Simplified financial statement.* Balance sheets, income accounts, and profit and loss statements provided in comparison with the figures of a year ago and with captions and explanations written for easy understanding. Footnotes should be avoided whenever possible, but if necessary, they can be printed in a typeface large enough to be easily read. The independent auditor's statement should be given adequate display to call attention to its importance.

9. *Background statistical comparisons.* Operating and financial statistics for a period of at least 10 years, and more if available, to indicate the long-term trend and operations prior to World War II and since. Here is where ratios and percentages will assist in interpreting the record. A chart cannot be regarded as a substitute for actual figures—both should be provided.

10. *Stockholder information.* Tabulations, charts, and maps to indicate average size of holdings, geographical distribution, and trend of holding by sexes, groups, etc. It is no longer enough to know how many stockholders there are: data on who and where they are should also be given.

The FASB. Since 1973, the Financial Accounting Standards Board (FASB) has been the organization in the private sector that has been charged with the responsibility for establishing standards of financial accounting and reporting which are, in effect, rules governing the preparation of financial reports. The FASB was conceived by a special study group headed by a former SEC commissioner and was carefully designed to carry out this responsibility.

The FASB's function is important because decisions regarding allocation of capital (investment) are based on financial information, much of which is the product of the financial accounting/reporting process. FASB standards are officially recognized as authoritative by the SEC and the American Institute of Certified Public Accountants.

The seven members of the FASB have diverse backgrounds, but they must possess knowledge of accounting, finance, and business and a concern for the public interest in matters of financial accounting and reporting. They serve full time, are compensated, and are required to sever all previous business or professional connections before joining the board. They are aided by a staff of 40 technical specialists plus administrative and other support personnel. The FASB issues statements of financial accounting standards, statements of concepts, and interpretations. Before it issues a statement, the board is required by its rules to follow extensive "due process" procedures which in many ways are more stringent than the requirements of the Federal Administrative Procedure Act.

Statements of financial accounting standards establish new standards or amend standards previously issued. Statements of concepts do not establish or amend standards they provide a guide to the board in solving problems and enable those who use financial reports to better understand the context in which financial accounting standards are formulated. Interpretations clarify, explain, or elaborate on existing standards. The FASB staff also issues technical bulletins to provide guidance on applying existing standards to certain financial accounting and reporting problems.

Among the significant and long-standing issues of financial accounting and reporting that have been resolved by the FASB are: accounting for research and development costs, self-insured losses, catastrophe losses incurred by property and casualty insurance companies, losses from expropriations of property by foreign governments leases, capitalization of interest cost, and defined benefit pension plans; reporting by development-stage companies; and segment reporting.

The board's conclusions on issues related to profit-making enterprises are based on the conviction that reported earnings should highlight differences in risk, not obscure them, and that similar situations should be accounted for in similar ways. While that conviction has emerged case by case, the board has perceived from its beginning the need to develop a consistent conceptual framework for financial accounting and reporting.

The Modern Trend Setters

True or false?
IBM (International Business Machines) was the father of modern annual reports.

The 1950s. Numerous sources cite IBM as the hallmark of the modern-day annual report as a result of its 1955 report. However, to be viewed in proper perspective, IBM's report must be placed in the context of American business history, the hundreds of thousands of annual reports generated, and the many events and actions which have had an impact on annual reports. The IBM report had no impact on disclosure; on interpretation of rules and regulations; on size, content, or color. It was an important influence, however, on an art form which was to last for the next 15 years.

Randall Poe, a public information officer at the Conference Board, aptly credited the IBM document with inspiring the Renaissance in annual reports, because for more than 40 consecutive years IBM's annual report had been a modest little libretto of some 20 pages, wrapped in a plain brown cover. Suddenly, in 1955, IBM delivered a sparkling, magazine-style model. It had hired Paul Rand, one of the world's leading graphic designers, who introduced lush paper and subtle typography, and brought in some of the country's leading photojournalists to capture IBM's mystery. Annual reports got hip.

Almost instantly, many other companies upgraded their annual reports. The rush was on to find top designers, photographers, chartists, and, as one executive put it, "a writer who had actually finished school." In the best-run companies, this period marked the beginning of the cerebral annual report—good-bye to smiling executives at company picnics and to factories belching smoke.

Through the 1950s, the annual report kept gaining momentum and style. CBS, Litton Industries, RCA, and Xerox, to name only a few, began using strong graphics to make their points. In some cases, fine art was not merely the medium but the message. "Make it pretty" became not a command but a standard. Many firms, of course, continued to produce dull annual reports, some because they lacked imagination, some on purpose. But a new trend was building. General Dynamics hired designer Erik Nitsche, and some of its annual reports quickly looked as if they had been made for the walls of the Museum of Modern Art. The reports included abstract designs of flying machines soaring through space.

The 1960s. While the 50s marked the Renaissance, the 60s brought us Annual Report Impressionism. Companies learned that they could influence public perceptions and forge instant images through their annual reports. "Use color," one designer used to say. "Just a little dab will do it."

The times seemed right. Profits were heady, and conglomerates were the rage. The stock market was humming, and accounting rules were positively lax by today's standards. Annual reports, which always mirror their times, turned beautiful and chick. Some read like business science fiction, and some were designed solely to hype the company's stock. But the game had changed.

The master, the one everybody began to watch, was Robert Miles Runyan. A disciplined rebel who made and lost $2 million in the stock market, Runyan helped Litton Industries quickly gain reputation as a powerhouse corporation. Runyan, together with an adroit communications pro named Crosby Kelly, transformed the annual report into a spectacular sales machine. Their approach: To tell the world that Litton was not simply honest and well managed by bursting with vision and creative energy. "Get aboard," their reports shouted to investors and the media, "and let's go." Which Litton did.

Litton's 1962 annual report seemed to have brought back Plato as consultant. It dealt with no less than the eternal quest for freedom, opening with a provocative shot of the Acropolis on the cover. Inside, photos and text trumpeted the freedom message. It was Litton's way of telling the world that it had ideals and was driving for higher stakes than those around it.

In 1967, Litton produced an annual report that may be *The Last Supper* in business communications (though Runyan was not involved). Designed by James Cross, a top West Coast designer, it meticulously reproduced 30 exquisite stained-glass windows dealing with business subjects. It lured the reader with a stained-glass window on the cover that the reader could peek through. The window, which symbolized business ethics in 15th-century Belgium, showed a man stepping forward to be sure a cask was honestly measured. Another window inside, from 13th-century England, argued the need for profitable investment.

Although the annual reports of the 60s brought drama and zest, they were very shy about company facts. Many were slinky lettuce sandwiches—pleasant, often tasty, but totally without substance. One annual report writer who asked a company to give him some hard figures on new orders was told: "Run a nice picture of them."

Since the early 1970s. Then, in 1974, came the collapse—of the stock market, conglomerates, and profits. This had an instant impact on annual reports. They turned cautious, and some veered back to the unthinkable: black and white. The forces impacting on the annual report since the early 1970s have brought about the Age of Seriousness, with the exceptions noted in the following section. The 1980s may well be known as the Age of Turmoil, as companies have been literally scrambling to comply with ever-mounting rules and regulations. Companies have been competing to do the best job of complying with regulations rather than the best job at obtaining shareholder readership. A few companies have even put covers on their 10-Ks and called them annual reports. But earlier influences are still making themselves felt.

WHAT IS AN ANNUAL REPORT?

Mirror, mirror on the corporate wall, who's the fairest of them all? "You are, you are," *says the modern annual report again and again.*
RICHARD A. LEWIS, President, Corporate Annual Reports, Inc.

From a publishing standpoint, the annual report is the most amateurish job undertaken by corporate management.
Public Relations Director of Large, Diversified Company

Most annual reports have turned into management showcases. With features and photographs, they hammer home whatever message the company's chief executive happens to have in mind.
Fortune

Now the annual report is into yet a new era. Yes, it is the age of the slick bureaucratic report.
WILLIAM DUNK, President, Corpcom Services

Annual reports should be telling, not selling, vehicles.
JAMES MIHO, Miho, Inc.

Its primary purpose is to inform a corporation's stockholders as to what transpired during the past year and the company's financial position at the end of the year.
KOLMAN GLICKSBERG and RICHARD F. KOTZ, formerly with the SEC

A Rose by Any Other Name

Numerous views, though they vary, accurately portray the status of the annual report. Like the rose, the annual report is beautiful to behold when it is in full bloom, but it is covered with thorns too. A highly influential factor is the effect that the general atmosphere of the 1970s and 1980s has on management's most important document. It was relatively simple to produce an annual report in the 1960s despite the prevalent go-go attitude. Regulations were minimal, and objectives were clearly defined.

At that time, the most important reasons for an annual report, apart from fulfilling legal requirements and informing shareholders, the most important reasons for an annual report, were to enhance corporate image and general identification, inform employees, improve the P/E, sell products or services, recruit employees, attract acquisitions, raise capital, serve as a "corporate calling card" overseas, and plan and analyze markets. A company wanted to give the impression that it was growth oriented, progressive, well managed, honest, aggressive, innovative, profit oriented, financially sound, diversified, an industrial leader, technological, modern, dynamic, and future oriented.

It can be detected quite readily that the annual report is no longer merely a report on business. Rather, it is whatever management or the annual reporter wants it to be. Waves of consumerism, activism, protestism, and numerous other isms have swamped some managements. Astute managements have found that they can use the annual report to honestly and accurately explain the corporate responsibility side of their business. Others have grasped at straws in an effort to be trendy or unique.

Impacting the Annual Report

Here are some brief examples of how social and economic changes have affected annual reports:

Esterline Corporation, to point up its successful "battle for productivity," devoted more than six pages of a report to an interview on the topic with a professor of advanced management.

Bowne & Co. devoted 10 pages of an annual report to interviews with former secretary of commerce Juanita M. Kreps and former assistant secretary of the Treasury Murray L. Weidenbaum on the topic of government regulations.

Coca-Cola Bottling Company of New York, and a host of other companies, used their final annual report of the 1970s to discuss strategies for the 1980s.

AT&T believed that it was being so wracked by contention in the regulatory arena and the court of public opinion that it issued a "new" statement of purpose and used its 1977 annual report to announce it.

In the early 1970s, numerous companies, including Eaton Corporation, Bank of America, INA Corporation, General Motors, TRW, and ITT, embraced the multilingual approach and issued their annual reports in various languages, such as German, French, Spanish, and Japanese.

Celanese Corporation devoted eight pages to reporting on its environmental and public responsibility activities, including the role of the Public Responsibility Committee of the Celanese board of directors.

Philip Morris tackled the antismoking issue by categorically stating that "despite the expenditure of hundreds of millions of dollars by government, the tobacco industry, and other research groups over more than 25 years, no conclusive clinical or medical proof of any cause-and-effect relationship between cigarette smoking and disease has yet been discovered."

Kimberly-Clark's 1979 annual report did double duty: (1) it spoke out against new financial guidelines on inflation; and (2) it presented "Fairness Goals" to "reaffirm the moral and ethical character of the company."

The Trendies

On the trendy side, consider the following items. While there are numerous examples, these items portray better than any commentary could the perspective from which some managements view annual reports.

When PERT, a complex system requiring a high degree of engineering knowledge on manufacturing production was introduced in the 1960s, who tried but failed to adapt it to annual report production? The annual report producer.

When the desk top computer was introduced in the early 1970s, who tried but failed to adapt it to annual report planning? The annual report producer.

When the word processor was introduced in the late 1970s, who tried but failed to adapt it to annual report planning? The annual report producer.

The timely approach. Every year, someone comes from out of the corporate woodwork to meet the challenge of creating something unique in an annual report. The record holder for the most expensive report is Gulf & Western. To commemorate its 20th anniversary and increase its visibility in the marketplace, the company reprinted its entire report—64 pages—as an advertisement in *Time* magazine at a cost of $5 million. Expecting 300 requests for more information, the company was overwhelmed to receive 3,000. With a price tag of $1,666.67 per request, Gulf & Western may hold the record for many years to come.

Uncommon scents in annual reports. Many companies put out good-looking annual reports. But how many put out good-smelling ones? McCormick & Co., producer of seasoning and flavorings, did. Its 1979 annual was scented with pumpkin pie spice, topping earlier reports that came with a whiff of vanilla and the fragrance of cinnamon. How's that for appealing to the scentses?

Report for Lilliput. Honors for the tiniest annual report easily go to Georgia-Pacific. It published a pocket-sized version which it mailed along with a full-scale edition. A company spokesman said that the pint-sized report, which covered the basics but dropped the footnotes, had become popular among shareholders, employees, and customers alike. "Of course, it doesn't tell the whole story," he admitted, "but it is good for people who like to have ready answers to questions about our company."

Heavy reading. It would be difficult to misplace Warner Communications' 1978 annual report. It tipped the scales at nearly one pound. Most analysts didn't mind the bulk, however. They said that the report offered valuable information, not only about Warner, but about the many industries in which the company operates. A Warner spokesman explained that "as the company grows, we have more to talk about." But he didn't expect future versions to be weightier. "There's a limit," he said.

Getting down to earth. In the belief that many shareholders don't read annual reports because they don't understand them, St. Paul Company issued a "plain English" report containing a seven-page summary of how the company prepared its financial statements. Included were a detailed explanation of such elementary accounting concepts as amortization and goodwill and a complete rundown of how the company filed its income tax return. A. Kent Shamblin, vice president of communications and public relations, said, "Before we simplified our report, a lot of us here didn't even understand the jargon."

Extra! Leonard Maxwell, vice president of communications for South Carolina's Liberty Corporation, believed that it was senseless to try to put out the most colorful annual report when so many investors didn't even bother to read it. Liberty, an insurance and broadcasting holding company, chose another technique to get its name known. In addition to its traditional report, it sent investors a six-page newspaper filled with articles on the company's many activities. "Virtually everyone reads a newspaper," observed Maxwell. He said that 94 percent of those who responded to a survey rated the overall multimedia report as "good to excellent."

A+ for effort. Michigan-based Bank of Commerce wanted to make sure investors didn't overlook its annual report. The report was fashioned after a school "bluebook." "Final Exam" was printed on the front cover; "Note from our Principal"—President Carl Weinert's message to shareholders—opened the text; and the financial tables were headed "Accounting" and "Economics." "We got a lot of publicity," Weinert noted.

As the twig is bent. "A very long-range investor relations tool," as Chairman Finn Caspersen described it, was Beneficial Corporation's report to the younger generation. Entitled *Susan, John, and the Company without a Factory,* the 44-page, four-color booklet attempted to spell out to children what a finance company was and how it raised money and created profits for shareholders. Beneficial distributed about 75,000 copies. Said Caspersen: "It gets your name out in a very nice way. And some over the age of 12 have read it too."

Taking stock in employees. Clorox publishes a separate annual report for employees. A company spokesman said that this report, written more simply and briefly than the regular annual report, had been a very effective instrument for communicating management's views to the company's workers.

Fighting the fluff. Texas Instruments and William Wrigley, Jr., have more or less left their annual reports in the hands of lawyers and accountants and have begun to use other documents to tell their story. TI mails out a comprehensive first-quarter report that includes the kinds of features most companies put in their annual reports. Wrigley has a separate mailing for a letter to shareholders, which it omits from the annual report.

The minnow swallowed the whale. David T. Kimball, the chief executive of Leeds & Northrup, used his company's 1977 annual report to help fight off a bid by Tyco Laboratories. The report, an unabashed testament to Kimball's leadership, described him as the company's "no-nonsense, analytical president and CEO," who had turned in a "solid performance under fire." Tyco lost its takeover bid, but the following year Leeds & Northrup was swallowed up by General Signal.

Consuming investors. McDonald's Corporation published a high-styled, 44-page, multicolor report befitting a consumer products company. But to make sure that its shareholders contributed to the company's profitability, it attached a 44-page directory of its restaurants—worldwide.

22 cents apiece. American Telephone & Telegraph, which has 3 million shareholders, prints 4 million copies of its annual report. The printing costs alone approximate $1.2 million.

The broad brush. Native-son artists have been used to enliven annual reports. Wyeth prints were used by Multimedia with the explanation, "We strive to make every message clear and meaningful. So does he [Wyeth]—and succeeds like no other artist we know of." Caland Holdings N.V. of Rotterdam thought otherwise. It used seven works of Co Westerik, a leading Dutch artist, and it made its report available in English, Dutch, and French.

Candor above all. Binney & Smith, whose Crayola crayons have been hard hit by the baby bust and the soaring prices of raw materials, began its management letter on the cover by stating that 1979 was a "difficult economic year."

All above candor. The Kemper Group said that it had had "good, but not great, financial results" and had its report signed by over 10,000 employees.

IS THE ANNUAL REPORT WORTH IT?

Each year, when a communicator sees the annual report heading for the U.S. Post Office, there is a concern about the value of the document. Was all the blood, sweat, and tears worth it?

Annual Report Readership

To help position the relevance of the annual report, the Advisory Committee on Corporate Disclosure of the SEC conducted a survey among 11,000 individual investors in 15 publicly held companies. Approximately 43 percent of the questionnaires were returned.

To the question "Do you generally make it a practice to read the company's annual report?" the answer was an overwhelming 90 percent yes to 9 percent no. To the question on the thoroughness with which they read the annual report, 26 percent responded "very thoroughly"; 51 percent, "somewhat thoroughly"; and 23 percent, "casually."

Table 9-1
Interest in parts of annual report (direct and street-name investors combined)

How thoroughly do you read the following parts of the company's annual report?

Parts of company's annual report	Read very thoroughly Number	Percent	Read somewhat thoroughly Number	Percent	Read casually Number	Percent	Do not read Number	Percent	Total* Number	Percent
President's report	1,810	46	1,231	31	787	20	112	3	3,940	100
Management description and pictorial presentation	1,310	34	1,518	39	977	25	83	2	3,888	100
Income statement	2,043	52	1,326	34	515	13	58	1	3,942	100
Balance sheet	1,553	40	1,300	34	850	22	171	4	3,874	100
Funds flow statement	869	23	1,090	29	1,231	33	540	15	3,730	100
Footnotes to financial statements	977	26	1,005	26	1,241	33	586	15	3,809	100
Auditor's report	741	19	805	21	1,376	36	906	24	3,828	100

* The number of questionnaires processed totaled 4,426; 233 of the respondents did not rate the parts of the annual report because they did not read the report; the remaining residuals represent nonresponses which vary for each part of the annual report.
Source: Individual Investor Opinion Survey, Advisory Committee on Corporate Disclosure, Securities and Exchange Commission, 1977.

There is a standing cliché that once a reader looks at the president's report and the income statement, the annual report hits the wastebasket. The Advisory Committee study, however, indicates a reasonable interest in all parts of the annual report, including the auditor's report (see Table 9–1).

Recipients of annual reports were asked why they did not read them. "Wasteful public relations" was at the bottom of the list, along with "boiler-plate language"; both of these reasons for not reading the annual report were categorized among "other miscellaneous" (see Table 9–2).

Table 9–2
Reasons for not reading the annual report

Reason	Number	Percent
Lack of time	121	33
Lack of interest	78	21
Difficult to understand	130	35
Information not credible	15	4
Other miscellaneous	23	7
Total	367	100%

Source: Individual Investor Opinion Survey, Advisory Committee on Corporate Disclosure, Securities and Exchange Commission, 1977.

Do Your Own Readership Study

Far too often, the annual report does not get readership because the communicator is content to convey management's message without giving any thought to what the reader wants to know beyond the information required by government regulations. Numerous devices can be used, ranging from expensive to cheap, to measure readership.

One year, I received necessary feedback through the reader survey, but such a survey presents pitfalls as well as opportunities.

For a large company with a broad shareholder base, the costs of printing, postage, and evaluation can make even a mail survey expensive. For a smaller company, a survey can eat up an inordinate amount of the budget. The greatest pitfall to avoid is improper structuring of the survey, which would produce useless answers.

To hold the costs down and in keeping with the format of the annual report, I decided to direct a mail survey to a key list of individuals. The list included financial analysts, bank trust officers, and other investment advisers who were vital links in the company's efforts to convey company information to potential shareholders.

Two basic types of information were sought.

The first was an evaluation of whether the company annual report fulfilled its objective of supplying sufficient information to professional investors and investment advisers. In this evaluation, participants were asked to approach the report with their own informational needs in mind.

The second was an evaluation of whether the annual report conveyed the essence of the company in a form understandable to new or unsophisticated investors. Here, participants were asked to approach the annual report in its role of educating new or potential investors about the company in such a way as to make it easier for the investment adviser to do his job of explaining the company.

It was my concern that "good, fair, poor," "yes or no," or "helpful or not helpful" ratings, while providing helpful generalities, would not secure the specific answers which were necessary to make the survey valid. This problem was solved by providing space for comments on each question.

The wisdom of adding a comments section for each question was evidenced in the returns. For example, while 98 percent of the respondents indicated that the annual report was well organized, the comments revealed that the respondents desired a one-volume report instead of the separate financial and text volumes that they had been given.

In the areas "overall description of the company" and "vital statistics," the respondents gave the company 89 percent ratings on quality, yet 25 percent of them added comments that were useful in planning the next annual report.

My concern that 15 tables of information might be too much was eased by comments like these: "Excellent, wish your competition did this"; "The tables were an excellent addition to the report"; "Very useful"; and "Would like even more data."

Although the respondents were busy people, they were interested enough in the company and its annual report to contribute 208 comments to help the company with this important communication device. This valuable information was gathered at a cost of less than $1,500—a very low investment for measuring the current annual report and planning the next one.

The Extra Value of Advertising

Following its annual NYSE annual reports section, *Barron's* analyzes responses.[1] A typical analysis showed 7,000 requests for 153,000 annual reports. From these responses, *Barron's* determined the effect which the annual reports received had had on investment decisions.

---

[1] "NYSE Annual Reporter," *Barron's.* Copyright © 1977, Dow Jones & Company, Inc.

More than 9 out of 10 of the respondents (94.99 percent) said that the annual reports had been helpful in their investment decisions; nearly one half (45 percent) said that they or their organizations had bought or recommended the purchase of shares in companies from which they had ordered annual reports; more than three out of five (73.6 percent) who had purchased or recommended shares had invested in two or more companies; and in addition to the shares that the respondents had already purchased or recommended, a significant percentage of them planned to make additional recommendations or purchases in the next six months.

To position the impact of advertising on the annual report, Doremus & Co. surveyed people who had requested copies of corporate annual reports offered in *Crain's Chicago Business*.[2] The survey was distributed with a cover letter from George Fischer, vice president and manager of the Chicago Doremus office, to individuals who had requested annual reports.

The purpose of the study was to determine investing habits and concrete actions of the respondents once they received the reports. The annual reports of five Chicago-area corporations were offered.

Of 405 questionnaires mailed out, 166 were completed and returned. The results showed that the persons who order annual reports through advertising are investors in common stock. This point has been proven in many studies done for Doremus clients and in studies conducted by *Fortune* in 1976 ("And Then What Did They Do?") and *Barron's* in 1977 ("Annual Report Advertising Works in *Barron's*").

The principal finding documented in the Doremus study is that of the persons who request an annual report, one out of eight actually buys common stock in one of the companies whose report was requested. A second person out of the same eight says that he or she plans to purchase common stock. Sending out the remaining six annual reports may be of some value, though these reports did not produce new or potential shareholders. Specifically, 12.5 percent of the persons who received the annual reports purchased stock as a result, while another 15.0 percent intended to purchase stock within the next six months.

Why You Need Results

A good reason for attempting to get results from annual reports is that the printing and distribution of these reports have become quite costly. By the early 1980s the top 500 companies were sending out 25 million copies of their annual reports, while all 11,000 publicly held companies in the United States were distributing 50 million reports at

---

[2] "A Survey of Those Requesting Annual Reports through *Crain's Chicago Business*," Doremus & Co., November 12, 1979.

a total cost of more than $120 million. This works out to an average cost of $2.40 per copy for production and postage. These costs will be increased by inflation. And the amounts given do not include the costs of the executive time spent on annual reports.

There is reason to believe many companies are not getting their annual reports into the hands of the right people. It is estimated that fully 20 percent of the money spent on these reports is wasted because of faulty distribution, primarily in the area of secondary distribution. This estimate takes into consideration all the reports whose distribution is not required by law. Typically, such nonrequired distribution has as a main goal an increase in the shareholder base, so companies tend to use a shotgun approach rather than zeroing in on the most productive targets.

It is also estimated that since fewer than 10 percent of shareholders read an annual report thoroughly, companies are paying $30 to $50 for every report that is actually read. This is a telling reason for doing readership studies on your reports to determine how to increase interest in them. As long as the annual report is required by law, build in the most value possible.

One sensible manager—and investor—said that an annual report should be regarded as an investment memo. Consider it as a memo asking the board of directors to commit $10 million for a new project. Just as such a memo should answer all the questions that the board might have, so an annual report should answer all the questions that investors might have before they commit large sums to the corporation. Your report should be full of answers produced by honest writers who are trying to provide information. If it is, it will be read.

Annual reports have always been difficult, but now they are under the tightening noose of government regulation—pursued by a posse of attorneys, accountants, analysts, and corporate critics. The demand for more and more disclosure is being coupled with the passion to make annual reports serve multimarkets. The reports are no longer aimed solely at investors and analysts, but also at regulators, employees, college students, customers, the media, and business-baiting outsiders. The result is that annual reports, which were once innocent little 16-page storybooks, are becoming encyclopedias running 80 to 90 pages and weighing a pound. Some people believe that the 100-page annual report is near. Unfortunately, the new requirements are not necessarily increasing the average shareholder's understanding of the company. But they are definitely increasing the profits of law and accounting firms, and of paper and printing companies.

As weight of the annual report increases, there are doubts that more tables, more charts, and more financial footnotes add up to more information. Disclosure is not necessarily communication. Much of the disclosure now required is deceptive. It gives the reader a false or confused picture of the company. Just because you keep adding details to your report does not mean that your readers will either understand them or even bother to read them. Readers simply refuse to wade through a volume of business pomposity, particularly dense financial material. Know what the reader wants.

OTHER FINANCIAL REPORTS

In addition to the annual report, the average corporation produces a myriad of other reports. Some of them, such as the 10-K, are required by law. Others, such as the quarterly report, are required, but with only minimal standards, giving the communicator relatively free reign. On the voluntary list is the fact book, which numerous companies produce for the professional investment adviser.

The annual reports prepared by private philanthropies have been brought under the required status in recent years. However, alert organizations discovered the advantages of annual reports for fund raising long before their reports were made mandatory.

The Quarterly Phases of Reporting

A number of factors account for the rise to prominence of the quarterly report. It is timely. It permits you to reach shareholders and audiences soon after events occur. You can report the effect on your company of inflation, a major management change, or a new product sooner rather than later. It is relatively uncluttered. The annual report has been mired down increasingly in accounting and legal restrictions and jargon. And top management's close involvement with the annual report tends to restrict it. But the quarterly report is usually the communications department's pet, so it can be used to tackle a wider range of communications objectives. It is comparatively inexpensive compared to the annual report. It is highly useful to professional investors who need its details and interpretation.

While many companies now provide a brief fourth-quarter report while the annual report is in production, the Financial Analysts Federation would like to see even more financial material, including surplus reconciliation, adequate discussion of "current developments," an explanation of any unusual charges or of any changes in accounting practices, and the adoption of the continuous reporting technique—giving figures for the latest 12 months in addition to results for the latest quarter and the year to date.

As a Matter of Fact-Book

"The fact book is the fastest growing alternative to the annual report." "Fact books are dead." These divergent views about fact books as a communications tool are not uncommon as communications professionals attempt to assess their future.

Fact books directed to financial analysts have enjoyed considerable growth, with more than 300 companies now producing them and also producing "rep books," stripped-down versions of the annual report, to be sent to brokerage houses and large individual investors.

Two reasons have prompted the growth of fact books. The first is the desire to produce cost-effective materials with specific messages directed to specific audiences. The second is that management can produce fact books outside the regulatory clutches of the SEC.

It is because of the growth of regulations governing the annual report and the 10-K, however, that some communicators predict the eventual disappearance of the fact book. These doomsdayers believe that as more and more information is mandated in required reports, there will be less and less need for alternative publications.

Most fact books are in the 24-to-36-page range, but the Gargantua is that of Gould, Inc., which produced a statistics-ladened 339-page tome, far beyond the comprehension or the absorptive capacities of financial analysts. Fact books have found the greatest favor among utilities, railroads, and oil companies, whose results readily lend themselves to unit breakdowns and analyses.

The fact book is designed to contain a concise summary of "hard" data, a collection of the basic facts of greatest importance to the financial analyst. Unlike the annual report, it does not focus on activities during the prior year but presents a factual overview of the company at the time of its formation.

There are two important points about fact books:

1. They are used by professionals who already have a basic understanding of a company and its industry.

2. They are used most, not by ultimate decision makers, but by people who do basic research and analysis and present ideas on which others take action. For example, a financial analyst at a brokerage firm uses the fact book to develop recommendations for brokers to relay to their customers, or for institutional clients. The fact book user at a financial institution is usually an analyst who prepares research reports that will be presented to an investment committee.

Thus, the fact book is essentially a briefing document. It provides basic background around which the analyst can build a story on a company. The annual report is useful, but it contains subjective material that the analyst must weed out to get to basics. The fact book has done that weeding out.

The goal is to make the analyst an emissary who will tell a story credibly to the investment decision makers.

Fact books generally follow this outline: statement of purpose, including name of company contact for analysts; table of contents; company description; company history; products and/or services section; facilities section; employee data; labor relations; stock data; financial data; listing of officers and directors, with key biographies; directory registrar, stock exchange listing; and auditor. Some fact books also present more subjective information, for example, management philosophy, diversification philosophy, research and development goals, and marketing strategy. Charts and graphs are useful in highlighting quantitative data.

A fact book has a small press run, normally not more than 1,000 or 2,000 copies, and is distributed to the company's small, close following of analysts. It must be updated frequently—at least once a year. Staff time and expense in preparing a fact book are heaviest for the "maiden" issue. Updates are relatively simple.

It makes sense to design a fact book with a low initial out-of-pocket cost and a low unit cost for updating. This argues against the glossy, four-color book—though for some giant, prestigious corporations, anything less might be inappropriate. But for many companies, the answer may be a simple black-and-white fact book, possibly a simple typed and multilithed document in a plastic cover or a spiral binding. With the glossy version, the unit cost is especially high since the fixed costs of typesetting, color separations, and press setup must be spread over a small number of copies.

A Profitable Book for Nonprofits

Limited budgets and concern for image put restrictions on the annual reports produced by nonprofit organizations, but these reports are a valuable resource, according to communicators in the private philanthropy field. The field is a major industry in America. The public gives billions of dollars annually to nonprofit organizations in the areas of religion, health and hospitals, education, social welfare, and the humanities.

But none of the thousands of organizations in the nonprofit field can afford to take their vital assets of public confidence and support for granted. Those with an urgent need to expand and strengthen their programs are sharply aware that the status quo can no more exist in philanthropy than in business and industry. For the nonprofit field, the annual report has become a key channel through which agencies reiterate their institutional case on their terms to their constituents. Competition for volunteers and contributions is getting keener. A more sophisticated and knowledgeable public is asking more questions about the role played by agencies in dealing with some of the nation's critical social and health issues. In turn, the federal government is expanding its activities at a faster pace into areas traditionally served by voluntary associations.

The annual report provides individual agencies with the opportunity to clarify their functions and purposes in current terms. It positions agencies honestly and fairly in the context of the broader environment in which they operate and demonstrates how agencies respond to change and developing needs. Obviously, a routine account of a year's work just will not do anymore. The annual report is becoming more and more the opportunity to deliver a "state of the art" message that will give readers insight into the dynamics of an agency's operations. This task cannot be dashed off lightly; it must be handled—and it is being handled increasingly—by skilled public relations staff members.

What are the physical aspects of the annual reports in the nonprofit field as compared with the annual reports of the business world? Most of these reports tend to imitate the traditional style of the reports produced by business and industry—large pages, good paper, color covers, perhaps a second or third color inside, contemporary typefaces in an airy layout, tightly cropped photographs providing dramatic expressions of the reality that the organization works in, charts and graphs to describe finances, and a much-massaged message.

If there is a significant difference, it arises because nonprofit organizations are usually limited by budget—not choice—to one-color black-and-white interiors, though many of these organizations limit the attractiveness of their reports to avoid antagonizing readers who might react unfavorably to expensive appearance.

Surprisingly, the Salvation Army published its 1973 annual report as an advertising supplement in the *Reader's Digest*. This report was underwritten by a number of major corporations which used their ads to tout the Army's work. And in a footnote the Army expressed its appreciation to the "Advertisers, the *Reader's Digest* and the J. Walter Thompson Co., our volunteer advertising agency who conceived this way of portraying the work of The Salvation Army and carried it through to execution." No doubt, the Army reached many more people and won many new friends by using this unique device. But, on the whole, agencies shy away from elaborate reports. The reasons are obvious. The fund-raising and administrative costs of nonprofit agencies have been subjected to critical attacks from time to time. Usually, the finger has been pointed at a small minority of abusers who operate outside the mainstream of private charity. But none of these organizations wants to risk being the butt of future charges.

The overall goal of an association's annual report is accountability to its membership, the companies that financially support the organization. If the annual report achieves its goal, it will play a positive role in membership retention and acquisition. It can also provide a forum for the president's report to the membership, information about association programs and services, background for the news media and others outside the industry, and a vehicle for determination of member attitudes.

The Institute of Scrap Iron and Steel, a relative newcomer to this area, published its first annual report in 1972.[3] The report provided a capsulized but comprehensive account of the institute's programs and services, but its use for secondary objectives was prevented by the limited size of the press run. However, as the institute's annual report has evolved, it has been possible to incorporate other objectives and to reduce the overall cost and staff time required.

With planning, the institute's annual report achieved a number of other objectives. In 1976, the annual report was the vehicle for a comprehensive membership evaluation survey, designed to determine how members felt about the association as a resouce and about its leadership and its positions on issues, programs, and services. Members were also polled for suggestions on how to make the institute more valuable. The results, generally quite favorable, were used by the institute's board of directors to enlarge its solid base of support.

Another objective of the annual report of associations is to recruit new members. Most associations prepare a printed piece of some kind, but many of these pieces appear to be extremely generic, and with minor changes they could be used by any association. The broad categories of association programs and services are outlined, but generally there is little specific information.

A trade association annual report is not subjected to the exacting reporting requirements of the corporate report. There is no law requiring a trade association to print one. In the sense that it helps retain existing members and encourages new ones to join, however, the report is an income producer. It can also be one of the most effective communications tools available to an association.

A hospital annual report to the community seems to be a simple question of public relations values, but it is a question with a lot of ramifications: Is there something positive to say? What information is of the greatest interest and value to the public? How can the information be presented best? How can the best audience be reached most economically?

To find out what other Colorado hospitals were doing about annual reports, Jerry Stremel, director of public relations, Poudre Valley Memorial Hospital (PVMH), surveyed 70 hospitals in the state.[4] Of the 61 that answered, 46 did not have a formal annual report. Among the remaining 15, 10 printed brochures and 5 used newspaper advertise-

---

[3] James E. Fowler, "The Many Facets of Association Annual Reports," *Public Relations Journal*, September 1977, pp. 20–22. Copyright © 1977, Public Relations Society of America.

[4] Jerry Stremel, "Should Hospitals Publish Annual Reports?" *Public Relations Journal*, September 1977, pp. 24–25. Copyright © 1977, Public Relations Society of America.

ments. The brochures differed from the ads in cost, format, and audience. There were also marked differences within each category. The cost of the brochures ranged from $20 to $9,450. The lowest cost per copy was 2.7 cents; the highest was 41 cents. The formats included the typed single sheet and the splashy layout.

There was also a wide variation in the newspaper ads. For one hospital, local businessmen sponsored the space. Other ads cost from $480 to $7,281. The lowest cost per copy was 0.0093 cents; the highest was 2 cents. The formats varied from a press release style to an eight-page color insert in the Sunday edition. The circulation of the newspapers used ranged from 11,000 to 368,000. Only one of the 26 Denver metropolitan hospitals reported using newspapers. (Almost 30 percent of the Colorado hospital beds and 25 percent of the Colorado hospitals are in the Denver area.)

Since 75 percent of the hospitals answering the survey did not have a formal annual report, Stremel wondered whether PVMH should publish one. The doubt vanished, however, when pollster Louis Harris reported that 66 percent of the American people did not know why hospital costs had gone up. He suggested, "Whatever a hospital does in its image building must be based on reality."

PVMH saw the annual report as an ideal way to build its image on a factual basis and began a study of the pros and cons of using the press versus a mailed brochure. A brochure would cost over $2,000, but for about $800 the hospital could purchase a full page with a circulation of over 45,000. Francis Bacon said that not every piece of writing should be consumed in the same way. Some pieces are to be merely tasted, others to be quickly swallowed, and still others to be chewed and digested. The same for annual reports. Nobody wants to eat a soggy pancake—dull, heavy, and tasteless. Like a birthday cake, the annual report should be colorful, fresh, and flavorful. Thinking this way, the hospital planned the format of its annual report. Its first step was to choose the theme that the hospital was helping people and that it was both responsible for and responsive to the needs of the community. The idea of incorporating the necessary material into a one-page ad was challenging, but Dick Albrecht, new director of the Chamber of Commerce, said, "As a newcomer, it was the best way for me to find out about the hospital without actually going there." This annual report coverage cost two cents per person reached. The hospital got its two cents worth—and a lot more.

Alphabet Soup

As discussed in Chapter 6, corporations are required to file reports other than the annual report. Most of these reports are produced by batteries of lawyers and accountants primarily for filing with the SEC and the stock exchanges. The most noted and the most controversial is the 10-K. It was mandated by the SEC to provide substantive information going beyond the annual report, such as the ages and backgrounds of corporate officers. Later the SEC mandated that the annual report and the 10-K contain substantially the same material. The SEC regulation also required that the 10-K be offered to shareholders upon request. I know a company with 15,000 shareholders that received three such requests, indicating the level of the individual investor's interest in the document.

ALL IS NOT SERENE

With new, liberalized approaches that permit the annual report to be used for any purpose, and with millions of dollars spent on it, the publication still has many critics. I am one of them.

Managements are maligned, "run over the coals," and "strung up by a rope" for the quality of the annual reports they produce. The largest body of complainers is composed of public relations personnel. The standard complaint is, "How can I get management to listen?"

I suggest, however, that the binoculars are focused on the wrong target. It is not management but the public relations person who is the real culprit. Annual report producers, I believe, are copycats, trendies, poor writers—and inept at dealing with management. There is a potful of creative crookery when a communicator borrows fragments from several sources and puts them together in a new annual report labeled "creativity." Give management a fresh, forthright approach that will increase public understanding and respect for the company, and management will buy it.

I think that many public relations practitioners do not view the annual report as a communications tool subject to the same canons of readability and pertinence that dictate other written communications. Instead of relating to their main audience, the broad financial community, they relate only to a select group—members of their own corporate boardrooms.

Yet, ironically, CEOs actually spend very little time on annual reports. One survey showed that the maximum time spent by a CEO on annual reports was 100 hours—enough to ensure an excellent product—but in most companies the CEO spends as little as 10 hours. So, most of the problems could be prevented at the outset if the company admits that an annual report can really speak for only one person—the one who runs the company. That person must be close to the project at the outset, and must delegate its execution to someone who has his complete confidence and backing.

Also, despite many improvements, annual report writing is still marooned on Cliché Island. Annual reports still ritually describe company earnings growth as "dramatic" and prospects as "promising." Negative events "impacted unfavorably on company operations."

The greatest problems seem to arise because companies and their communicators do not fully understand the expectations of those for whom they are issuing their annual reports. I believe that public relations executives should start telling management unpleasant or unwelcome truths. If we are not telling our managements what the public and the market think of us and expect from us, then who will? How long can the communicator remain satisfied without knowing the desired impact of the annual report on the reader, whether the reader is a shareholder, a potential shareholder, or an investment adviser?

How to produce your annual report will be discussed in Chapter 10.

CHAPTER TEN

How to Produce Your Annual Report

Amateurs read annual reports from front to back, and professionals read them from back to front, beginning with the footnotes.
Wall Street Saying

THE ANNUAL REPORT IN PERSPECTIVE

The annual report obviously means different things to different people. Some view it is a torturous exercise mandated by the Securities and Exchange Commission. Others see it as a chance for top management to pat itself on the back for a job well done. Still others see it as a vehicle to apologize for a poor performance.

The annual report is a tool that can serve a multiplicity of communications. It can have multiple objectives and reach multiple audiences. Its primary targets, of course, are the financial community, shareholders, and potential shareholders. Its secondary targets are customers, employees, suppliers, and the general public.

More than 11,000 publicly held U.S. corporations produce annual reports. Unfortunately, far too many communications people at these firms have become satisfied with going through zombielike motions at annual report time. As a result, annual report readers have become satisfied with going through the motion of leafing through the report and then depositing it in the nearest circular file. With the millions of dollars spent each year on annual reports, this whole "going through the motions" syndrome is a very expensive way of supporting the paper recycling effort of the nation.

Unread annual reports fall into several categories. But all of them have one common denominator—lack of consideration for the informational needs of their audiences. A blatantly one-sided or glossed-over account of a company's performance is a sure way to turn off a reader. This is true whether the account is a glowing tribute to management's own adeptness or a transparent litany of excuses for declining or nonexistent profits. In either case, the corporate communications manager strangely loses sight of what communications is. Simply stated, *it*

219

is the transference of meaningful information from one party to another. Without this consideration, a report may as well be written in hieroglyphics.

I have always been amazed at how communications people can do an exemplary job of marketing a product or service through advertising, promotion, and publicity and then stumble over themselves when it comes to annual reports. I contend that the annual report is also a marketing tool. In this case, it helps market an impression, or the *corporate image.* With capital shortages reaching an estimated $25–50 billion a year, this marketing job has become more important than ever. As a communications tool, the annual report is subject to the same principles that guide other such tools.

What a Good Report Can Do

First, let's define what a properly conceived, well-executed annual report can do. Plenty. For the professional analyst, it can provide information going beyond the form 10-K requirements; it can heighten the interest of potential shareholders; it can reinforce the faith of present shareholders; it can give customers and suppliers a good reading on the company's depth and scope; and for employees, it can be a source of personal identification and pride.

To do these things, the report must probe *below* the surface facts. This means including a discussion of the inputs that go into day-to-day management decisions—why these decisions are made and how they are executed. It means going beyond generalities into specifics such as market position, marketing environment, and strategies for growth. In determining content, there should be a sincere effort to synergize copy and graphics. In other words, these must work together instead of clashing.

If your major message is that the company is a strong marketer of products, it makes no sense to reinforce the copy with pictures of production workers. If your theme is the importance of people to your operations, avoid static pictures of products and machines. These may seem like basic points. But I assure you that what many annual report producers lose is the *basics.* Once you have these basics in place, you are ready to produce the annual report. Correct? *Wrong.*

You need research. There is no substitute for research and more research—to determine the content and theme of the report. Once again, I come back to the concept of the report as a marketing communications tool. You would not dream of developing an advertising campaign without audience research. Nor would you attempt to place an article in a publication without understanding the editorial needs of both the publication and your company. The same principle applies to developing an annual report.

FUTILITY IN DEVELOPMENT

Before we produce the annual report, let us examine some of the major problems that impede the proper development of this major communications effort. The two biggest problems are:

1. Because of the differing personal purposes of the various sectors of senior management, senior management does not fully understand, or make allowance for, the needs and expectations of its varied audiences.
2. Due to lack of experience or lack of management clout, the public relations manager fails to clearly and accurately counsel senior management on the company environment and on changing audience attitudes.

Pleasing Everyone

Managements get cross-eyed at annual report time. While they focus one eye on a report of stewardship for the previous 12 months, they keep the other eye on the new first quarter so that they can say things are going great and will stay that way—or, conversely, that they see the light at the end of the tunnel, after a bad year.

The vice president of marketing wants a beautiful brag piece that he can use with new and existing customers to push his sales. The human resources executive wants lots of employees pictured to help maintain the camaraderie of the work force and to show equal opportunity in action. The public affairs executive wants to show how all the vital aspects of social responsibility are being met. The investor relations executive wants the report loaded with fiscal minutiae for his financial audience. The chief financial officer wants the report, particularly the financials, to be a fashion plate reflection of solid financial management. Every general manager of every subsidiary or division wants lots of space to show that operation's importance and contribution to the company. And, finally, the public relations executive wants to make a contribution while coping with everyone else's ego.

The problem is to satisfy everybody. The corporate communicator knows that the annual report must represent a long time span and must appeal to many audiences. Both management and the annual report writer are at fault for dwelling on the past. Nearly all annual reports tend to tell readers what they already know: what happened during the last year. They do not tell readers what they really want to know: what the company expects to happen during the coming year or years. A lot of the money that shareholders put into a company's stock will be invested according to how they think the company will perform in the future.

There are good reasons, however, why managements do what they do. First, no company has ever been singled out for providing shareholders with an information overload during the year. Thus, the annual report is a good recap. Second, companies are still fearful of forecasting, at least until the federal government has more definitive ground rules. Yet, a discussion of the future, in moderation, can provide general guideposts on operations. For example: What problems does the company see ahead? What opportunities are looming on the horizon? How much capital will be needed for investment? What rate of return is being targeted on that investment?

Can you imagine the impact of credibility that would have flowed to the U.S. auto companies had they reported the impending influx of foreign car sales instead of being eternal optimists? U.S. Gypsum did an exceptional job in its 1978 annual report by giving its shareholders a sense of what the company's plans were. In a 16-page section, the company had a presentation "Changing markets/new opportunities" in which it explored in detail, with statistical support, the trends in its four major markets.

At Trans Union, I have used history to project the future. "As we invest, so shall we reap" was the major thrust of the historical view. Investing in leased assets for a decade at the rate of 11 percent resulted in a compounded growth rate which was also 11 percent. A detailed explanation was given of the investment process and the calculations for determining investment priorities, so that shareholders could readily determine future growth in the general range of 11 percent.

The Report Is Not Cost Effective

Another believer in the futility of annual report development is Alfred B. Smedley, group vice president of the Burson-Marsteller public relations agency, who contends that the cost-effectiveness ratio of the average annual report is the worst in the free enterprise system. Says Smedley,

> Most corporate executives would be fired if they ran their businesses the way they put out their annual reports. Hundreds of thousands—maybe even millions—of high-cost executive hours are spent in the annual rites of agonizing over what to say and how to say it, comma juggling, and generally wasteful and/or duplicated effort.
>
> Lest you think I'm biting the hand that feeds me or trying to establish a we versus they situation, I hasten to add that I think many of these people agree with this evaluation. In addition, it's apparent that people in our business and the others who play an important role in helping corporations issue their annuals are obviously still part of the problem. That's because, despite our efforts to become part of the solution, we seem not yet able to make a major breakthrough in turning the publishing of annual reports into a better and much more cost-effective part of the American economy.

William Braznell, an investor relations consultant in Tiburon, California, attributes annual report failures to the "drag factor." Braznell says:

> It's the biggest source of frustration among young writers and veteran annual report editors, and the principal reason why so many reports are flops. All annual reports are alike. They are as ritualized as a Japanese tea ceremony. There is no opportunity for creative expression or originality. There is no point in doing a real reporting job, because all the good material you dig up will be red-lined. Good writing is an unacceptable affectation in annual reports. Besides, no one is going to read the damned thing. Ergo, editing the annual report is a drag.[1]

An anecdote about General John Pershing also illustrates a problem with annual reports. In 1927, when an aide rushed in to inform the general that Colonel Charles Lindbergh had successfully crossed the Atlantic, the curt reply was: "Don't bother me with that. One person can do anything. When a committee crosses the Atlantic, then let me know."

When it comes to corporate annual reports, the committee approach is a fact of life. Why? Because, in the mind of management, no other corporate communications tool is by nature so many things to so many people. The end result is frequently stated another way: Never have so many said so little to so few.

Report by Committee

I doubt whether anyone who has ever written or edited an annual report has not been hindered by the drag factor or the committee approach. Overcoming these hindrances is not just a matter of thinking positively; it is also a matter of thinking creatively and analytically. It is getting unhooked from convention.

Convention and sometimes regulations dictate that every annual report shall contain exactly the same elements in essentially the same order—financial highlights, a description of the company, a two- or three-page management letter, an operations review with photos, a five-year summary and management analysis, the financials, and a listing of officers and directors.

It is true that reports *must* contain certain financial and operating data. The SEC reporting requirements say you must briefly describe the nature and scope of the corporation's activities and present cer-

[1] William Braznell, "How to Overcome the Annual Report Drag Factor," *Public Relations Journal*, August 1978, pp. 22–29. Copyright © 1978, Public Relations Society of America.

tified financial statements for the last two years. But they do not say how or where this information has to be presented. And there is no rule that says you *must* have an operating review, a letter, or a table of financial highlights. That is purely conventional. What I'm suggesting is that we have more freedom in the way we organize and develop our reports than many annual report producers seem to realize.

The starting point is to place one person in charge of the annual report. That person is *not* the chief executive officer. There is only one person who is suited for the task by training, experience, knowledge, skill, and a broad overview of the company and without having a little piece of ego at stake. That person is the chief communications executive—or designee—who has writing and editing skills; is knowledgeable in design, photography, finance, public relations, research, and the management thought process; and has an objective overview of all functions in the company.

My experience has been that since so many of the activities involved in the annual report are alien to most members of the management structure, they are inclined to divide up the responsibilities rather than place trust in one individual. Bringing in the marketing and/or investor relations person, they believe, will strengthen the annual report. But since even these knowledgeable people have their own interests, this directive can only lead to confusion, waste of time, and an unnecessary add-on to the production budget.

The annual report is like a battle. It is a pretty straightforward job for one individual to develop a highly creative annual report concept: graphics that communicate; a crisp, definitive writing style; and compelling photography. But the astute public relations professional knows that developing the concept is only the first skirmish in a lengthy war. Preparation of the annual report takes on all the characteristics of a full-fledged battle: logistical planning, skirmishes, strategic withdrawals, tactical pursuit—and that's just in-house. It is not that the corporate officers involved in annual reports enjoy doing battle. It is simply that each has his or her special interest to protect. Thus, the success or failure of the communicator will determine whether the corporation will communicate effectively with the many audiences it must reach.

The members of a committee will sit around a conference table and argue for hours about whether the annual report is going to talk about people, feature new products, show brick and mortar, or talk about what good people or neighbors they are. Finally, in disgust, they may agree to a rundown on operating divisions, rather than trying to reach agreement on a central theme. And if a weak person or a person who lacks a clear mandate is handling the report, he or she can get pushed in many directions and be unable to order or control costs.

Where to Begin

We can begin with two fallacies about annual reports:

1. The annual report begins with a theme or layout.
2. The annual report is a six-month job.

In regard to fallacy 1, the beginning step in the annual report process is research. You must know your audiences and what they need to know about your company. To me, management and communications executives display an air of arrogance if they proceed with production not based on audience research. And it is also arrogant to rely only on the input of one audience, say, the financial analyst, at the expense of the individual shareholders. Many a CEO has ignored the feelings and desires of the individual shareholders only to wonder why the company gets no loyalty and only little support from this vital group.

Burson-Marsteller's Smedley agrees. The communications expert knows where to begin—with planning. Smedley suggests: Determine and value-weigh your audience; find out, if possible, what your most important audiences most want to know; decide whether that's what *you* want to and can say, and determine how to say it; and then say it in the most informative and interesting way you can with a strong *visual* and *verbal* cohesiveness.

Your audiences, in order of importance, are:

1. *Shareholders.* You need to make the distinction between the truly sophisticated shareholders and the Aunt Janes and Uncle Charlies in terms of their interest and understanding, but not in what you tell them.
2. *Key security analysts and other important members of the financial community.*
3. *Employees.* Ideally, at all levels and in all countries. If you have employee shareholders, they are obviously in category 1.
4. *The management of the company.* Starting right at the top with the person or persons signing the shareholder letter, and going down through the corporate hierarchy.
5. *Everybody else.* Customers, vendors, dealers, the press, government, plant city influentials, and so on.

The very thought of asking the above what they would like to see in the annual report is enough to cause apoplexy in some executive suites. But not enough of American's best companies do it. A big plus in asking is that the feedback turns a one-way street of communication into a two-way street. A company can discover that the people it is surveying are interested in company areas, product lines, or whatever that management thought they were either well aware of or uninterested in.

Fallacy 2, that the annual report is a six-month project, also is tied into research. Once a theme or creative approach is approved by management review, the remaining work may only take six months. However, the proper execution of research and theme or creative development will add several months to the front of the schedule.

WHEN THE PLANNING STARTS

When an annual report is off press, the work of the public relations executive in charge is just beginning, not ending. There may be time for accolades on a job well done, but the executive is still on the hook to make sure the annual report is deliverable and readable.

Begin with Research

The research begins immediately. What are the initial reactions of senior management, of line management, of employees, customers, financial analysts, and shareholders? Conversations may cover the first three groups. Contact with your marketing department and your chief financial officer will clue you in on reception by customers and analysts. Then, watch for letters from shareholders to the CEO and the corporate secretary. Meet with your staff and your suppliers to critique their efforts and the quality of their performance.

These steps should give you a quick, reasonable overview as to whether or not your dream of September turned out to be the ides of March. The most complete input, of course, will come from formal research, which I have used with shareholders, financial analysts, and even key bankers with whom my company does business. Surveys have been used before annual report production to help determine a direction and after the annual report has been mailed to measure the effectiveness of the final product against the original goal.

One year, for example, I asked financial analysts informally at luncheon meetings and a visitation tour: What information do you need to better understand the company? What information should the annual report contain to make it easier for you to interest a prospective investor in the company?

As a result, 25 information bits were plugged into the next annual report. One month after the report was mailed, a lengthy questionnaire covering each segment of the annual report was sent to the analysts on each of the above questions. A 96 percent positive response indicated that we had fulfilled their original information concerns and needs.

If you have neither the need nor the money for detailed information, you can continue with your informal research. A focus group of six to eight analysts at a luncheon can bring in a wealth of information, even though that information may not be ironclad statistically.

Here are some other informal research suggestions:

1. Always keep your "ear to the ground" for questions that analysts and other investors ask your company's chief financial officer. Constant contact with the financial executive should enable you to build a file of pertinent information.

2. Review every financial analysts' report, newsletter, market letter, and commentary on your company. That includes Standard & Poor's reports, Value Line, and other regular investor reports.

3. Review internal management reports. Most large corporations require brief monthly narrative and financial reports from each operating division. In our company, the controller summarizes these reports to brief the company's top-management and directors. Corporate planning documents, capital budgets, and marketing plans are among the other important source materials you may need to review.

4. Review current and prior reports issued by the company, such as back issues of annual reports, 10-Ks, 10-Qs (quarterly reports to the SEC), and prospectuses.

5. Reread all press releases issued during the past year, not only at the corporate level but at the division level too. The same applies to the employee magazine, the clipping file, and industry and trade publication articles about the company.

6. Interview top staff executives and line management with a general questionnaire covering the broad areas of interest to shareholders. This checklist ensures coverage of all the bases.

For shareholders, research can be as simple or as elaborate as you want. Surveys can be done over the telephone, for example. Obviously, such surveys should be constructed so that you are truly attempting to gather pertinent information and not just slanting your questions to justify a predetermined point of view.

Here is a typical telephone questionnaire for shareholders:

> What is your general opinion of the company? What are its strengths and its weaknesses in your opinion?
>
> Which areas of the company offer the greatest growth opportunities? The least? Why?
>
> What would you like to know about the company that you don't now know?
>
> Is there any aspect you don't fully understand? How can the company correct this?
>
> What is your impression of the members of the management team? You can tick them off by name if you think it will help.
>
> Does the annual report tell you all you need to know? If not, what are your suggestions? Any other comments?

Most readers of the annual report are shareholders who do not know one footnote from another and couldn't care less. But these people are just as much owners of the company as the big institutional holders, and they are entitled to your respectful attention. Your objective should be to make every item in the report intelligible to them, even the financial notes. Every item of information contained in the report should be somehow related to their interests, their need to know.

Yet, numerous annual report producers write primarily for the professional investor—for the small number of institutions that own or control the majority of the company's stock. I'm sure they have good reason for doing this. But it seems to me that printing 55,000 annual reports, as we do, just to reach an audience of a hundred key professionals is doing things the hard (and expensive) way. In advertising, that is a lot of wasted circulation.

Research accomplishes several goals. It gives you an accurate reading of your audience's concerns. It also helps you build a documented case for a specific theme. In other words, it's not your concept pitted against management's concept. It's facts with a strong mandate. Without such groundwork, management will find it easy to dictate what it wants in the report. For example, our management was enthralled one autumn when we introduced a new railroad tank car. However, in the cold light of February, other events had preempted the car. Research supporting the importance of these other events led to putting the car in proper perspective. It was mentioned in the report, without full-blown treatment.

As for selling management on a new idea, you won't find it all that difficult, provided the idea is a good one and you have all your research material as ammunition. The CEO may not have artistic sensitivity, but he can recognize a surefire investment when he sees it. Show him an annual report that will increase public recognition and respect for his company, and he will buy it.

It helps greatly to have a solidly established financial relations program in place. Each year, my company sponsors analyst and banker seminars where top management is exposed to a "firing line" situation. This serves two purposes. First, it showcases our management. Second, the experience gives our management a firsthand idea of what key issues should be addressed in the annual report. Armed with this arsenal of information, you are ready to proceed into the minefield of annual report production. Although pitfalls abound, ample professional advice is available to you.

Be Aware of Pitfalls

Let us look first at some of the problems and common criticisms you will encounter. First, be aware and beware that at annual report time the CEO will become a semantics expert. The legal department will have visions of legal plums with every word. The marketing department will regard each page as a full-page ad. And, finally, the finance department will want the cover looking like a bank facade. Among the common complaints are:

1. Annual report writers don't use readership-building devices used by communications professionals. Too often, they use sterile, legalistic phrases.
2. Everything a company does is "important," "major," "significant," or "substantial." Operating efficiencies are always "optimated." Any organizational change involves a "thorough restructuring." And selling your losers is called "asset redeployment."
3. Many annual report producers don't take full advantage of good charts and graphs and other illustrative devices to catch the reader's attention and hold it.
4. Many companies use overly impressive color photographs which overpower the reader and detract attention from the text.
5. Annual reports are written for the professional, so that they are meaningless to "mom" and "pop."
6. All annual reports look alike.

Part of the problem lies in the fact that, despite all that planning year after year, one of the greatest dangers in report preparation is routinism. Plans are laid so perfectly and things go so well that after a while too little effort goes into innovation and inventiveness.

Graphic designer Roger Cook, Cook and Shanosky Associates, Inc., calls it "automatics," saying:

> Put half a dozen annual reports in front of us—unopened. Ask us to write the contents of each one, and even the order in which things will appear. And we'll bat at least 750. . . . Each year's crop creates a case of near-terminal déjà vu. Annual report design has reached the era of the automatic. And as soon as something becomes automatic, not only can it become dull, but it can also become dangerous—today's problems are not solved with yesterday's solutions.

While much of the annual report's content is required by law, a lot is not. It is not mandatory that the board of directors be pictured, that a report be split up into a chief executive's message with narrative and the financial section, that you lead off with financial highlights, that you show a picture of the chief executive, or that you use aerial pictures of plants. What is mandatory is that each report have a strong central idea and an objective against which performance can be measured.

When you ask practitioners to list the principal reasons why annual reports so often fail, high on the most lists will be the lament, "There was confusion over the audiences."

Meeting the Needs of Audiences

Reports have many audiences, and the needs and interests of these audiences vary. Obviously, the interests of retired shareholders are quite different from those of the security analysts.

The problem can be covered this way:

1. Provide a statistical briefing of highlights. The analyst will read this immediately and, if satisfied, will set the report aside for later reading.
2. The president's letter should be directed to the majority of individual shareholders. Preferably, it should be no longer than two facing pages, so that no turn need be made.
3. Cover the past year, and expand on any opinions for the year ahead. Any changes in accounting procedures and company or industry conditions and any significant financial or operating changes that have occurred or are expected are treated fully in this section.
4. Show detailed statistical exhibits near the end of the report. There should be, in addition to statistics covering the past year, comparative data for at least 5 years and preferably 10.

The last two sections are used by financial analysts in their yearly reviews, so full disclosure, completeness, and consistency of methodology are important.

Improving the Report

Over the years, numerous recommendations have been made for improving the annual report from the financial analyst's point of view. Among them are:

1. *The discussion by management.* This section should lay an adequate base of information and explanation on which investors can make independent judgments. It should be objective in tone, candid in exposition, and devoid of promotional comments.
2. *The SEC-mandated "management discussion of operations" should be combined with management discussion.* In most cases, this discussion is routine and merely states the obvious. The chronicle of events should provide perspective, for example, by indicating what contribution a new product is making to total sales or how a new plant adds to capacity.
3. *Discussion of financial results.* This section should have analytic content, explaining the causes and the significance of developments and relating results to general economic, industry, and regulatory trends when possible.
4. *Corporate objectives and strategies.* This type of information is

fundamental to projections of future earning power. Analysts need to have an idea of how goals will be achieved and what obstacles or constraints must be overcome.

5. *Investors should be given forward-looking information.* A company should explain how its specific plans, such as capital expenditures, plant construction, and new production, relate to its longer range goals and strategies.

6. *Reporting on segments of diversified companies.* Since each segment has a different market, each segment's rate of growth and degree of risk should be analyzed separately in relation to specific economic environments and a composite projection should be built from the separate analyses.

7. *Foreign activities of multinational companies.* More attention should be given to financial data regarding these activities, including sales, operating expenses, income taxes, net income, dividends remitted, and principal balance sheet items by principal countries or geographic areas, based on materiality to the company as a whole.

8. *More operating statistics.* Typical information sought includes output of major products, selling prices, plant capacity, and mineral reserves. These data are used to compare the company with the industry and to project potential sales growth without additional capacity.

9. *Historical data.* Analytic data for the preceding 10 years could be added to improve understanding. These data include profit margins, earnings rate on shareholders' equity, fixed-charge coverage, preferred stock dividend coverage, capitalization ratios, and compound growth rates in sales, expenses, net earnings, and assets.

10. *Pension costs and funding.* The impact of future expense on profits can be projected from the funding of accrued liabilities to date, the interest assumption, the actuarial method, and, if there is an unfunded liability, the amount and rate of amortization.

11. *Effects of inflation.* Investor understanding can be improved by a discussion of the method by which the data were prepared and their significance for the business.

12. *Readability.* The needs of varied audiences can be met in one document by the use of a summary review with key financial data, followed by the comprehensive report. A statistical supplement, intended for financial analysts but available to all shareholders, is desirable for some large companies. Annual reports can be made more readable with good typography, organization, and editing. A news style of writing, charts, and suitable pictures can engender reader interest. Analysts and potential investors want straightforward information applicable to the corporation alone.

To some extent, the investor is asking for simple answers in a complicated world. The answers could be much simpler and more informa-

232

tive if management were freed from regulatory shackles and could deal with its investors in simple business terms. Given the real world, however, we need to go on trying to help the investor in the frustrating effort to read the future.

GETTING THE JOB DONE

Your most bruising relationships will be with executive egos. Though you are armed with research and know you are right, you cannot be rigid and inflexible.

Dealing with Management

You can help your cause with the following advice:

1. Keep senior management informed of your ongoing research. This will precondition executives for later developments.
2. Get a unanimous agreement on your initial concept. Any person with approval or rejection powers can destroy you later.
3. Keep decision makers to a minimum. The fewer executives involved, the greater the clarity, and, conversely, the bigger the team, the poorer the quality.
4. Know executive tastes. Don't propose a concept or plan that will blatantly bruise executive tastes or egos. A liberal approach in a conservative company, for example, will get you a walk to the dugout instead of first base.
5. Know when to fight and when to give. Critical points are the management letter, graphics, and textual clarity. Try to hold steadfast in these areas.
6. Keep all areas in perspective. Domination by an executive in one area, marketing, for example, can be devastating to the overall tone of the report.
7. Picture yourself as an editor. The publisher, i.e., the CEO may have veto powers, but a strong personal relationship can water down the veto. Others may make suggestions, so accept the good.
8. In particular, hang tough with the lawyers. Public relations counselors occasionally get challenged about practicing law without a license. But more often than not, lawyers should be challenged for practicing communications under the guise of legal advice.
9. If you lose the major battle, live with it. You will be dealing with the same adversaries next year, so don't burn your bridges.

Dealing with Suppliers

The economics of producing an annual report have little relationship with the quality of the final product; the financial public relations man who is ignorant of them—or simply ignores them—can run up costs needlessly. Therefore, every supplier involved in your annual report, from creative director through mailer, must be a member of your team. Have these team members work with you, not for you, or against you.

I believe that it is vital for you to have a working knowledge of the services performed by suppliers. But there is no way for you to become an instant expert in each area. You may know typefaces, but your creative director will tell you what the final product will look like and your typesetter will tell you whether the type is handset, machine-set, or available on a computer. The latter determination can involve tens of thousands of dollars. A fatal mistake that many companies make is to throw away the team concept and go for the low bid. Millions of dollars were lost when a spaceflight was aborted because of a low-bid part costing pennies.

My experience with the development of a team is that each supplier is neither the low nor the high bidder. But I know the capabilities of my suppliers, the extent of their service, and the limitations of their staffs or equipment. Is each segment of your supplier team geared to giving the required around-the-clock service, or do your suppliers close up shop at 5 P.M.? Does the printer have the right presses in the colors necessary to get the job done, or will the job be farmed out to a third party? More important, my suppliers are attuned to my needs, so they can save me bundles of money. For example, a creative director familiar with my annual report may create the layout so that some printing signatures—16-page units—will only require a two-color press on what is essentially a four-color product. Or a creative director and a printer knowing the type and layout of the photography may be able to recommend a less expensive grade of paper stock. That stock can then be ordered early, before paper takes its traditional price jump on the first of the calendar year. And a lighter weight stock will translate into postage savings at mailing time.

Among the items which your team can work out, even long before the final concept has been developed, are:

1. *Scheduling.* Key dates and deadlines can be established for each supplier activity.

2. *Design elements.* The use of embosses, die cuts, gatefolds, and end sheets can be determined.

3. *Color.* One, two, four, or more colors can be agreed upon for inclusion in the design concept and the photographic direction.

4. *Photography.* The number, sizes, and color of photographs can be established.

5. *Cover.* You can decide whether this will be a self-cover of the same weight as the body paper or a separate cover of heavier weight.

6. *Size.* Will it be a standard 8½ by 11 inches or an odd size, and

234

what impact will this have all the way down the creative and production schedules?

7. *Envelope.* Secure the right envelope for the right size and weight of annual report. Also, make a determination on the utility and the cost effectiveness of the Federal Two-Envelope Piggy-Back system, the Federal Self-Mailer Piggy-Back system, and the Bi-Pac method.

8. *Type.* Agreement can be reached on the face, size, and production method, such as machine-set or computer. Considering having the type set with a ragged right margin, so that minor changes can be made without resetting entire paragraphs.

9. *Proofs.* Who will get "readers," inexpensive preliminary proofs, and who will get "etches," expensive final proofs, and how many copies of each? Decide now to save money. Etches, for example, may be totally unnecessary until final keylining and paste-up by the creative director.

10. *Printing plates.* Determine whether the printer has an in-house facility. If not, find a platemaker that is open 24 hours a day. It will kill your production schedule if a plate change is required on a press at 3 A.M. and your platemaker's shop does not open until 9 A.M.

11. *Ink.* Determine whether you can get by with standard inks or whether you will need quick-dry or reflective types.

12. *Dummies.* A blank mock-up of the report will get you mentally attuned to the task ahead and help you determine envelope size and postage. A mock-up of the accepted concept will be your working document through the entire creative and production schedules.

13. *Bindery.* Determine whether, once the annual report is off press, the document will need special folding, stitching, or collating or a varnish or plastic finish. Can the printer handle this work, or will the work require another supplier and thus extend the schedule? Will the annual report be boxed or skin-packed, and will drop shipments be required?

14. *Mailing.* This element will be discussed in the section on scheduling.

THE PLAN

Emerging from all your research, your management discussions, and your meetings with suppliers, you will have your plan. The traditional date for planning is September—not because summer vacation is over but because it does take a full six months to meet the March mailing date for the majority of publicly held companies.

The plan includes all of the input that you sort out and the common objectives that are to be addressed by words and pictures. You decide what kind of annual report you are going to do by developing a plan that spells out the purpose and procedure and becomes the marching orders for the rest of the project. You turn your momentary attention to these special elements.

Design

I consider myself a communications executive. I am not a designer. Therefore, I give the designer complete freedom for creative responsibility, based on certain key elements. First, I share with the designer all the input from my research, details of the management discussions, major changes in the company's direction, and then, most important, a description of the personality of the company as an entity and of senior management members as individuals. I try to obtain access to senior management for the designer so that he or she can make a personal evaluation.

Copy

No words in modern history have been more maligned than those appearing in annual reports. Good annual report writing, like any form of writing, requires common sense and good judgment in the selection and ordering of detail. Once you have clearly established the interests of your readers, it will be relatively easy to select, assemble, and order your facts in a way that makes them meaningful. Do not omit important information because it doesn't fit into your theme or your space allotment. That is called "omission of material fact," and it can be considered fraudulent.

Be concerned, however, about detail that clutters rather than clarifies—the sort of useless information that some editors use simply to pad out their text. Words should be strong enough to stand on their own without design. Design should enhance communications, not get in its way. A few years ago, the Pullman Corporation had an excellent management letter. But it was so proud of its new logotype that it used the logotype more than 100 times in its annual report, including its use as emphasis points in the letter. The result was jumbled jargon.

Simple, direct statements are great values to adopt. Use them to explain the major accomplishments, problems, and outlook of your company, sans the editorializing, exaggeration, and adjectives. Be consistent with what you said last year. Remember that a portion of your audience is new every year; do not assume prior knowledge.

Place yourself in the position of the reader. What does the copy mean to that person? Let's look, briefly, at a few examples.

In one annual report, the American Broadcasting Companies, Inc., had this caption: "At Weeki Wachee Spring, performing birds roller skate, do card tricks, and play basketball." What does that tell the shareholder? ABC has smart birds? In management?

American Bank Note Company, in a caption, reported: "Shown at the left are some of our sophisticated new high-speed presses. Clockwise from upper left: a multicolor intaglio press, a multicolor lithographic press, a numbering press, and a modern multicolor offset press." Is American Bank Note in the printing press business? What is the significance of the various presses? How do they differ? How do they contribute to growth and profits? What are they *really* for?

Now, compare these captions with a typical caption in an annual report from Abbott Laboratories:

> David Quach, born at the 27th week of pregnancy, weighed only 1,000 grams (2 pounds 2 ounces). David's short life has been full of complications. Still, he hangs on and grows. He is fed *Similac* Special Care Formula whenever he is hungry or every hour. His father, Luong, is proud of David's progress. "In Vietnam, they would have let him die," he said. Their older son was born in Vietnam, and they had a house and a good life before communists took over. Many friends were killed, and Luong was drafted into the service for 13 years. Eventually, the Quach family spent six months in a Vietnamese refugee camp before coming to the United States by boat. They now live in Los Angeles, where Luong is learning to become an auto mechanic.

The caption tells who is in the photo, what his and his family's special circumstances are, and what use he makes of the company product. Lengthy, perhaps, but planned that way and effectively executed! In its text, Abbott uses its name for medical products, but it proceeds to tell what they are, what they are used for, what their market penetration is, and where or how additional growth is planned. The reader can overcome the natural resistance to complex brand names by receiving capsulized, but descriptive, explanations about them.

There is a school of thought that says the chief executive officer should write the annual report, or at least the chairman's letter. I agree with the latter under controlled circumstances, but I vehemently disagree with the former. First, writing the entire report is a poor use of executive time. Second, it is rare indeed that a CEO has either the training or the natural ability to perform that function.

The most efficient method I have been able to devise for having the CEO write the management letter sounds simple, but it involves considerable work. The chief financial officer and I independently develop lists of what we believe were the financial and operating highlights of the year. In a series of meetings, we arrange the major events in the order of their importance and discard the lesser events. We then present an outline to the CEO for his agreement. This becomes our working document, and his working document, through all of his revisions.

Photography

It is interesting to note that while passionate pleas have been made for good, solid writing, in annual report "how-to" articles more has been written about photography than about all the other aspects put together. And there have been instances where pictures have replaced, or almost replaced, text. In 1973, the Philip Morris annual report had no text at all in the divisional sections, while in the late 1970s, Itel used two-page, four-color spreads with single paragraphs of copy. One wag noted that the editor of the annual report was probably the most underutilized spokesman on the payroll.

Photography is used to project a personality or style that encourages trust in the words and numbers; to show officers who are warm, sensitive, and dynamic; to reveal exciting, dramatic moments in the corporate growth adventure; to display fine taste and design, suggesting sophistication throughout the business; and to create moods that touch people and make them want to read the text.

Another school of thought expresses the idea that although annual report photography has been upgraded in recent years, the improvements have generally been cosmetic rather than substantive. The depth is superficial, the content literal, the presentation predictable. The subject matter remains the same, year after year: posed executives; glossy, carefully composed views of products, plants, facilities. The result is competent commercial illustration. Little more.

The Professional Photographers of America surveyed the annual report photography of the Fortune 500. The survey showed a trend toward "candid" shots in place of "formal" shots. It established that, in an effort to transform corporate goals of growth, diversity, and service into believable realities, corporations are relying as much as ever on the power of the picture to show off new products; tie together diverse product lines, services, and locations; and educate the public on social concerns such as ecology, minority employment, community action, and consumerism.

Most of the annual report photos I see do not convey information to the reader beyond the most superficial levels. Many are literal, for-the-record shots—this is our building; this is our product; this is our president; this is someone using our product. The photos say nothing else. The fault lies, I believe, with the responsible public relations executive for viewing photography as a separate, rather than integral, element in the annual report. Photos do not fit into or reinforce the basic theme and may not even fit into the design or copy in a particular section. Far too often, the copy discusses a new manufacturing process for left-handed widgets, while the photo shows a customer with a new ribless umbrella.

Some annual report editors have explained to me that their big problem is that they are out shooting photographs in the summer—before brown leaves and snow—while the copy is not being hammered out until January. A well-conceived game plan may not eliminate this problem, but it surely can reduce its occurrence.

There is one other simple but effective device that I use to overcome this problem—and enjoy other benefits as well. The device is to track all photographs from advertisements, brochures, promotional publicity, and employee publications from various divisions and build a library at the corporate level. While small companies spend $2,000 and large companies pay $20,000 or more for annual report photography, my annual report photography bill is in the $300 range for 18 to 20 photos—and most of that expense is incurred in reprocessing existing library material.

Every annual report producer knows that photographs, per report copy, don't cost much. But most annual report readers don't know that. They have no perspective for judging the costs of color photography. So they think they are being denied huge dividends because the chairman has his color photograph in the annual report. Complaining shareholders are overwhelmed when I explain that the entire photographic bill is less than 2½ cents per investor and less than 0.005 cent per copy. Someday, a brave editor is going to print something to that effect in the annual report.

The Role of the Communicator

As you refocus on your plan, firmly implant this advice in your mind:

1. You are not a design expert.
2. You are not a photographic expert.
3. You do not know all of the techniques and nuances of production.
4. You may be an excellent copywriter, but throw pride of authorship out the window; too many people are involved.
5. You may be good, but don't let your ego get in the way any more than you must; stifle others—gently, of course.

Your major role, by knowing something about everything, will be that of editor, arbitrator, compromiser. It will be your responsibility to make sure that as many good ideas as possible flow into the annual report and that as many poor suggestions as possible wind up in the wastebasket.

On egos, the chief financial officer of one of my employers felt totally frustrated after we lost a long and heated battle with the CEO over one point in the annual report. My philosophical statement to him was, "OK, we lost the battle, but we won the war." We had won indeed, for, while the CFO felt frustrated because the CEO killed 2 percent of the plan, the CEO did approve 98 percent!

Scheduling the Work

Considerable advice is available on scheduling the work flow of an annual report. That work flow ranges from simple to complex, but, whatever the schedule, it must be flexible above all else, to accommodate the greatest need of all—management decisions. What is the best way to make sure your report touches all bases? By getting an early start. This is a typical flowchart to help plan and produce a company's annual report:

Week 1:	Start analysis of previous books. Develop goals/themes. Contact division/department heads for ideas/copy. Circulate timetable with delivery date.
Week 2:	Begin rough design exploration. Begin copy outline.
Weeks 3–4:	Continue design and copy outline.
Week 5:	First design review and copy outline.
Week 6:	Start photography. Develop copy and comprehensive design.
Weeks 7–8:	Continue developing copy and comprehensive design.
Week 9:	Begin production and type estimating.
Week 10:	Final review of comprehensive with photos. Copy review.
Week 11:	Start retouching. Develop charts, illustrations and typesetting, if possible.
Weeks 12–13:	Typesetting and mechanicals.
Week 14:	To printer. Check silver prints.
Weeks 15–17:	Printing and binding.
Week 18:	Delivery.

For the neophyte facing his or her first annual report, or anyone else desiring valuable basic tips, paper companies produce excellent materials. Among these materials are:

Preparing the Annual Report, from Potlach Corporation, Northwest Paper Division, Cloquet, Minnesota 55720. This booklet contains a guidebook and a working calendar, along with hints on format, graphics, photography, and paper selection. Potlach also has available the *Annual Report Guidebook*, which gives tips on assigning responsibilities, research, objectives, content, and graphics.

The Annual Report, from S. D. Warren Company, a division of Scott Paper Company, 255 Franklin Street, Boston, Massachusetts

02101. This booklet includes the history and purpose of the annual report, along with tips on establishing objectives and themes and ideas on writing, designing, and printing. Also available from S. D. Warren is *Making Points with Your Annual Report,* which gives numerous points that the annual report producer can use in an annual report.

Taking Stock of your Annual Report, from Appleton Papers, Inc., P.O. Box 359, Appleton, Wisconsin 54912. This booklet contains a working calendar, along with suggestion charts and graphs and samples of how companies have used varying cover designs.

Annual Report Kit from Mead Paper, Courthouse Plaza NE, Dayton, OH 45463. The three parts of this kit are broken down as follows: (1) for those in top management who have corporate responsibility for the report; (2) for those who carry out the directives of the top executives; and (3) the paper samples most frequently specified for annual reports.

Planning is no gimmick or momentary thing. Like research, it spans the entire year. On a wet, cold April day, it is not unusual for me to doodle over the past annual report and then to make an outline on how to improve certain elements for the forthcoming year. On a hot, sticky summer day, while reviewing midyear results, it is not unusual for me to research and mentally review rough thematic and design approaches. To develop a working schedule, the first move I make is to contact the corporate secretary. From him, I learn two important things: (1) the annual meeting will be held the fourth Thursday of April, but (2) he wants the report out in sufficient time to make a double solicitation of proxies, so that there is excellent voting representation at the annual meeting.

My next move is a meeting with the mailing house. The account supervisor will advise me on the number of days required for mail processing in-house and the number of days required for postal delivery. From this information, I know that the mailing house needs the completed report on the first weekend of March. Month 3, weekend 1, is the target date. From there on in, everything flows backward on the calendar. Week 1, therefore, is not theme development week but printing and binding week. Other major steps are factored into the schedule, including such items as the release of financials from the controller's department, the length of time for typesetting and platemaking, and the CEO's annual skiing trip in late January.

From the delivery date, my schedule works like this:

Weeks 1–2:   Printing and binding.
Week 3:   Final revisions and platemaking.
Week 4:   Sign-off by controller and outside auditor on silver prints.

Week 5:   Final keyline and paste-up of copy.

Week 6:   Author's alterations on type and addressing of mailing lists.

Week 7:   Typesetting of all financials and management letter.

Week 8:   Delivery of financial text and type specifications by designer.

Week 9:   Type specifications and setting of text materials.

Week 10:   Delivery of preliminary color proofs for checking and color correction.

Week 11:   Completion of photo layouts and retouching.

Week 12:   Finalize working layout with approval by CEO.

Week 13:   Production of final text copy and photos.

Week 14:   Completion and approval of preliminary copy drafts.

Week 15:   Order paper stock and envelope.

Week 16:   Comprehensive layout for management approval.

Week 17:   Discuss financials and footnotes with controller, and allocate space.

Week 18:   Review photography. Reshoot or secure new photos as needed.

Week 19:   Select type.

Week 20:   Select paper by size, weight, color. Have blank dummy made to figure postage.

Week 21:   Present preliminary format to senior management.

Week 22:   Have designer working on preliminary layout.

The next step is to extrapolate the schedule backward on the calendar, so that I know the entire process must be well underway by the end of September. The time from Labor Day until Week 22 is devoted to a final review of research materials, copy, and the photo file; a preliminary meeting with senior management; and direction to the designer.

The most frequently committed fatal mistake made by the public relations executive occurs in the last three weeks before mailing. A full year's work can be jeopardized if you sit in your office from the time of the outside auditor's sign-off until your copy of the annual report arrives fresh off the press. Each year, I camp out at the engraving and printing shops, reviewing each piece of film and each printing form as it goes on press—whether that is two o'clock in the afternoon or three o'clock in the morning. It is truly amazing how you can control quality and scrub last-minute errors.

From time to time, annual report producers have tried to explain how to control costs. The most effective means that I have found are simply these: do your homework, conceptualize well, rely on expert suppliers, think each step through thoroughly, follow your schedule, and don't panic.

Opportunity for Excellence

The annual report is a source of pride for the corporation, the shareholders with a stake in the corporation, employees working to make the corporation grow, and the person responsible for putting the report together.

Do not think of it as a yearly burden. Think of it as an opportunity—an opportunity for excellence.

CHAPTER ELEVEN

Corporate Advertising

A VAGUE AND INDEFINITE ART

Mr. X, the CEO of a Fortune 300 company, was sharing the dais at a New York black-tie affair with his counterpart of a Fortune 5 company. Mr. X smarted under the collar when the president of the larger company could not readily grasp the many products, or even the major line, of number 300. Upon his return to the Midwest the next morning, Mr. X ordered his public relations department to start a $250,000 corporate advertising campaign—immediately!

In 1940, Texaco, caught illegally selling oil to the German Air Force, was in deep trouble with the public. It responded by sponsoring the Metropolitan Opera on radio every Saturday afternoon—and it kept sponsoring the Met for over 30 years!

What a vague and indefinite art we practice!

Corporate advertising can be best characterized by the CMC factor: Controversy, Misunderstanding, and Contradiction. These outcomes are not unexpected. There is no reliable record of early corporate advertising expenditures. There is no fully documented record of objectives or achievements. Only recently have there been repositories of outstanding campaigns.

Corporate advertising, as a communication form, is in its infancy compared with other communications techniques, such as product advertising. People refer to it in many ways. And, to paraphrase Winston Churchill, "Never has so little done so much for so many." Despite its aging, maturing, and growing success, corporate advertising is still veiled in a shroud of mystique. Why?

Much of the responsibility, intentional or unintentional, falls on advertising practitioners. Aren't product advertising agencies abdicating their responsibilities when, armed with their knowledge of advertising, they throw up their hands at the thought of dealing with the intangible corporate image? Wouldn't it be worth the investment to secure talent knowledgeable in the maze of the financial community to produce corporate advertising?

Agencies know a good deal about what works in brand advertising,

243

but they are amateurs when it comes to corporate advertising because such advertising is only a marginal part of the business of most agencies. Most of the account executives in agencies nowadays come out of business schools and are trained in marketing, not in public relations or communications. Creative people in advertising agencies know how to talk to housewives about toilet paper, but they're over their heads when it comes to corporate advertising.

What about the public relations agencies? Do they assume full responsibility? Aren't there some that prefer to keep corporate advertising a mystery, and thus ensure the life of the goose that is laying the golden egg? What about the failure of managements to follow the three C's—credibility, consistency, and continuity? Aren't there some that are inclined to snort loudly in a bull market and to hibernate in a bear market? And what about our educational system? Aren't there educators who stress form rather than substance? Aren't there others who try to slot students into specific disciplines?

Corporate communicators are not faultless. There are some who wrap themselves smugly in a cloak of mystery so that they can occupy an office in corporate row while their product advertising counterparts practically sit in a closet. Wouldn't it really be better for the company to have unity rather than friction among its communications people? With so many negatives, how can anyone be convinced of the value of corporate advertising? More important, how can management be convinced of the value in corporate advertising? This chapter will explore the CMC factor to determine "what a vague and indefinite art we practice."

FROM THE BEGINNING

"The trade of advertising is now so near to perfection that it is not easy to propose any improvement." This was written by Dr. Samuel Johnson in 1758. Over the years, the skills and artistry of those who purchase space or time to sell a product have attained a high level of sophistication and effectiveness. Product advertising has been superbly effective. It has informed and persuaded people, moved goods and services, stimulated economies, and made enormous contribution to personal well-being.

But Dr. Johnson was writing about perfection in advertising 150 years before corporate advertising appeared on the American scene. Credit for the oldest continuous corporate advertising program in America goes to American Telephone & Telegraph Company. In the summer of 1908, Theodore N. Vail commissioned the N. W. Ayer & Son advertising agency to launch five advertisements for the company. Vail, a pioneer American industrialist unique in his time for having a sense of social responsibility, had taken over the AT&T presidency during the previous year, at the age of 61. He wanted a national campaign to persuade the American public that AT&T provided excellent service, that its rates were fair, and, above all, that the telephone industry could serve the public best if it were a monopoly.

Vail dreamed of AT&T controlling the telephone and telegraph industries in America. To accomplish that dream, he knew he had to change public opinion. Although Americans then accepted the U.S. Post Office and utilities as monopolies, many favored competition in the telephone business. Ayer's S. A. Conover convinced Vail that mass circulation magazines were the best platform for the sort of persuasive advertising effort Vail had in mind, and that Ayer was the best agency to handle the job. Ayer decided to try a series of advertisements that would sink deep into the hearts of all classes of people that used the telephone—giving them facts and explaining all the problems experienced in running a big telephone company in any part of the country (see Figure 11–1).

The campaign was neither planned nor written to directly increase business. Its objective was to make known and understood the purposes, problems, and policies of the telephone system. It educated people in the use of the telephone and in how to get the best service from the system. The institutional nature of the first ad was apparent immediately. The ad made a strong plea for the public to accept the telephone industry as a monopoly like the Post Office.

The advertising not only accomplished its overt public service objectives admirably, but it also packed considerable sales wallop. During the first five years of the campaign, the company gained over 2 million new subscribers. Soon this strange new phenomenon of public service companies assuming a friendly, public-spirited attitude and using advertising to increase public understanding and goodwill became quite common. Streetcar companies advertised to teach the rules of the road and to allay prejudices. Power companies interpreted electricity as a public service. Railroads promoted "safety first." Among the other pioneers with more than 40 years of corporate advertising were such notables as Container Corporation of America, U.S. Steel, and General Electric (see Figure 11–2).

The two world wars temporarily molded corporate advertising strategy. During these times of world conflict, many products and services were nonexistent or in extremely short supply. Corporate advertising concentrated mainly on "keeping the name before the public" and interpreting the corporation's role in the war effort. After World War II, gradually at first and then with increasing momentum, more and more corporations launched corporate advertising efforts. The objectives of this kind of advertising grew along with the numbers of

246

Figure 11-1
An early AT&T advertisement (1906)

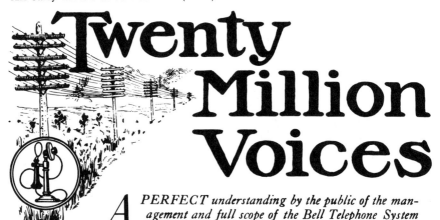

Twenty Million Voices

A PERFECT *understanding by the public of the management and full scope of the Bell Telephone System can have but one effect, and that a most desirable one —a marked betterment of the service.*

Do you know what makes the telephone worth while to you—just about the most indispensable thing in modern life?

It isn't the circuit of wire that connects your instrument with the exchange.

It's the Twenty Million Voices at the other end of the wire on every Bell Telephone!

We have to keep them there, on hair trigger, ready for you to call them up, day or night—downtown, up in Maine, or out in Denver.

And to make the telephone system useful to those Twenty Million other people, we have to keep *you* alert and ready at this end of the wire.

Then we have to keep the line in order— 8,000,000 miles of wire—and the central girls properly drilled and accommodating to the last degree, and the apparatus up to the highest pitch of efficiency.

Quite a job, all told.

Every telephone user is an important link in the system—just as important as the operator. With a little well meant suggestion on our part, we believe we can improve the service—perhaps save a second on each call.

There are about *six billion connections* a year over these lines.

Saving a second each would mean a tremendous time saving to you and a tremendous saving of operating expenses, which can be applied to the betterment of the service.

The object of this and several succeeding magazine advertisements is *not to get more subscribers*. It is to make each one of you a better link in the chain.

First, give "Central" the number clearly and be sure she hears it. Give her full and clear information in cases of doubt. She is there to do her utmost to accommodate you.

Next, don't grow fretful because you think she represents a monopoly. The postmaster does, too, for the same reason.

The usefulness of the telephone is its *universality, as one system.* Where there are two systems you must have two telephones—and confusion.

Remember, the value of the service lies in the number of people you can reach *without* confusion—the promptness with which you get your response.

So respond quickly when others call you, bearing in mind the extensive scope of the service.

The constant endeavor of the associated Bell companies, harmonized by one policy and acting as one system, is to give you the best and most economical management human ingenuity can devise. The end is efficient service and your attitude and that of every other subscriber may hasten or hinder its accomplishment.

Agitation against legitimate telephone business —the kind that has become almost as national in its scope as the mail service—must disappear with a realization of the necessity of universal service.

American Telephone & Telegraph Company

And Its Associated
Bell Companies

LOCAL AND LONG DISTANCE TELEPHONE

One Policy—One System
Universal Service

UNITING OVER 4,000,000 TELEPHONES

Figure 11–2
An early energy conservation advertisement (1916)

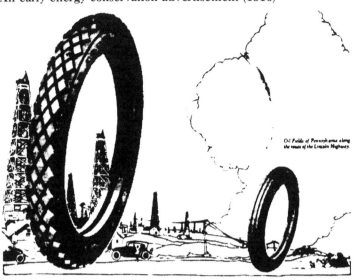

CUTTING DOWN THE NATION'S FUEL BILL

Anything conserving the natural resources of this country is a national asset

We claim this distinction for Goodyear Cord Tires

They conserve one of the most precious energizing forces of this era, gasoline

And it needs to be conserved

If the scientists tell us truly, the gasoline supply of America at the present rate of production and consumption will be exhausted in 27 years more

But were every one of the three million American cars equipped with Goodyear Cord Tires, this supply would last seven years longer, or 34 years

For Goodyear Cord Tires actually effect a saving in gasoline of approximately 25 per cent over ordinary canvas tires

They cut the fuel cost of the nation—in direct and positive proportion to their use

They cut the fuel cost of the individual—paying a separate return, literally in dollars and cents, to every Goodyear Cord user

Nor does their economical advantage stop there

It is so broad, so comprehensive, it affects almost every phase of car operating expense

Goodyear Cord Tires cut general maintenance costs, because any motor works easier and smoother with these lively, athletic tires underwheel

They cut car-parts costs because they ride more comfortably, absorbing road shocks, saving springs and structure

They cut eventual tire cost, because while priced a little higher, they wear longer and go farther

Every advantage to be found in Goodyear Cord Tires traces straight back to their peculiar construction—a construction combining extreme flexibility with extreme strength

They are built up of thousands of cords placed side by side in diagonal layers, without cross-weave each cord and each layer being cushioned in springy rubber

They are master tires—strong and supple both

Their quality makes them higher-priced and better

They come in No Hook and Q D Clincher types, in both All-Weather and Ribbed treads, for gasoline and electric cars

Goodyear Tires, Heavy Tourist Tubes and "Tire Saver" Accessories are easy to get from Goodyear Service Station Dealers everywhere

The Goodyear Tire & Rubber Company, Akron, Ohio

GOODYEAR
AKRON
CORD TIRES

corporations involved, as did the corporations' skill in the strategy and execution of such advertising.

With the economic downturn of the late 1950s, many companies, pressed for communications dollars, discovered the budget-stretching value of corporate advertising. Considerable correlation and even overlapping between corporate and product advertising began to develop. Companies realized that overall corporate objectives could be interwoven with product advertising and that corporate advertising could sell products.

With the dawn of the 1960s came a ground swell that was to change the role of corporate advertising forever. First came the ABC–XYZ craze, with companies changing their long, no longer descriptive, corporate names to initials. Along came the "merge-surge" and the "conglomerate urge." Some companies were advertising that they had power and growth because they were conglomerates. "Buy our stock" was the stock thrust beyond their advertising. Other companies flashed their peacock feathers in search of takeover candidates. Their attitude was, "Hey, get married to us. Look how wonderful we are."

Finally, corporations were besieged with a series of unrelenting and unending shock waves. Some of the issues are still vivid, while others blur in the minds of advertisers and consumers. Do you remember the supersonic transport, the oil import quota system, recycling centers, effluents, emissions, catalytic converters, electrostatic precipitators, and phosphate detergents? How about minority rights, equal employment opportunity, the ERA, black power, product labeling, civil rights, cyclamates, mileage labeling on new cars, the energy shortage, drug addiction, the Pinto gas tank, television advertising, and grade labeling on tires? Will consumers need to tell the dealer they want a number 80 slant 3 star slant B polysteel belted AH 78 dash 15 radial with whitewalls?

There were Ralph Nader, women's liberationists, student and minority dissidents, consumer advocates, rights advocates, and disenchanted consumers—all with a sense of frustration and alienation. Then, there were the business issues—capital formation, foreign trade, overregulation of business, business concentration, productivity, international payoffs, OSHA, nuclear power and hazardous waste disposal, and FTC.

The 1980s have been described as the "dangerous decade" and a time of turmoil. Issues on the scene were fractionalized publics, inflation, rising expectations and the sense of entitlements, lack of credibility of any institutions, the decline of the United States as a world power, the reemergence of black rights, energy, the increase of self-centeredness, and the aging of the public. The impacts have stemmed from economic, social, and political bases. They have changed the business situation dramatically. Business managers are being forced to deal with issues that heretofore were considered the domain of politics. It is truly unfamiliar—and uncomfortable—territory. The corporation must cope with a galaxy of external, seemingly extraneous, forces. Few of these forces are under corporate control. Few of them ever will be.

WHAT'S MY LINE?

The nature and extent of corporate product advertising is far easier to document than the nature and extent of corporate image advertising. To begin with, image advertising is very hard to define. And defining this communication form is no more difficult than trying to find a name for it. First, it is known by many names: advocacy advertising, capability advertising, competence advertising, corporate advertising, corporate image advertising, correctional advertising, general promotional advertising, goodwill advertising, idea advertising, identity advertising, insitutional advertising, issue-oriented advertising, paid message advertising, public relations advertising, public service advertising, strategic advertising, and umbrella advertising. Add to this more recent specialty names such as crisis advertising, economic education advertising, controversy advertising, and consumerism advertising, and then add your own term.

In 1958, Publishers Information Bureau began a classification of corporate advertising as general promotion. In broad terms, general promotion advertising may be defined as devoted primarily to selling the corporate personality; its first objective goes beyond the direct sale of a single product or service. For an advertisement to be classified as general promotion, PIB says that it must fulfill one or more of the following qualifications: to educate, inform, or impress the public with regard to the company's policies, functions, facilities, objectives, ideals, and standards; to build favorable opinion about the company by stressing the competence of its management, its scientific knowhow, manufacturing skills, technological progress, and product improvements; its contribution to social advancement and public welfare; on the other hand, to offset unfavorable publicity and negative attitudes; to build up the investment qualities of its securities, or to improve its financial structure; and to sell the company as a good place to work such advertising is often designed to appeal to college graduates or people with certain skills).

PIB includes aerospace advertising in general promotion advertising. The PIB definition and reason are that all advertisements whose major emphasis is on corporate participation in the space program are considered aerospace advertising. In the broad sense, this includes spacecraft, satellites, space communication systems, missiles and rockets, radar, control systems, Polaris submarines, and components and materials used in these. In no case does PIB consider consumer product advertisements as aerospace advertising.

Business Week has described corporate advertising thus:

> Corporate advertising is an important tool in building a favorable reputation in the selling process. As product advertising promotes product advantages, corporate advertising promotes reputation—what people

think of the company behind the product or service. Corporate advertising has many audiences: Customers, the general business community, sales and distribution channels, the plant community, bankers, brokers, investors, employees, stockholders, labor leaders, thought leaders, special-interest critics, politicians, government and—the general public. Corporate advertising takes many forms. It may be a simple display of the complete product line or a complex statement of a controversial matter. It may be designed to introduce directly a new corporate name or mark. Or it may seek a more subtle objective by building a political constituency to influence legislation. Ultimately, corporate advertising's purpose centers on one goal: to build an identity and a reputation which will improve a company's prospects for sales, growth and profits.[1]

Many communicators really have no set definition as to just what corporate advertising is. For some, it is advertising that doesn't sell anything. For others, it is a quasi-political effort, aimed at wooing the goodwill and favor of legislators and assorted government officials. Still others view corporate advertising as a way to jack up the market price of the company's stock, or improve a company's community relations, or open doors for a company's salespeople.

The truth is that corporate advertising is none of these and all of these, for corporate advertising is what you mean it to be. It begins with a long-range corporate objective separate and distinct from, but essentially related to, the marketing of a product or service.

Consider this simple definition: Corporate advertising attempts to explain a corporation—to whatever audiences may be important to that corporation's future. It is a company talking about itself. For this reason, the preparation of such advertising can involve more executive suite fireworks than almost any other form of corporate communications.

Many corporate controllers define corporate advertising as a frill that represents a very inviting target during any budget-cutting program.

CORPORATE ADVERTISING VIEWPOINTS

Institutional advertising is something like peeing in the pants of a blue serge suit. It gives you a nice, warm feeling, but no one else notices it.
LEO BURNETT, Leo Burnett Company, Inc.

One major mission in corporate advertising is to reach, inform, and we hope to impress the investment community—analysts, fund managers, individual investors, stockholders, bankers, and others in a position to offer or confirm investment advice.
WILLIAM T. YLVISAKER, Chairman of the Board, Gould, Inc.

---

[1] "ABC's of Corporate Advertising," *Business Week*, undated.

If you're in the brand business, you have to go for brand advertising or your brand dies. Very few of the big brand advertisers do have corporate advertising.
DAVID OGILVY, Director, Ogilvy & Mather International, Inc.

I submit that there is no such special breed as "corporate advertising." There is only one kind of advertising. It's just plain old advertising, a highly pragmatic method of getting people to do something.
PAUL C. HARPER, JR., Chairman and Chief Executive Officer, Needham, Harper & Steers, Inc.

The Professional View

While the above statements on corporate advertising are not diametrically opposed, they do reflect varied interpretations on the subject. Further, the variances would grow with each name added to the list. Vagaries persist. Among the views that have been expressed within the profession is the view that preparing corporate advertising requires more attention than developing a campaign for a national packaged goods brand. How much easier it is for a consumer to grasp hold of a can of orange juice, even enjoy the taste, than to grasp and retain a corporate image, let alone be convinced of its credibility. Because corporate advertising is comparatively new and subordinate to the direct promotion of products and services, surprisingly little is known about this form of paid communication—what is expected of it, who can best use it, or how it works.

My own view is that a company has many elements to work with in the development of the corporate personality, whereas the product advertising person may have only one element—a sense of taste, or smell, or sight, or sound—with which to give his product a personality. Moreover, that the same techniques of research, objective setting, evaluation, copy writing, and creativity are available to both. Thus, the development of corporate advertising can be as simple as, or easier than, product advertising.

Even Leo Burnett, as years passed, was to modify his opinion of corporate advertising by saying, "If it accurately reflects the company's deeds, corporate advertising can enhance the public's perception of the company. But if corporate advertising is contradicted by a company's deeds, it is worse than useless." He went to the heart of *all* communications with that bit of philosophy.

The Management View

Because of the growing acceptance of corporate advertising, one might conclude that it is a universal subscribed to by all but the extremely shy or naive. That certainly would be the impression of corporate leaders based on a *National Geographic* study.[2]

The top managements of Fortune's 500 were surveyed on corporate advertising attitudes. One of the major findings was that regardless of product line, sales volume, or ad dollars spent, top management generally regarded corporate advertising favorably (see Table 11–1).

Table 11–1
Are corporate ads highly regarded?

Yes	72%
No	25
No opinion	3

Source: William S. Sachs and Joseph Chasin, "How Top Executives View Corporate Advertising," *Public Relations Journal*, November 1976, pp. 20–21. Copyright © 1976, Public Relations Society of America.

The preponderance of favorable attitudes in the survey was surprising in view of the fact that the influences of corporate advertising are long term and subtle, that measurement is difficult. Communicators no longer face an unsympathetic or uninformed management, according to the survey. Rather, current conflicts, when they exist, arise from a sophisticated management's understandable insistence on greater efficiency from campaigns. This was evidenced by management's contention that some corporations could use corporate advertising to better advantage than others, depending on the products marketed (see Table 11–2).

These highly encouraging results were not shared, however, by the *Gallagher President's Report*, which showed that not many company executives saw the worth of corporate advertising since 78.8 percent did not conduct corporate advertising campaigns. Moreover, 65.1 percent of the respondents without corporate advertising programs thought that such advertising failed to affect the market price of stocks. The same survey revealed that 87.2 percent of the respondents viewed product quality as a key concern of consumers, yet only 49.9 percent had programs to measure consumer satisfaction with goods and services!

[2] William S. Sachs and Joseph Chasin, "How Top Executives View Corporate Advertising," *Public Relations Journal*, November 1976, pp. 20–21. Copyright © 1976, Public Relations Society of America.

Table 11-2
Who benefits most from corporate advertising?

| | | Management of Companies whose main product line is: | | |
| | Percent of executives | *Consumer goods* | *Producer goods* | *Both equal* |
Product				
High-priced consumer goods	79%	74%	84%	73%
Packaged goods	61%	51%	67%	68%
Industrial products	72%	72%	72%	64%
Base	618	234	249	105

Source: William S. Sachs and Joseph Chasin, "How Top Executives View Corporate Advertising," *Public Relations Journal*, November 1976, pp. 20–21. Copyright © 1976, Public Relations Society of America.

Another study revealed that what business executives want most from corporate advertising is the feeling that the advertiser is an honest company. But this attribute isn't coming through. Attributes which executives would have liked to see but were not seeing in corporate advertising were "honesty," which placed first, beating out "helps control inflation," "quality products," and "truth in advertising." Such traditional corporate ad themes as "pays good dividends" and "leader in its field" finished low on the list, but "competent management" was a close second to "honesty."

Why don't more managements use corporate advertising? Other than the general disbelief of some in its effectiveness, no specific reasons have been uncovered for not using it. One interesting facet is why managements *stop* corporate advertising, even after having conducted successful programs. There were, of course, a great number of dropouts during the 1973–74 market plunge. Many companies never resumed despite the disclaimers that their advertising had many noble objectives; that the advertising was not merely to push the stock price.

But there have been dropouts even in the 1980s, for some very unusual reasons. One company said that it had ceased corporate advertising because it started a commission plan for its salespeople and needed the money for the commissions. Another company suspended its program, after several years, because it was building a new plant and needed the money for that purpose. Two other companies stopped regular space programs in order to sponsor the Winter Olympics. A Wisconsin firm said that it wanted to look good before the residents of the state, where the North American speed skating qualifications for the Winter Olympics were being held. Then there was the company that underbudgeted the furnishings and open house for its new corpo-

254

rate office building. It is easy to guess the source of the necessary funds.

The "Street" View

Studies of how investment professionals rank their most important sources of information provide a clue to the credibility problem facing corporate advertisers, because corporate advertising always ranks last behind all other forms of communications. Realistically, not many communicators expect advertising to rank "on the Street" as the most important source of information, because a company would be in trouble if an analyst had to rely on advertising to get significant facts and figures about it.

Therefore, the *Barron's* "Money Manager Survey" is quite revealing (see Table 11–3). Its results are interesting because very few people—especially financial professionals—want to admit that they are influenced by advertising or public relations. Yet, in candid discussions with analysts, I have found many who were surprisingly familiar with advertising themes that they were supposedly avoiding. Some admitted that their curiosity had been stimulated by ads, while many had even requested reprints of ads so as to have them available in their offices. Keep in mind that money managers are human. They read, watch TV, hear speeches, read the business press, and see ads. They absorb all of these.

The Trade View

Many professionals within public relations have a low regard for corporate advertising. They point with disdain to statements about "making things better" or "serving you in a variety of ways" or "are with it" or "doing amazing things." They also note that the following surface time and again:

Photos of the factory	Sales and earnings graphs
Bogus heartiness	Exclamation points
Ponderous humor	Trite graphics
List of products	Founding dates
Fake humility	Tired ideas
Photos of the sales force	Photos of the founders

Gleaned from the communications community are such descriptions as bland, platitudinous, irrelevant, blatantly self-serving, completely sterile, safe, dull, boring, counterproductive, stolid, unimaginative, hardly worth investing money in, belligerent, aggressive, attacks its audience, as exciting as jumping off a pancake, pompous, dull generalities instead of specifics, boring hard-sell copy or vague

Table 11–3
Money managers' views on corporate advertising

Do you consider a "corporate image" important?

	Percent
Yes	90.1%
No	9.1
Not stated	0.8
Total	100.0%
Number of respondents	(373)

Has so-called corporate image or institutional advertising ever served to call your attention to or led you to look into a company's investment qualifications?

	Percent
Yes	78.3%
No	21.4
Not stated	0.3
Total	100.0%
Number of respondents	(373)

In your opinion, does such corporate image advertising favorably affect the value of a company's securities?

	Percent
Yes	75.9%
No	20.9
Not stated	3.2
Total	100.0%
Number of respondents	(373)

Source: "Money Managers Survey," Barron's, 1977.
Copyright © 1977, Dow Jones & Co.

soft-sell copy, distracting graphics, lack of credibility, condescending or cute copy, and phony claims about corporate responsibility.

The buffeting of corporate advertising appears to have reached a peak in the mid-1970s, a few years after the debacle in ecology advertising. What disturbed many was the apparent assumption underlying some of the environmental advertising that creating an appearance of environmental consciousness could substitute for the reality of action—form over substance. The Council on Economic Priorities Report on Corporate Advertising and the Environment concluded that many environmental ads were false and some "subtly co-opt . . . the public's right to free and informed decision making in this area of vital concern."

One critic claimed that advertising "now owns the word *ecology*." That same critic also claimed that "most of industry still sees pollution and environment questions as more of a public relations problem—in other words, an image problem—than as anything fundamentally related to the way they are doing business." Typical substitutions which sprang up were "prostitution" for "pollution" and "ecopornography" for "ecology."

A second buffeting of corporate advertising occurred in the early 1980s with the outpouring of advertising by the oil companies. Opinion polls showed that more than 50 percent of the population did not believe there was an oil crisis. The "safe" advertising concentrated on gasoline conservation, with the result that the use of oil dropped 2.7 percent in 1980.

Several oil companies, however, spewed forth messages about the billions of dollars they were spending on finding oil resources at "home"—in the good old U.S.A.—so that the country would not be dependent on foreign oil. This was when the *Oil and Gas Journal*, the industry trade book, was reporting that 1980 domestic oil production was approximately 8.5 million barrels a day compared with the 1970 figure of 9.6 million barrels a day. And the industry was wondering why it had a credibility problem!

Public relations professionals, while admitting to the "corporate ego" and the poor quality of some campaigns, took vehement exception to running oil company corporate advertising for either of the above reasons.

Corporate advertisers indicate strongly that there must be a need to communicate. That need is determined by extensive research. Research will identify the problem. With knowledge of the problem, a company can establish goals or objectives. These goals or objectives are then translated into an action plan. Once the action plan is placed in motion, research is used to determine its effectiveness.

Who Runs the Show?

One of the side battles that continuously rages around corporate advertising is over who is the power on the throne of decision—the public relations executive or top management. Many public relations professionals believe they play a major role in shaping corporate advertising policies and practices. Certainly, they are involved significantly in concept, theme, budget, and media selection, according to numerous surveys among leading advertisers. Corporate advertising originates in the public relations department 58 percent of the time compared to only 14.5 percent for the advertising department, 13 percent for top management, and 14.4 percent for public relations in advertising agencies.

But another school of thought believes that corporate advertising, or at least its purpose and strategy, lies in the realm of top management, with execution being the province of the public relations department. This school sees corporate advertising as a function of senior management, and no longer as merely an element of marketing or as wordsmiths for the president's office.

Ogilvy states,

> In my judgment, which is also the judgment of my great hero, Marvin Bower of McKinsey, it is the inescapable duty of the top man in every corporation to define its purpose, and to define it in a way that will be relevant far into the future. It's rare for anybody in a corporation to think more than six months ahead, except sometimes the head of the corporation. Unlike product advertising, corporate advertising is the voice of the chief executive and his board of directors.[3]

Philip S. Boone, senior vice president, Dancer-Fitzgerald-Sample, Inc., goes a step further. He calls the "I Imperative" the condition upon which the success and quality of corporate advertising depends. He explains that there are three elements which must function as one throughout every stage of planning, execution, and administration. These are the corporate chief executive and his immediate management team, the corporation point man, and the agency team. He adds, "Corporate advertising is a tool of corporate management. To make it work it must accurately reflect the attitudes and thinking of top management, and that means that top management must be involved."[4]

Still another school of thought believes that some corporations treat corporate advertising as a kind of safety valve which permits the chief executive to let off steam about his own pet peeves and opinions. And too often corporate advertising is, in fact, a plaything of management—a yo-yo on a string. It does go up and down in importance according to the whim of the CEO. If the corporate pocket is brimming over with excess profits, then the CEO benevolently decides that it's time to throw a few extra bucks in the direction of corporate advertising. But if a recession begins looming on the horizon, the zipper on the corporate pocket closes like greased lightning.

Ideally, management should make a commitment to corporate advertising for a minimum of three years, with a promise that budgets will never fall below the first year—that they will only increase—and that both content selection and creative strategy will be determined for

[3] David Ogilvy, "Creating Corporate Advertising," *Fortune 1978 Corporate Communications Seminar/Europe*, p. 13. Copyright © 1978, Time Inc.

[4] Stuart B. Upson and Philip S. Boone, "The I Imperative," *Fortune 1977 Corporate Communications Seminar*, p. 60. Copyright © 1977, Time Inc.

each 12-month period in advance, because effective corporate communication is not the result of frantic brainstorming sessions.

It is interesting that as the ideological battle for control swirls around corporate advertising, little is said about the role of the advertising executive. The main reason, apparently, is that public relations, unlike the advertising department, has a pipeline into management. The latter is often subordinate to the marketing or sales department. A survey of 108 companies revealed that 65 communications executives, or 60 percent, reported directly to the CEO, 28 percent reported to another key officer such as the executive vice president, and only 12 percent reported to the marketing head. On the other hand, only 30 percent of advertising executives reported to the CEO, while 46 percent reported to the marketing head.

Arguments as to the best person to handle corporate advertising could go on ad infinitum. The real test is to determine the best fit in your organization so that programming and talent fit like a glove on a hand.

The Inner Workings

Corporate advertising is second only to the annual report in ego involvement, misconceptions, unclear ideas, and lack of measurement. Undoubtedly, this is because it gets the same kind of management attention and involvement as the annual report.

Yet, corporate advertising is subject to the same type of research, planning, objective setting, execution, and measurement as the annual report and other forms of communication are.

The Three C's

Any discussion on corporate advertising will bring forth the three C's—credibility, consistency, and continuity. Credibility is uppermost in the minds of corporate communicators because they read survey upon survey showing the decline of faith in our institutions, with advertising faring poorer than the rest. Research indicates that only 5 percent of Americans associate the word *trust* with the word *business*. Too much corporate advertising falls on deaf ears because people do not trust its source.

Corporate advertising must be credible. It is not easy to jump over this hurdle. What may seem totally credible to the advertiser may be anathema to the audience. The advertiser must test advertising for credibility at the inception stage. Otherwise, the advertising could be a waste of money. It is ironic that one of the big movements in corporate advertising—advocacy—is steeped in the lack of trust, or the mistrust, of business in one of America's institutions—the media. As a result, one of Mobil Oil's targets has been the reporting technique of print, television, and radio.

The need for a message, or basic theme, receives harmonious agreement from most advertisers because it means rifling in on targeted objectives rather than using buckshot. The message should be changed only as research calls for change in basic objectives. A new calendar year or a new budget year is an insufficient reason for change. Conversely, if the need for a change is evident in midyear, the change should be made even if the budget boat is rocked.

It appears that more company managements are recognizing what good communications people have tried to tell them for years—that if the objectives of a program are important and sound, it takes time and consistency to achieve them. And if the objectives are not important enough to stick with, every dollar spent on achieving them is sheer waste. Communicators recognize that it takes up to 18 months for an advertising program to make its full impact. They strive, basically, for a three-year program with increasing budgets so that the full potential impact of the program can be achieved.

One study of long-term corporate advertisers showed that 78 percent of the companies used their basic objective for three or more years, with 51 percent using the objective for five years. Only 15 percent directed their advertising at the prime objective for less than two years, and only 7 percent for less than one year. These are the pluses of continuous advertising: it increases remembrance; it improves individual ad readership and cost efficiency; it improves reader attitudes toward a company; it increases product recognition and brand preference among readers; and it lowers selling costs. On the other hand, decreased advertising reduces awareness of brand and company name . . . over both the short and the long run.

One highly important reason for a long-term commitment to corporate advertising is the "churn-over" of your audiences. *Time* magazine produced a study indicating that 78 percent of upward-mobile multinational executives changed titles during a five-year period. As these executives moved up in management positions, they often moved to different companies as well.

Tracking my own mailing lists has disclosed an even higher rate of churn-over in highly desirable audience components. Over a five-year period, I tracked a rate of 35 percent turnover—*annually.* A McGraw-Hill study confirmed that the most important buying influences are often mobile—the ones most likely to move up, over, or out to better jobs. The job turnover of 35 percent of managerial and professional subscribers to McGraw-Hill publications is 2½ years or less; for 5½ years or less it's 60 percent.

Lining Up the Message

The approach toward corporate advertising should be along these lines:

1. The unique nature of your corporation's identity is where the advertising should start. You must learn what that unique nature is and try to project it. Then, you must make sure that by doing homework, the audiences peculiar to your corporation are correctly identified. What worked yesterday may not automatically work today. So, the more work, the greater the rewards. To keep up with change, you must continue the study. There are many corporate communication challenges that simply can't be met by short-term solutions.

2. The secret of successful corporate advertising is simple. Start with the problem, not with the message. Start with the audience, not with the factory. Just as any successful product campaign starts with the consumer, so any successful corporate campaign starts with the segment of the public where action is required.

3. Planning for successful corporate advertising programs starts with the recognition that paid space advertising may not be useful at all. There may be far cheaper and more appropriate ways to reach necessary audiences. Four questions must be asked:

a. What change or action do you desire to bring about—and where?
b. Can the desired change or action really be accomplished by advertising?
c. How much money is this change or action worth to your company?
d. Assuming that advertising is appropriate to the problem, what is the cost-benefit relationship between dollars spent on advertising and dollars spent on other means of persuasion, such as public relations, industry-wide activities, sales promotion, and lobbying?

4. It's a hard fact of life that the only way a corporation gets to be thought of as being a "good guy" is by being a "good guy." Deeds still speak louder than words—performance is the payoff! Verbalizing an intention without taking corresponding action can do more harm than good.

5. When the people responsible for corporate advertising do their homework; when they subject themselves to the same disciplines that are second nature to good marketing people; when they ask, and answer, the same kinds of fundamental questions that invariably precede the execution of effective consumer goods advertising—then corporate advertising can become an important influence on the public's perception of a company.

6. Good corporate advertising derives its effectiveness from clear-cut, attainable objectives. You must know what it is supposed to do if you are to know whether it is accomplishing its purpose.

7. Corporate advertising is supposed to project a corporation's identity in order to reinforce or change the corporation's image. It makes good sense, therefore, to find out what the existing image is before trying to change that image or to communicate a new one.

8. Likewise, corporate advertising that is intended to change people's minds must be preceded by probing, objective analysis of what people really think as opposed to what we think they think. Once who thinks what has been determined, intelligent approaches to changing opinions become possible.

9. The most important decision you will make is how to position your company. You should make that decision before any advertising is written or even attempted. Positioning is how you describe your company to the target audience. These three criteria must be met: your positioning must be distinctive; your positioning must distinguish your company from the great blur of corporate slogans; and your advertising must stand out.

10. Because "image" is difficult to define, it is even more difficult to evaluate. One way to avoid these difficulties is to avoid using image in your corporate advertising. Instead, think in terms of something that can be evaluated, such as an awareness on the part of your audience—about your growth, about your diversity, about your new name or corporate symbol, or about the people who work for you.

Nearly all corporate campaigns appear to be generated by one of two attitudes of management. The first attitude can be stated like this: "We believe that a condition or state exists in the minds of the public that we would like to change, correct, or modify." And the second attitude can be stated in this way: "We would like to tell the public more about our company—what we are, what we're trying to do, what our corporate philosophy is."

While there is considerable soul-searching and wrestling with the corporate image prior to a campaign, there is unanimity that corporate performance is a precondition of successful advertising. Take the example of a company that was in the *Fortune* top 40 in the early 1970s. Its $70 million advertising budget nearly exceeded its profits. By the end of the decade, the company had plunged more than 20 places on the *Fortune* list, and despite massive infusions of advertising dollars, it was struggling to maintain its image. The simple fact was that its basic industry was in a state of decline, and so were company profits—from a margin of 4 percent in the early 1970s to 1 percent a decade later. Advertising was challenged to do the impossible—and couldn't.

What Do You Say?

The person to whom you direct advertising comes tailor-made with his or her beliefs. Advertising goes into the intake valves called senses, with the result that beliefs cause behavior. If you don't know what kinds of human behavior you are trying to affect, you should not spend money on corporate advertising. The key is to find out the beliefs, so that you know how to address them.

In the 1950s and 1960s, corporate advertisers talked about the benefits of bigness, profits, diversity of interests, new products, dedication to research and development, and technological leadership. Corporate advertising featured the corporation as the hero. In the early 1970s, the American public considered a good company to be one that was reliable, was fair to employees of all races, made quality products, gave good value for the money, and paid good wages. In the late 1970s, many companies went on the attack with advocacy advertising, responding to consumer and legislative criticism as it arose. In the early 1980s, companies stayed away from the big issues of inflation and regulation to again talk about dedication and leadership. Thus, when queried on their overriding objective, 50 top advertising executives said that it was awareness.

In a study by Bozell and Jacobs, themes in corporate advertising were ranked in order of their impact on stock prices (see Table 11–4).[5] Bozell and Jacobs used an index score of 100 for the average for all corporate advertising.

Who are the primary and secondary target audiences for the major programs? Relatively few corporate advertisers are reaching for Nirvana—the entire population. Most are after specific segments: upscale economic or education demographics, the "movers and shakers," social and consumer activists, and governmental or political segments.

Pumping the P/E

At the end of a seminar on corporate advertising at which I was a speaker, a participant remarked, "Gee, this is a strange meeting. Two days of talking, and nobody said anything about pumping the P/E." At another seminar, an attendee stated, "My guess is that roughly 98 percent of all corporate advertising is aimed at giving the stock price a massive kick in the pants. Don't let anyone tell you different." And at yet another conference, the president of a Fortune 150 company measured his company's corporate advertising thus: "The program has been successful, since our stock appreciated 11 percent during the two years of our campaign, while the Dow Jones average went down 26 percent."

Concern with reputation in the financial community is one of the

---

[5] Jaye Niefeld, "Corporate Advertising . . . and the Wall Street Payoff Guide for Bottom Line Results," *Industrial Marketing*, July 1980, pp. 69–74. Copyright © 1980, Crain Communications, Inc.

Table 11–4
Effective themes

Theme	Index score
Productivity of labor	116.3
New product announcement	114.8
General puffery	113.1
Product description/claim	111.0
All other	109.6
Basic industry/we're essential	108.5
Need for national policy	106.8
Annual report	106.4
How company helps ecology/conservation	104.4
Sales/earnings growth	102.2
How company helps solve energy crisis	101.5
Bad news about company	101.1
American economic system/free enterprise	99.8
Who we are/diversification	99.3
Company strength/reliability	99.2
Earnings consistency	98.9
World hunger/food production	98.7
Good works by company/employees	98.2
Antigovernment restraints	97.6
Nonfinancial brochure	97.6
Technology/R&D	96.6
Capital formation/shortage	93.8
Number of different themes	93.0

Source: Reprinted with permission from July 1980 issue of *Industrial Marketing.* Copyright © 1980 by Crain Communications, Inc.

reasons most frequently given privately, but least often mentioned publicly, for launching corporate campaigns. But any company which announced that it was embarking on corporate advertising because it wanted to influence its stock price upward would be certain to attract unwelcome attention from the SEC. So companies don't say that. They know, however, that a low P/E ratio will put them in a favorable position for expansion through acquisition or merger, since most such arrangements are based on exchange of stock.

To answer the P/E corporate advertising question, Eugene P. Schonfeld, assistant professor of advertising, and John H. Boyd, Jr., assistant professor of finance, Northwestern University, conducted a massive computer-oriented study of 721 companies over a three-year period.[6] The annual sales of these companies had to be more than $200 million.

---

[6] Eugene P. Schonfeld and John H. Boyd, Jr., "Does Corporate Advertising Affect Stock Prices?" *Fortune 1976 Corporate Communications Seminar,* pp. 67–78. Copyright © 1976, Time Inc.

264

Among the companies were 265 corporate advertisers that spent an average of $90,000 per year. The conclusion drawn by Schonfeld and Boyd: a firm *maybe*.

They confidently concluded that corporate advertising *seemed* to have a positive statistically significant effect on stock prices. Other conclusions, equally forceful, were as follows. The impact of corporate advertising *seemed* greatest in an up market. *Perhaps* the market was in a speculative mood, and *if* you drew attention to yourself, a broader range of investors would consider you. *They really didn't know.* But there was *some* evidence that ad impact was greater in an up market. Many firms could *probably* benefit from spending significantly more on corporate advertising than they now did, if their intention was to affect the price of their stock. There was *some* evidence that firms which *could* report stable earnings growth had more favorable results from their corporate advertising. (Surprisingly, most of the other message effects tested by Schonfeld and Boyd, such as growth in earnings per share, were not consistently significant.)

One of the more forthright views of the impact of corporate advertising on the P/E comes from Carol J. Loomis, of the *Fortune* board of editors. "My advice would be to stop being self-conscious, to stop being at all defensive about any honest, straightforward, law-abiding steps you may take to try to improve the public's opinion of your stock. There are just too many good reasons why you should be doing exactly that."[7]

Advocacy or No?

Capability, whether it is product, technology, or progress, is undoubtedly the backbone of corporate advertising. Across this base have fluttered numerous themes of "with it" advertising—ecology, cyclamates, economic education, and dozens of others.

The latest corporate advertising technique, and because of the money behind, the most powerful, is advocacy advertising. This technique has been used sporadically for decades. Its origin is traced to Carl Byoir, in the late 1930s, when he worked with Great Atlantic & Pacific Tea (A&P) in the company's defense against the national "Death Sentence Bill" which had a discriminatory tax designed to put chain stores out of business. Byoir created an advertising campaign, stressing the stake of consumers. The bill was killed in committee amid overwhelming public opposition.

Starting in the mid-1970s, advocacy advertising was finely honed by the oil companies in response to consumer criticism of their practices, policies, and pricing. Numbers tell the story. At the end of the 1950s,

[7] Carol J. Loomis, "Should a Company Promote Its Own Stock?" *Fortune 1973 Corporate Communications Seminar*, pp. 50–52. Copyright 1973, Time Inc.

the top three oil companies spent only $750,000 on corporate advertising in print. This rose to about $5 million at the end of the 1960s and to about $13 million at the end of the 1970s. The magic of the electronic media has been discovered by the oil companies. They pour more than $50 million annually into network and spot television! But, because advocacy advertising can be used to influence political and legislative processes, it has come under intense scrutiny in both houses of Congress and, at the urging of consumer activists, at the FTC, the Internal Revenue Service, and several state public utility commissions as well.

There is an aggressive, reform-minded regulatory presence in the federal bureaucracy amid the public outcry for fairness, honesty, and informative value in advertising. The fallout for both product and corporate advertising has included these decisions: the FTC granted a Ralph Nader–inspired consumer group free air time to counter the oil industry's well-financed advocacy advertising campaign on energy issues; the FTC imposed a series of stringent restrictions on children's television advertising; and the U.S. Supreme Court ruled that guild restrictions on professional advertising were unconstitutional—setting a precedent for lawyers, doctors, certified public accountants, and other professionals.

The advertising industry generally recognizes that a strict monitoring system is necessary, but the industry argues that it is providing that supervision voluntarily through its highly respected CBBB National Advertising Division and the National Advertising Review Board. Despite the excellent record of these bodies, however, it appears that the advertising industry will have to play a more active and visible role in policing itself and in persuading the public of its good intentions and its intrinsic value. Individual advertisers and their agents will have to step up their self-policing activities and convey their commitment to the public or bear the burden of additional stringent regulatory dictates.

Still, social critics are concerned about the potential domination by business of the public communication space denied to groups that are unable to match the financial resources of the large corporations. These critics are calling for reform of the tax laws dealing with the deductibility of corporate expenditures for advocacy advertising. They are critical of the FTC's failure to impose its advertising substantiation requirements on advocacy advertising. They are prepared to regulate and limit, even to prohibit, corporate communication of ideas in order to avoid possible distortions and biases in advocacy advertising.

U.S. Supreme Court decisions, however, have affirmed the right of corporations to speak publicly on issues that they consider vital to their interests and to expose falsehoods through public education and discussion. Corporate managements contend that they are exercising their right to protect their interests, present their understanding of and solutions to complex social issues in which they have a vital stake, and refute the allegations of corporate critics. They argue that they are performing a vital public service by expanding the scope of the public dialogue on crucial social issues.

The protection of First Amendment speech by corporations is not absolute. While the Supreme Court has affirmed the corporation's right to speak, it has not exempted the corporation from punitive governmental action if the corporation's commercial speech is deceptive, nor has it recognized an absolute right of management to engage in political speech on behalf of the shareholders.

At first, advocacy ads were defensive, coy, and meek, if not timid, about the subjects they discussed. The ads emphasized noble sentiments, for example, in campaigns for blood donations, energy saving, and sobriety. Later, advocacy advertising became more aggressive and militant. By far the most aggressive advertising—discussing such controversial matters as inflation, energy, conservation, environmental protection, nationalism, and the balance of trade—has been run by the big oil companies. While Exxon has been using television, with superbly executed color commercials, Mobil has spent large amounts on a continuing advocacy campaign. Mobil's headlines have become increasingly aggressive, especially in bewailing the fact that no one has been listening.

This trend has become so marked that organizations which never advertised have been galloping into the fray, fighting mad. But the recognized leader is Mobil. Its coordinated program works on several levels. On one level is the company's support of much of the best in public broadcasting. For a company that claims a social conscience, this is visibly putting money where the mouth is. Detractors point out that the results are highly subjective. Mobil is feistier in print. Interesting, provocative, and with a point to make, Mobil uses very direct counterattacks against the adversary. An increasing number of its ads have been treating subjects broader than energy.

Herbert Schmertz of Mobil rationalizes his company's expenditures on advocacy advertising by saying that to finance a point of view is also an indication of whether that point of view has a constituency to support it. Schmertz is on solid ground with regard to Mobil's constituency. Since Mobil began advocacy advertising, its stock has outperformed the market and the oil industry average and the company declared a 2-for-1 stock split.

Measuring effectiveness is the most disputed area of advocacy advertising. The International Advertising Association (IAA) claims that the only research results given to it have been favorable, indicating that a controversy campaign was successful in one or more of its objectives. Some advertisers have been using syndicated services, or doing research themselves, to measure the attitudes of various audiences to controversial issues before and/or after they have undertaken controversy advertising campaigns.

However, IAA notes that advertisers scrupulously avoid any claims that a shift in public opinion about broad issues can be directly traced to their campaigns, and generally take the position that the information about such shifts is confidential. And even more telling, most companies report that they have made no effort to pretest the effectiveness of their controversy campaigns and that they have not attempted to measure the impact of these campaigns.

S. Prakash Sethi was quite direct on this issue. He said,

> An extensive analysis of most of the recent advocacy campaigns has led me to conclude that advocacy advertising, as it is currently being practiced by major corporations and industry groups, with some notable exceptions, is of largely questionable value and doubtful effectiveness on economic, sociopolitical, and ideological grounds. This conclusion is further supplemented by intensive interviews with corporate executives, professionals in advertising agencies and public relations firms, journalists, news editors, academicians, and governmental officials.[8]

A major problem is that corporate campaigns about energy, oil prices, and the environment appear in business media, not mass media. Despite corporate complaints about the unfamiliarity of dissident youth and university professors with corporate endeavor, advocacy advertising does not appear in the so-called radical or intellectual press. This reluctance to run in the right media to reach the target audience raises some questions about the real objective of advocacy advertising, especially when few advertisers express interest in measuring the impact of such advertising through market research. But some advertisers even go so far as to deny that research is possible.

Despite all the advocacy advertising, the public image of business continues to decline. In a survey of public attitudes, business continues to receive low scores for pollution control and for dealing with shortages. The lowest marks go to conservation of natural resources. Among the industries ranked, electric utilities, gas utilities, and oil and gas companies have placed 12th, 13th, and 17th, respectively, though oil and gas companies and utilities have been the heaviest users of advocacy advertising.

The situation is no clearer for campaigns dealing with specific issues and companies. Strangely enough, no company executives admit to conducting tracking studies to evaluate the effectiveness of advocacy campaigns.

Even opinion leaders sympathetic to businessmen's problems have been critical of the approaches taken by various companies in their

---

[8] S. Prakash Sethi, "Advocacy Advertising and the Large Corporations," *Public Relations Journal*, November, 1976, p. 42. Copyright © 1976, Public Relations Society of America.

advocacy campaigns. For example, Professor George C. Lodge of Harvard Business School has said that it is naive for Mobil to think readers will believe a paid advertisement in which an oil company self-righteously proclaims its virtues and hurls blame on those who dare to differ with it.

The problem is not that the public does not believe in the free enterprise system, its misconceptions and misunderstandings about that system notwithstanding, but that people have come to feel that companies put their own interests first at any cost. Americans believe in the free enterprise system. However, campaigns to educate the public about free enterprise are loaded with clichés, so nobody listens.

The bottom line is that despite the millions spent by oil companies on advocacy advertising, more than one half of the people in the United States did not believe there was an energy shortage in the 1970s. The failure of advocacy advertising is traceable to the failure of advocacy advertisers to do their homework.

There are several organizational reasons why advocacy advertisers do not attempt opinion research:

1. Because of top management's remoteness from research procedures, it will not understand or it will tend to misinterpret shifts in attitude scores and scaling procedures.
2. Unfavorable results reported to top management could have serious repercussions without the company, owing to the high level of emotional involvement that is often present.
3. Research scores reflecting favorable results could, in the long run, pose problems by encouraging researchers to base their estimates of future advertising impact on the first round of successful scores.

A number of executives admit that attempts at impact measurement might have negative internal repercussions, discouraging the use of advocacy advertising.

THE PRICE TAG AND WHERE TO USE IT

One billion dollars. That is the price tag which has frequently been attached to corporate advertising at seminars and in numerous articles on the subject since the late 1960s. Facts belie this claim, however.

The True Amount

Each year, the *Public Relations Journal* conducts a broad survey of advertising expenditures by companies and associations. The survey covers consumer magazines, Sunday magazines, network television, spot television, radio, and outdoor.

The latest survey had corporate advertising by companies at approximately $429 million and by associations at about $198 million, for a total of $627 million. Of that amount, companies spent $222 million in magazines.[9] This was a record. Thus, the $1 billion figure is wrong. This is not to say that corporate advertising expenditures have not grown. Quite the contrary. Such expenditures grew 122.8 percent from 1970 to the end of the decade and showed a strong resistance to the mid-70s economic recession (see Table 11–5).

Table 11–5
Growth in corporate advertising expenditure (in $ millions)

	Company advertising	Association advertising	Total	Change
1970	$149,547.3	$ 70,757.0	$220,304.3	—
1971	157,575.8	72,635.5	230,211.3	4.5%
1972	181,810.7	85,859.2	267,669.9	16.3
1973	226,977.5	90,331.6	317,309.1	18.5
1974	224,336.2	87,482.9	311,819.1	(2.0)
1975	210,130.6	95,221.9	305,352.5	(2.1)
1976	292,724.9	117,717.5	410,442.4	34.4
1977	329,268.0	145,086.1	474.354.1	15.6
1978	330,716.3	160,090.7	490,809.0	3.5
1979	393,864.8	187,258.6	581,123.4	18.4
1980	429,267.8	198,228.2	627,496.0	7.9

The energy situation in the 1970s had an obvious impact on the corporate advertising expenditures of the oil companies. At the end of the 1950s, only two companies, Standard Oil (New Jersey) and Shell Oil were in the top 10 corporate advertisers in business publications—7th and 10th, respectively. The others were General Motors, General Electric, Boeing, General Telephone & Electronics, Borg-Warner, American Telephone & Telegraph, International Nickel of Canada, and Lockheed Aircraft.

By the end of the 1960s, Shell Oil and Standard Oil were still the only two oil companies in the top 10. Shell Oil had moved up to fourth place, but Standard Oil had dropped to ninth. The other familiar names from the previous decade were General Motors, General Electric, and AT&T, with International Paper, Chrysler, International Business Machines, Ford, and North American Rockwell replacing the other five companies. With the sharp focus on energy in the 1970s, 7 oil companies were among the top 10 by the end of the decade. Joining Shell Oil and Exxon were Gulf Oil, Texaco, Phillips Petroleum, Atlantic Richfield, and Mobil. The only nonoil survivors from earlier lists were AT&T, General Motors, and IBM.

Is the Medium the Message?

We have looked into television and radio advertising, but we cannot use it because of cost.

Television is an area in which I frankly don't know very many answers, and I don't know who does.

These are typical responses given by small and medium-sized corporate advertisers when they were queried about looking beyond print advertising. These advertisers appear to have been justified from the standpoint of measurement effectiveness and cost. Bozell and Jacobs did not include electronic media in its study, with the simple explanation that the state of the art wasn't up to doing content analyses of television commercials in a way that it found totally satisfactory. However, the firm did feel fairly confident about doing content analyses of print ads.

McGraw-Hill made a study on the use of television to sell industrial products in Philadelphia.[10] It contacted 315 buying influences with these results: phone not answered, 32.1 percent; buying influence not home, 21.6 percent; buying influence not watching television, 34.3 percent; watching other television program, 9.8 percent; watching program in question, 2.2 percent; and could identify sponsor, 0.6 percent. The Yankelovich, Skelly and White study for *Time* magazine tended to corroborate these results, though giving television much higher scores. The *Time* study stated that affluent, well-educated men and women did more reading than viewing. The average score for reading print was 37 percent, while the average score for watching television was 31 percent.

Each medium communicates in a different way and has something different to offer. The broadcast media project a "now or never" message form, while the print media provide longer lasting information. The long life of magazines, the advocates of this print medium will argue, is especially important for corporate advertising, which seeks to build and maintain a psychological franchise with target publics. The Magazine Publishers Association (MPA) scrutinized the inherent ability of magazines, television, and radio to concentrate impact on prime targets.[11]

MPA divided the exposure to each medium into three segments—

---

[10] *Laboratory of Advertising Performance*, no. 1055.2, pp. 1–6, McGraw-Hill Research.

[11] *Newsletter of Research*, March 1974, Magazine Publishers Association.

the heaviest two quintiles (40 percent) of U.S. adults, defined as *heavy* exposure; the third, or middle, quintile (20 percent), termed *moderate* exposure; and the lightest two quintiles (40 percent), classified as *light* exposure. On this basis, MPA examined the three primary demographic target groups: *graduated college, professional/managerial, and $25,000 and over household income.*

The results showed that 84 percent of all advertising dollars invested in a radio campaign were consumed by the heavy listeners, which accounts for only 38 percent of U.S. college graduates, 40 percent of all professional/managerial men and women, and 42 percent of adults living in households with $25,000 or more income. It was obvious from these facts, MPA contended, that radio placed too much emphasis on the heavy listeners and too little emphasis on both the moderate and light listeners to effectively communicate the corporate advertising message.

Television, too, was sharply out of balance in reaching the three primary demographic target groups. Only 23 percent of college graduates, 27 percent of professional/managerial people, and 28 percent of the $25,000 and over group were heavy viewers of television. According to MPA, advertisers were placing far too much emphasis on television, given its subpar penetration of the target groups.

Corporate advertising in magazines, however, was right on target, said MPA, placing corporate ad dollars in near-perfect balance with the parallel concentration of key target demographic groups, as illustrated in Table 11–6.

Many advertisers feel that no matter how effective television may be, the fact remains that it is overcrowded and overpriced. Why, then, in spite of the evidence, do corporations put their advertising dollars into television over print at a spending ratio of 5 to 2? Why is 40 cents out of every corporate advertising dollar plugged into television? Why has advocacy advertising, conceded by some people to be unmeasurable, become the darling of the tube?

Apparently, broadcast has its place. Radio, for example, is instrumental in reaching commuting businesspeople and shareholders during morning and evening drive time. Television is big, powerful, magical, and it can provide immediate national impact. The feeling is that TV may not be the right corporate advertising medium for every company, but for the company that wants to make a significant impact quickly, television can carry a heavy communications load.

For the average corporate advertiser, the stumbling block of television is cost. Corporate advertisers can buy a full year's program in print for less than the cost of six commercials on a "soap," 45 seconds on a topflight comedy, and 30 seconds on the Super Bowl—and forecasts already in hand predict a 300 percent increase in the cost of television commercials by 1990.

272

Table 11–6
Primary target shares by magazine reading (adults)

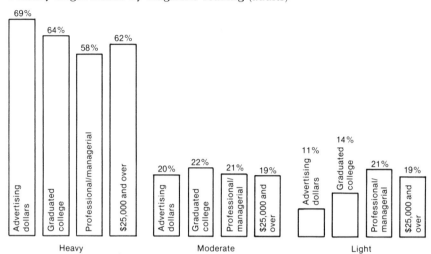

Heavy   Moderate   Light

Source: W. R. Simmons; *Newsletter of Research,* March 1974, Magazine Publishers Association.

IS CORPORATE ADVERTISING EFFECTIVE?

We get a lot of coupons back, so we know that our corporate advertising is successful.

This sole measure of effectiveness from an advertising executive in a multimillion-dollar company would stun communicators from companies a fraction of the size. But the statement was made, and it merely fans the flames for those who believe that corporate advertising measurement is elusive.

Deterrents to Effective Use

The most comprehensive study on the effectiveness of advertising was conducted by Arthur D. Little, Inc. Although Arthur D. Little concentrated on industrial advertising, it evaluated 1,100 research studies and came to conclusions that are appropriate as guidelines for corporate advertising research.[12] In general, Arthur D. Little saw four deterrents to the effective use of advertising research, none of them valid. In brief, they were as follows.

1. *The world will not stop turning.* New forms of marketing effort come along constantly. Each can distort data being gathered in existing

---

[12] American Business Press, Inc., "The Arthur D. Little Report: An Evaluation of 1100 Research Studies on the Effectiveness of Industrial Advertising."

efforts to measure advertising effectiveness. To avoid this distortion, one must, as the statistician terms it, remove "nuisance variables." When these variables are removed, the world, in effect, does stop turning. With sophisticated statistical analysis techniques, you evaluate the effectiveness of advertising in the presence of your own or your competitor's activities. It can be done with "historical data," as in the Morrill Study.

2. *The buying cycle is too long.* This problem is overcome by modifying the research design. An industrial goods advertiser cannot afford the luxury of waiting for the brand-switching phenomena to occur; he must monitor significant shifts in buying patterns. Methods for carrying out such monitoring have been described in numerous studies on purchase influences. One procedure consists of interrogating recent purchasers in a given product category along the following lines: Which brands did you consider buying? Which brand did you buy? Why did you *not* buy brand U? V? W? The information thus gathered permits analysis of what is important and leads to corrective action.

3. *Our business is different.* Another deterrent at work is the belief that the results of one company's study cannot be applied to another company. This belief is erroneous. Studies done for certain clients and their findings may be fully useful only to those clients. However, the results surely are applicable in part to other situations.

4. *Global and small-bite approaches.* Many advertisers are caught on the horns of a dilemma—whether to undertake "total research" or "piecemeal research," the latter being intended to answer specific problems. Total research means tackling the entire problem of allocating marketing funds among forms of marketing effort on a company basis. Piecemeal research means tackling day-to-day issues on a brand-by-brand basis. (How much in this medium? Which vehicle? What creative campaign?) As a result of this dilemma, some advertisers become immobile and do neither. There are always risks of "suboptimization" in tackling only a piece of a problem, but these appear to be outweighed by the risk of attempting the impossible. Thus, the solution to the dilemma is to accurately gauge the smallest "bite" that will yield useful results.

The Global Approach

Large corporate advertisers have no problem budgeting for continuing, large-scale studies by the leading research firms—the global approach. When United Aircraft changed its name to United Technologies, it directed an extensive advertising campaign to the financial community and its customers. This was followed by an in-depth study which showed that its key audiences were aware of the change, so United Technologies did not have to shout so loud about it. Rather, it directed the company and its agency, Marsteller, Inc., into *why* it changed its name.

The Small-Bite Approach

For some advertisers, the small-bite approach can be a valuable means for getting ongoing measurements. Each small bite may be inconclusive, but a useful pattern may emerge from adding different small bites together. Pitney-Bowes, for example, looks to its own 2,500-member sales force for part of its research, in the belief that among the more accurate barometers for measuring the impact of its advertising is the person who carries the bag from day to day, making calls on customers and prospects. For added measurement, the company conducts an annual survey of the value of advertising leads, since in one year it delivered to its salespeople over 350,000 leads resulting from communications.

Lead qualification can also aid in tracking actual orders and in evaluating various phases of an advertising program. For example, the water and wastewater group of Trans Union Corporation generated almost 10,000 leads from advertising, compared to only 87 leads generated when Trans Union featured its finance leasing group in its advertising. Tracking these leads turned up one very surprising piece of information. It was found that the 10,000 water and wastewater treatment leads were converted into $3 million in sales but that the 87 finance leasing leads were converted into $10 million in sales!

Another small-bite approach is to measure the response to literature offerings. One insurance company advertising department had a big surprise when this measurement tipped the scale in favor of advertising. Advertising department members were using standard research and various other types of feedback, but management didn't "feel" any effect. Then a literature offering brought in more than 400,000 requests. Management was sold. For both the global and the small-bite approach, the key to it all is to do as good a job with your corporate advertising planning as you do with your product advertising. Then you'll be able to measure your results.

The Benchmark Study

There is an implicit need for a benchmark study prior to corporate advertising. The benchmark study proved vital in the success of the "Come to Shell for Answers" campaign sponsored by Shell Oil Company.

Shell employed survey research in the conduct of its advertising and its public affairs. At various times, it participated in multiclient syndicated studies as well as proprietary tracking surveys of public attitudes and behavior. In these ways, Shell amassed a substantial body of information on the concerns, perceptions, and beliefs of American society.

These studies showed with remarkable unanimity the low credibility of the oil industry, whose representatives rated comparatively low, while oil company issue advertising was among the least believed forms of public communication. Shell concluded that if it was to use corporate advertising to address the electorate about concerns, it would have to begin by improving its credibility. Shell decided that it could do so by directing advertising, not to its own problems, but to those of the general public. Since the United States is a nation where 83 percent of the people over 16 are licensed automobile drivers, almost all of the electorate have done, or will do, business with Shell or its competitors.

Examining research data, Shell found that public concerns included environmental conservation, consumer needs, and economic anxieties. It decided to match consumer-oriented corporate policies and an advertising program responding to the needs of American drivers for better information on the care, maintenance, and use of their automobiles. Thus, "Come to Shell for Answers" came into being.

From that benchmark, Shell used diagnostic research to apply the budgeted expenditures in the most effective manner. For example, it learned early in the program that although the program was being extremely well received, it was not improving public attitudes toward Shell as much as had been hoped. Data showed that sponsor identification in the television advertising was weak. Corrective changes were made in the ads to improve the visibility of Shell's sponsorship and to associate Shell more effectively with the good results that were being achieved.

Research and Measurement

The extent to which companies research their corporate advertising was studied by Dr. William Sachs and Dr. Joseph Chasin, of the College of Business Administration, St. John's University, Jamaica, New York (see Tables 11–7, 11–8, 11–9, and 11–10).

Yankelovich/Phase I[13]

The most massive, prestigious, and telling research on corporate advertising was done by Yankelovich, Skelly and White, Inc., in stud-

---

[13] *A Study of Corporate Advertising Effectiveness Conducted by Yankelovich, Skelly and White, Inc. 1977 for Time Magazine*, Report no. PR. 1206.

Table 11–7
Evaluation of effectiveness of corporate advertising

Are your corporate advertising objectives specific
enough to be measured as to effectiveness?

	Percent
Yes	84
No	23
Don't know	7

Have you conducted such research?

	Percent
Yes	84
No	30

If yes, how frequently is it conducted?

	Percent
Continuously	28
Annually	21
Biannually	12
Irregularly	10
No answer	13

Source: William S. Sachs and Joseph Chasin, "How
Top Executives View Corporate Advertising," *Public
Relations Journal*, November 1976, pp. 20–21. Copy-
right © 1976, Public Relations Society of America.

Table 11–8
Monitoring of corporate advertising

Frequency of monitoring	Percent of all corporate advertisers
Regular basis	48
Selective basis, individual programs	35
Did not monitor	17
Base	(208)

Source: William S. Sachs and Joseph Chasin, "How
Top Executives View Corporate Advertising," *Public
Relations Journal*, November 1976, pp. 20–21. Copy-
right © 1976, Public Relations Society of America.

Table 11-9
Information sources used in assessing
corporate advertising

Sources of information used	Percent of companies assessing corporate advertising
Market research	90
Letters from public	49
Officers' opinions in own company	48
Feedback from sales force	38
Comments in media	23
Stock prices	11
Sales, shipments, billings	5
Other	2
Base	(173)

Source: William S. Sachs and Joseph Chasin, "How
Top Executives View Corporate Advertising," *Public
Relations Journal,* November 1976, pp. 20–21. Copy-
right © 1976, Public Relations Society of America.

Table 11-10
Types of measurement used in evaluating
corporate advertising

Type of measurement	Percent of use
Awareness of company/products	80
Company "image"	76
Recall of advertising	75
Changes in attitudes toward company/products	71
Number of inquiries, requests for brochures	47
Changes in attitudes toward point of view expressed	32
Sales, orders	7

Source: William S. Sachs and Joseph Chasin, "How
Top Executives View Corporate Advertising," *Public
Relations Journal,* November 1976, pp. 20–21. Copy-
right © 1976, Public Relations Society of America.

ies commissioned by *Time* magazine. The study methodology of the first Yankelovich study involved personal, in-home interviews with 700 business executives in the top 75 markets. All of those interviewed had individual incomes of $25,000 or more. Ten corporations were studied—five that currently did corporate advertising and five that did not.

The first study found that corporate advertising had a real and measurable effect on the attitudes of this key target audience. Even holding constant each of the four background factors—total advertising expenditures, gross revenues, earnings per share, and recent stock price—the conclusion remained the same. Yankelovich/Phase I produced very impressive findings. But, like any good research, it raised as many questions as it answered:

1. Would the initial results hold up against a broader target audience and across a wider spectrum of corporations and industries?
2. Were the results applicable when applied to consumers versus industrial corporations? Larger versus medium-sized corporations? Big-budget product advertisers versus small-budget or nonexistent product advertisers in borad-based media?
3. Did corporate advertising result in potential supportive behavior—something that was not measured in the previous study.

Yankelovich/Phase II[14]

More than twice as many personal, in-home interviews (1,533) were conducted in Yankelovich/Phase II. An equal number of men and women were interviewed. All of the respondents were college graduates, and 34 percent had postgraduate degrees. All had household incomes of $30,000 or more.

Sixty-four corporations in nine major industries were measured individually. The sales revenues of these corporations totaled $440 billion and ranged from $60 billion to $1.5 billion. For the first nine months of 1978, the corporations invested $786 million in advertising in broad-based media: $107 million for corporate advertising and $679 million for product advertising—a spending ratio of 1 to 6 in favor of product advertising.

Yankelovich purposely selected companies that did various amounts of corporate and product advertising. Using a split-sample technique, Yankelovich divided the 1,533 participants into five groups. Each respondent was asked to rate 13 corporations. Each cor-

---

[14] *Corporate Advertising/Phase II: An Expanded Study of Corporate Advertising Effectiveness Conducted for Time Magazine by Yankelovich, Skelly & White, Inc.* Copyright © 1979, Time Inc. All rights reserved.

poration was rated by approximately 300 respondents. A random sorting technique was used in presenting the companies to respondents. There's a theory of communications in the advertising industry that works this way. High advertising expenditures produce a reaction that causes high advertising recall. High advertising recall produces high familiarity. This leads to high association with specific traits and then to high favorable overall impression. When the theory is applied to a product advertiser, the end result, of course, is the purchase of products or services.

In Phase II, Yankelovich applied this same chain reaction effect to corporate advertising. Unlike product advertisers, corporate advertisers may have intermittent goals such as high association with specific traits, or high overall impression. In corporate communications, the final reaction is potential supportive behavior. Getting people to the ultimate goal is not always easy. It implies not only great effort, but greater expenditures as well.

Because potential supportive behavior was a new measurement, a new questionnaire was developed. In using phrasing such as "I would write," "I would take," "I would buy," and "I would recommend," Yankelovich was looking for an *action* response. This is one of the most important aspects of *Corporate Advertising/Phase II*. Potential supportive behavior represents what many companies are looking for—a tangible return on their corporate advertising investment. The advantages speak for themselves, not only in terms of impact on investors and the financial community, but also in terms of marketing support for products and services.

The study showed that advertisers with corporate advertising budgets of $5 million and product advertising budgets of $14.5 million had supportive behavior of 20 percent. This dropped to 14 percent when corporate advertising was $0.1 million and product advertising was $15.9 million. But when product advertising dropped to $0.4 million and corporate advertising rose to $1.6 million, supportive behavior stayèd at a strong 13 percent. When corporate advertising dropped to $0.4 million and raising product advertising rose to $1.4 million, supportive behavior went down to 11 percent.

Corporate advertisers outperformed light or noncorporate advertisers on all five key measurements of effectiveness studied. The high advertising recall advantage was 58 percent; high familiarity, 48 percent; high association with specific traits, 29 percent; high favorable overall impression, 30 percent; and high potential supportive behavior, 33 percent. Quite clearly, there was a distinct advantage for corporate advertisers in key measurements whether their product advertising expenditures were high or low. Yankelovich went through this same exercise for both high and low sales revenues and high and low

P/E ratios, and the results were exactly the same—a distinct advantage for corporate advertisers.

Conclusions

The following conclusions were reached from the second study:

Conclusion 1. Corporate advertising works. Yankelovich, Skelly and White found a significant advantage for corporate advertisers on all five key measurements of effectiveness, across a wide range of companies in nine major industry classifications.

Conclusion 2. Product advertising alone cannot be relied upon to build a strong corporate image. Dollar for dollar, corporate advertising was more efficient, and it registered a positive effect regardless of company background factors, such as product advertising level, sales volume, and P/E ratio.

Conclusion 3. In addition, corporate advertisers realized a tangible return on their investment in terms of personal behavior directly supportive of a company.

Conclusion 4. By every measurement, corporate advertising directed to an affluent, well-educated audience was effective in communicating a company's role in the business community, as well as its responsiveness to the needs of society at large.

CHAPTER TWELVE

Meetings

FACE TO FACE

"No, sir, I don't believe it."

So said Donald B. Romans, executive vice president—finance, Trans Union Corporation, when external public relations counsel and I advised him that financial analysts did not like meetings at resort areas. We produced surveys, including one made of analysts who followed the company. These analysts said such meetings ranged from low on the priority list to a "waste of time."

At Romans' vehement insistence, the company's 1979 meeting was held at a Florida resort location. The results? The meeting drew the largest attendance and the most enthusiastic responses of any of the company-sponsored meetings in over a decade! Who was right, and who was wrong? Perhaps the surveys were right in their time among those surveyed, but certainly Romans was right too.

Typical comments in a premeeting survey were:

> I prefer smaller informal meetings such as the splinter group sessions. A few formal remarks with plenty of time for questions and answers is a good approach.

> Frankly, it is hard for me to justify spending three days at a resort with one company.

Among postmeeting survey remarks among the same analysts, this one was representative:

> That kind of meeting is extremely worthwhile for analysts. It allows analysts to meet a company's various operating heads more informally than by visiting the company by yourself.

This mind set of financial analysts disliking resort area meetings, but attending and enjoying them, is one of the many problems that are encountered and must be solved by the CEO, the CFO, and the communications officer, for sessions with analysts are the most frequently held type of meeting in corporate face-to-face encounters. While the CFO, the investor relations officer, or the communications executive may see individual analysts frequently, companies still desire to hold numerous group sessions. These can be breakfast or luncheon sessions, meetings of investment societies, and company-sponsored meetings. Contrast this to the annual meeting, which, of course, is held once a year under federal government mandate. Some companies consider the annual meeting an anachronism that should be shelved. Other companies put on a virtual three-ring circus.

MEETING WITH THE FINANCIAL ANALYSTS

The success of Mr. Romans in taking financial analysts to a resort area was not a matter of blind luck. Rather, it resulted from a thorough knowledge of the analysts who follow the company and confidence in the in-house communications staff and external counsel to present an outstanding seminar.

The successful execution of such an event requires research, planning, hard work, and attention to detail. I am presenting the outline of one of the many successful meetings I have conducted to indicate the scope required to achieve that success. The outline will help you to do the same. Planning for the event, which was to be staged during the second week of May, began the preceding October, after the company's third-quarter results were known and its one- and five-year plans were determined to be on target.

Step 1 was the determination within management that the seminar should be held, and where. Step 2 was to determine audience interest in attending and the major program thrust. First, the analysts said yes, they would be interested in attending. Second, after meeting corporate management and having the complex financial structure of the company explained at previous meetings, the analysts said they were interested in meeting operating management. The emphasis, they indicated, was on market situation, risk management, and growth strategy.

The outline below was created by the communications department, based on management needs and the analysts' input by mid-February. The department was responsible for all program development and execution.

PROGRAM OUTLINE

The following questionnaire was issued to operating managers prior to visits by speech writers beginning March 1. The questionnaire made it possible to do ample research, have necessary material available, and greatly reduce the time that managers and speech writers had to spend with each other.

Financial Analyst Meeting Questionnaire
Trans Union Corporation

The following questions give the starting points and are meant more as a guideline for discussion. Any unique perspective the speaker can bring to his presentation—even if it strays from topics addressed in these questions—certainly should be pursued during discussion.

Introduction

1. What is the scope of products and/or services offered by your group?
2. What products or services of yours are in biggest demand?
3. What is the average sale price of your products? Range?
4. What new geographic areas and markets are served?

Market Situation

5. What is your share of the overall market?
6. What is its total size?
7. What is the growth rate of each market? Your potential?
8. Who are your main competitors? What are their market shares and sales volumes?
9. Are you considered competitive?
10. What competitive changes do you see in the immediate future for both your competitors and you?
11. What are your major competitor's main strengths and weaknesses?
12. What does the market think about your company and its products?

Management Strategy

13. What are the overall management emphases?
14. What special product, marketing, or service capabilities set your business line apart from its competitors? What management strategy sets you apart?
15. Do you have gross margin protection?
16. What is your policy governing accounts receivable management?
17. What technical innovations have been introduced in the last two years? How have they affected your business line?

Growth Strategy

18. What are the growth goals (percentage of compounded growth in sales, IBT, or both)? Have they been met consistently?
19. How have acquisitions been handled (criteria for evaluating candidate company, perceived responsibilities of both parties)?
20. Why did you acquire [company name]?
21. What are your plans for it?
22. Why don't you acquire certain companies?
23. Have past acquisitions been successful?
24. Will you continue to pursue growth through acquisition?
25. What other avenues will you pursue for more growth internally than through acquisitions?

Corporate "Fit"

26. The overall corporate strategy fits into these categories: growth through investment, aggressive marketing, and balance to offset external economic forces and cyclical down trends. How does your business line relate to these goals?
27. How is your business line like or unlike other Trans Union business lines?
28. How does your business line fit Trans Union's investment monitoring policies (optimum rate of return, investment continuity, sound debt leverage)?
29. How does your business line fit Trans Union's "leadership" marketing policy? How is this business line a leader?
30. How does your business line provide taxable income to apply against tax deductions and investment tax credits?
31. How is your business line protected against risk (wide customer base, proprietary products and services, firm order backlogs, long-term contracts)?
32. How is your business line protected against cyclical down trends? Are its activities "balanced" to provide protection?

Future

33. What is the future for the markets served? in the next year? five years?
34. What is the future for the competition? in the next year? five years?
35. What is the future for your business line? in the next year? five years?

Arranging the Work

Simultaneously, I met with L. James Lovejoy, the account supervisor for our public relations agency, Burson-Marsteller. We assigned the work flow for in-house and agency personnel. The following assignments were made:

	Analysts meeting	
Speakers	Company contact	Agency contact
Rail Car Leasing Services and Sales		
S. H. Bonser, chairman	Durack	Lovejoy/Anderson
J. R. Kruizenga	Durack	Lovejoy/Collins
K. Jagger	Durack	Lovejoy/Collins
Information Services		
W. J. Devers, chairman	Smith	Lovejoy/Green
G. J. Zvonecek	Smith	Lovejoy/Green
N. C. Jensen	Johansen	Green
S. L. Mularz	Johansen	Green

	Analysts meeting	
Speakers	_Company contact_	_Agency contact_
Finance Leasing		
D. B. Romans, chairman	Johansen	Lovejoy/Strauss
R. D. Ringe	Smith	Lovejoy/Collins
J. D. Dolin	Smith	Collins
K. Jagger	Durack	Collins
Shipping—to come	Durack	Collins
Distribution Activities		
R. J. Conroy	Johansen	Carr
W. A. Johns	Graves	Carr
Water and Waste Treatment		
T. P. O'Boyle, chairman	Wiberg	Lovejoy/Anderson
R. L. Hoard	Wiberg	Lovejoy/Anderson
G. T. Shannon	Wiberg	Carr
D. D. Welt	Wiberg	Carr
Corporate		
D. B. Romans	Lorino	Lovejoy/Strauss
C. W. Peterson	Graves	Tremulis
W. B. Moore	Graves	Tremulis
B. S. Chelberg	Graves	Lovejoy

A/V coordination: Green/Taylor

By April 1, all program participants were interviewed, first drafts of speeches were written, and recommended audiovisual materials were presented to the speakers and to the director of corporate communications for preliminary approval.

During the next month, all final speech drafts and visuals were approved ,by the speakers and the communications department. All speakers were given speech training on their materials. This permitted last-minute changes prior to arrival at the meeting site, where all participants were given dress rehearsals. As part of the speaker training, typical questions, which proved very accurate, were posed to the speakers for response training.

Notification to Attendees

Financial analysts and program participants were given preliminary notification of the meeting mid-December so that they could block out the appropriate general dates on their calendars. When the outline and work schedule were developed in mid-February, a tentative schedule was issued to the same groups. By May 1, once speeches were timed, a definitive schedule, including meeting rooms, was forwarded so that secretaries would know at all times the locations of their bosses.

Financial Analyst Seminar

Sunday May 6, 1979	6:30 P.M. Cocktails and dinner
Monday May 7, 1979	7:00 A.M. to 8:00 A.M. Breakfast buffet
	8:00 A.M. to 10:00 A.M. Rail Car panel: Bonser, Kruizenga, Jagger Sidney H. Bonser, chairman
	10:00 A.M. to 10:15 A.M. Coffee break
	10:15 A.M. to 11:15 A.M. Information Services panel: Zvonecek, Jensen, Mularz William J. Devers, chairman
	11:45 A.M. to 12:45 P.M. Luncheon buffet
	1:00 P.M. Recreation
	6:30 P.M. to 7:30 P.M. Cocktails
	7:30 P.M. to 10:00 P.M. Dinner Bruce S. Chelberg
Tuesday May 8, 1979	7:00 A.M. to 8:00 A.M. Breakfast buffet
	8:00 A.M. to 10:00 A.M. General Leasing and Rental panel: Ringe, Dolin, Jagger Donald B. Romans, chairman
	10:00 A.M. to 10:15 A.M. Coffee break
	10:15 A.M. to 11:30 A.M. Distribution Activities panel William A. Johns, chairman Robert J. Conroy, chairman

---

Financial Analyst Seminar (*concluded*)

11:45 A.M. to 12:45 P.M.
Luncheon buffet

1:00 P.M.
Recreation

6:30 P.M. to 7:30 P.M.
Cocktails

7:30 P.M. to 10:00 P.M.
Dinner

Evening speaker, Jerome W. Van Gorkom

Wednesday   7:00 A.M. to 8:00 A.M.
May 9, 1979   Breakfast buffet

8:00 A.M. to 10:00 A.M.
Water and Waste Treatment panel: Shannon, Welt, Hoard
Thomas P. O'Boyle, chairman

10:00 A.M. to 10:15 A.M.
Coffee break

10:15 A.M. to 11:15 A.M.
Perspective, Donald B. Romans

11:45 A.M.
Lunch

Arranging Amenities

With the wheels set in motion on the program, definitive travel, lodging, and food arrangements were started. Forwarded to all attendees with the preliminary program were an information response form and literature on current events in the resort area. This permitted planning for company-sponsored or personally desired activities.

Once flight times were known, pickup arrangements could be made and guests preregistered. Golf and tennis information was necessary in planning tournaments. The arrival times of speakers were also needed, so that dress rehearsals could be staged.

Machinery also was set in motion for the normal food and libation, highlighted by a poolside lobster cookout. One word of advice here is to work closely with the resort catering staff, which can supply special foods and wines at a reasonable cost over published menus.

Information Response Form

Trans Union Analyst Meetings
May 2–May 9, 1979

You are welcome to attend all or any part of the meetings and may arrive or depart at any time prior to or after the conclusion of your scheduled appearance.

Please arrange lodging (indicate single or double occupancy) for the following nights: _____

I will be arriving at the following date and time: _____

I will be departing at the following date and time: _____

I would like my name tag to read: _____

I would like to participate in the following tournaments:
Golf _____
Tennis _____   Tennis rank: A_____ B_____ C_____

I would like to play the following on Friday, May 4, or Tuesday, May 8:
Golf _____   Tennis _____   Partners _____

Name _____
Title _____
Wife's name (if attending) _____

Please complete and return to the company no later than March 30th.

Staffing and timing are vital to make the amenities work as well as the programs, so a work flow schedule was developed similar to the speech and program schedule. Persons assigned to the original speech contact and writing, for example, were responsible for coordinating audiovisuals, speech training, the speakers' schedule, and dress rehearsal.

Homeward Bound

Once everyone is homebound—and you have your big letdown—how do you know the impact of the program? As analysts were returning to their offices, waiting for them was the accompanying survey, which, in this instance, had a 75 percent response vote.

Financial Analyst Seminar Survey

1. What was your general impression of the seminar?
    Outstanding___ Excellent___ Good___ Fair___ Poor___

2. What was your opinion of the various presentations?

    Rail Car panel—Bonser, Kruizenga, Jagger
    Outstanding___ Excellent___ Good___ Fair___ Poor___
    Comments:

    Information Services panel—Devers, Zvonecek, Jensen, Mularz
    Outstanding___ Excellent___ Good___ Fair___ Poor___
    Comments:

    J. W. Van Gorkom
    Outstanding___ Excellent___ Good___ Fair___ Poor___
    Comments:

    General Leasing and Rental panel—Romans, Ringe, Dolin, Jagger
    Outstanding___ Excellent___ Good___ Fair___ Poor___
    Comments:

    Distribution Activities panel—Johns, Conroy
    Outstanding___ Excellent___ Good___ Fair___ Poor___
    Comments:

    Bruce S. Chelberg
    Outstanding___ Excellent___ Good___ Fair___ Poor___
    Comments:

    Water and Waste Treatment panel—O'Boyle, Hoard, Shannon, Welt
    Outstanding___ Excellent___ Good___ Fair___ Poor___
    Comments:

    Donald B. Romans
    Outstanding___ Excellent___ Good___ Fair___ Poor___
    Comments:

3. Meeting facilities
    Outstanding___ Excellent___ Good___ Fair___ Poor___

    Meals
    Outstanding___ Excellent___ Good___ Fair___ Poor___

    Timing of events
    Outstanding___ Excellent___ Good___ Fair___ Poor___

Financial Analyst Seminar Survey (*continued*)

Presentation contents
Outstanding___ Excellent___ Good___ Fair___ Poor___

Handout material
Outstanding___ Excellent___ Good___ Fair___ Poor___

Personal aid and attention
Outstanding___ Excellent___ Good___ Fair___ Poor—

Question periods
Outstanding___ Excellent___ Good___ Fair___ Poor___

Order of presentation
Outstanding___ Excellent___ Good___ Fair___ Poor___

Morning and evening sessions
Outstanding___ Excellent___ Good___ Fair___ Poor___

4. What improvements would you suggest for future meetings?

5. Do you feel anything important was omitted?
   Yes___ No___ No comment___
   Yes:

6. Would you be interested in a seminar conducted on a specific segment of Trans Union's business?
   Yes___ No___ No comment___
   Which segment would interest you most?

7. What type of location would you prefer for future seminars?
   Resort___ Company operating facility___ Either___
   Comments:

Impressions of Trans Union

1. How do you rate Trans Union management? Is the company well managed?

2. How does Trans Union rate on profitability . . . does the company show a good return on invested capital . . . do you feel it has shown a better-than-average earnings record?

Financial Analyst Seminar Survey (*concluded*)

3. How do you view Trans Union's outlook in terms of earnings potential? Do you feel its future (three to five years) growth rate in earnings will be better than average?

4. How would you rate Trans Union's various phases of business activity in terms of their ability to contribute to company growth and earnings in the future (three to five years)?
   Rail cars and related services—United States and Mexico
   Rail cars and related services—Canada and United States

5. Is there any specific information about Trans Union that you would like to receive?

Upon receipt of responses, scores were tallied and both typical positive and negative responses were recorded. These were analyzed by the corporate staff and external counsel on a project-by-project basis within the overall program. The results showed that there were no areas of weakness, as a result of the planning and attention to detail, but they did reveal areas where even greater strengths could be built into the program.

Speech Training—A Hidden Plus

Equally important was the fact that results were issued to all programs participants so that they could see the measures of performance given to them by the audience. Worthy of mention is the score received by each person on actual presentation. All of the corporate executives who participated in the program received a score one point higher, on a scale of 1 to 5, than they had received at earlier meetings, for which they had not been given speech training. Needless to say, it is now a requirement, with the speakers' concurrence, that such training be given for all major meetings of this type.

Speech training was only the proverbial tip of the iceberg in preparing managers for the presentations. From the moment they received their outlines, they started to think about being on stage. Interviews with the speech writers aided them in focusing on major points and eliminating material known to analysts, or fluff. The rehearsals also gave the managers stage presence, a relaxed attitude, and a firm manner in responding to questions—no hedging, no beating around the bush. Answer them! Along with their higher presentation ratings, all of the speakers showed an improvement in credibility over the previous meeting. This was a positive result of the speech training. The other improvement can be explained thus: As a manager, not an orator, trying to explain a complex topic before a strong audience, how do you keep your knees from knocking? All of the speakers expressed appreciation for the help they got and asked that such help be given to them the next time they made an appearance.

GAMES PEOPLE PLAY

Following are ingenious ploys used by companies to woo the financial community, as gathered by Laurie Meisler, of *Institutional Investor*. It is important to remember that analysts want meetings that are all-business at convenient nonresort areas.

Lobster Tale

"Don't eat for three days before Congoleum's annual outing," advises a security analyst who made the trip. Congoleum, a company involved in such areas as home furnishings and shipbuilding, took 25 of its closest followers to Booth Bay, Maine. For dinner, it hustled them aboard an excursion-like tugboat and provided hors d'oeuvres and drinks while they steamed toward a restaurant for a feast of lobster and steak. Upon leaving the following day, participants were presented with two lobsters as mementos of the trip. Ralph Reno, Congoleum's director of corporate communications, says the food has generated almost as much enthusiasm as the information imparted: "Maybe these people don't get to eat real Maine lobster very often."

Briefings with a Baedeker

Director of corporate communications Gerard Griffin insists that the two field trips Louisiana-Pacific schedules for analysts each year are intended for business and not pleasure. "There's very little boondoggle," he states emphatically. Yet Griffin admits that L-P has a reputation for doing "everything" first class and that its 2½-day outings are so popular that the company has had to make room for more analysts. For example, participants happily recall their travels to L-P operations in Alaska, where they got around by boat and helicopter, and to Northern California, where they spent time contemplating the redwoods. "We try not to make the trip burdensome," says Griffin. Adds an analyst: "They hit your pleasure button."

Bring Your Own Popcorn

Like most companies, Midland-Ross once relied on slide presentations to demonstrate its products and markets. But the multi-industry, complex company wanted to develop a larger following among security analysts, portfolio managers, and registered reps, so it opted for a more sophisticated approach. It sent three camera crews around the country to film its products in use—rather than the conventional manufacturing sequences—and commissioned Louis Rukeyster of "Wall Street Week" to narrate the documentary. Jerome Isham, vice president of public relations, is confident the 10-minute film, *Making*

Things for the Better, will have a noticeable impact. "It is as good as, and perhaps better than, anything I've ever seen," he boasts.

Building Contacts

"All us frustrated kids in the sandbox," as one analyst refers to himself and his peers, had an opportunity to play out their fantasies during a Tenneco trip. A group of 40 brokerage and institutional analysts were taken on a tour of four plant locations to examine construction equipment, a shipyard, and a packaging mill, among other things, and then learned for themselves what it is like to be at the controls. They were each encouraged to try their hand at driving a bulldozer and tractor. It is the kind of trip a company can't stage too often because of the expense involved, reports a Tenneco spokesman, but it was a definite attention-getter. Was a good time had by all? "You bet," he replies.

Warming Up the Analysts

After each meeting, IC Industries likes to give analysts a little memento. While it has handed out such items as a transistor radio inside a soda can—to remind recipients of IC's Pepsi bottling company—one analyst speaks most fondly of the gifts she received during the company's Midas Muffler promotion. She reports that she has made good use of her Midas "muffler," an orange and black striped scarf, and enjoyed her Midas beach towel as well: one side depicts the underside of a car; the other conveys the message, "Muffle your tired body."

A Day at the Races

Kendall Motor Oil is one of the sponsors of the Grand Prix automobile race at Watkins Glen, New York, and Witco Chemical Corporation, its parent, doesn't let analysts forget it. Each year, a Witco-chartered airplane picks up about 10 of them and their spouses on Saturday morning and delivers them in time for lunch. A festive dinner dance is scheduled for evening. Early on Sunday, a motorcade brings them to the track, they are given passes to go into the pits and see the cars being prepared, and a police escort whisks them away at the finish. Witco director of corporate communications Harvey Golubock points out that the mission does have a message: Everywhere analysts encounter signs and posters—not to mention actual cans—of Kendall Motor Oil.

Putting On Airs

The T-shirt "war" being waged by two television networks gives some indication of their (mis)fortunes. It started when ABC offered broadcasting analysts T-shirts emblazoned with a chart showing its stock price. "It was kind of low quality," recalls a recipient, "and a little bit tacky." Top-rated CBS followed with a somewhat classier item: an all-white sport shirt decorated with a discreet network logo. "Now, *that* was suitable for a country club," says this analyst. But ABC stock continued to climb, and CBS was not as lucky. ABC, currently number one, still sends out its unsophisticated shirt, adorned this year with its "Still the One" motto, while its competitor's handout, now almost indistinguishable in quality, has "Looking Good" printed on the front.

Bringing the Mountain to Muhammad

The problem with annual meetings, according to Emhart's vice president of public relations John Budd, is that they've become "privileged sanctuaries for those who are closest." So, for the shareholders unable to attend Emhart's annual meeting, the company, a diversified multinational manufacturer, brings the meeting to them—by loaning out 25-minute videotapes of the proceedings. Asserts Budd: "Slides are pedestrian, and films give the impression of trying to educate. Videotapes offer freshness and credibility, rather than canned propaganda."

PRESENTING . . .

"Our speaker for today needs no introduction. Then there was a long pause, and I think that he forgot my name." So reports an executive of a financial analysts meeting in Hartford. The day was saved, he says, when someone down at the front table called up to the podium in a loud stage whisper—"Bernie Cornfield."

But it is the face-to-face encounter that is most important to the investor relations practitioners in reaching their investor relations objectives. More than one half of practitioners say that the most important contribution in reaching investor relations objectives was made by annual personal meetings in analysts'/portfolio managers' offices, while 36 percent said the most important contribution was made by semiannual/quarterly meetings in those offices. Although the importance of written materials is stressed by some investor relations people, written materials are clearly overshadowed by personal contact.

Management Reachout

In light of this, let us look at some ORC findings on company practices regarding personal contact and meetings with the investment community.

On the average, management personnel in the companies ORC surveyed spent 77 days—close to three working months—either in preparing for meetings with analysts and portfolio managers or in actually meeting with them (see Table 12–1). This was only an estimate, of course, and my bet would be that it was an *under*estimate, but you can readily see that it represented a significant commitment of dollars and management time to the personal contact side of investor relations by management.

ORC findings on presentations by companies at analyst society meetings are shown in Table 12–2. About one fifth of the companies surveyed made no appearances at analyst society meetings in the prior year. About one fourth made one or two presentations, three to five

Table 12-1
Time spent by management personnel on
analysts and portfolio managers

	1979	1981
Average number of working days spent by management personnel in . . .		
Preparation for meetings with analysts and portfolio managers	37	27
Face-to-face meetings with analysts/investment decision makers	40	36

Eugene E. Heaton, Jr., "How Wall Street and Business View Investor Relations Practices" (ORC Executive Briefing on Investor and Financial Relations, New York, December 7, 1981).

Table 12-2
Number of appearances at analyst society meetings in last year

	1977	1979	1981
None/not reported	24%	22%	21%
One or two	25	26	24
Three to five	30	27	27
Six or more	21	25	28

Eugene E. Heaton, Jr., "How Wall Street and Business View Investor Relations Practices" (ORC Executive Briefing on Investor and Financial Relations, New York, December 7, 1981).

presentations, or six presentations or more. The median number of presentations was thre a year for both 1977 and 1979.

There had, however, been some increase in *company-sponsored* meetings (see Table 12-3). In 1979 as compared with 1977, somewhat fewer companies said that they did not utilize this communications medium, and the proportion of companies that reported having sponsored six meetings or more per year increased from 18 percent in 1977 to 27 percent in 1979. The median number of such meetings thus increased from two per year in 1977 to three per year in 1979.

Stockbroker societies are springing up around the country. They invite corporate chief executives to speak at luncheon meetings, and companies are seizing this opportunity to deliver a firsthand account of operations. Many companies also see the meetings as an opportunity to

Table 12–3
Number of appearances at company-sponsored
meetings in last year

	1977	1979	1981
None/not reported	33%	27%	25%
One or two	28	27	26
Three to five	21	19	21
Six or more	18	27	28

Eugene E. Heaton, Jr., "How Wall Street and Business View Investor Relations Practices" (ORC Executive Briefing on Investor and Financial Relations, New York, December 7, 1981).

clarify what kinds of information reps need and want most. The speech can be a teaser, and, hopefully, some brokers will want to know more.

Some companies believe that registered representatives like to be courted, especially by the company chief executive. A meeting with the president or CEO is often the spark that turns a broker on to a company and gets him out selling its stock. And it's an added selling tool if a broker can tell his client firsthand what an executive has to say about company operations.

What kinds of meetings do the registered representatives attend? In a New England study, the representatives attended their own firm's meeting the most (see Table 12–4).

The New England representatives generally participated in meetings arranged by their own firms and meetings arranged by individual companies as a means of getting current information about specific companies. The frequency with which they attended is shown in Table 12–5.

Table 12–4
Types of meeting attended (for company information)

Type of meeting	Percent
Meeting by representative's firm..................	78%
Meeting by individual companies	68
Stockbroker clubs	39
Private meetings arranged by representative	28
Analysts groups	18
All others	6

Base: 211.
Source: *Study of Stockbroker Registered Representatives in New England, 1978,* Lowengard & Brotherhood and Marketing Services, Inc., Hartford, Conn.

Table 12–5
Frequency of attending meetings (by type of meeting)

Frequency of attending	Representatives's firm	Individual companies	Stockbroker clubs	Private meetings	Analysts groups
More than once a month	49%	14%	45%	—	45%
Once a month	24	38	41	50%	41
Every three months	7	11	6	13	6
Every six months	20	31	8	24	8
Once a year	—	6	—	13	—
	100%	100%	100%	100%	100%
Base	(165)	(143)	(82)	(59)	(38)

Generalization: Representatives attend stockbroker clubs and analysts group meetings more frequently than any other types of meetings.

Source: *Study of Stockbroker Registered Representatives in New England, 1978,* Lowengard & Brotherhood and Marketing Services, Inc., Hartford, Conn.

The registered representatives ranked all of the meetings high in usefulness, and they were generally favorable to a variety of formats (see Tables 12–6 and 12–7).

Table 12–6
Opinion of usefulness of meetings (weighted ranking)

Type of meeting	Index
Representative firm's meetings	89
Individual company meetings	84
Private meetings (arranged by representative)	84
Stockbroker clubs	84
Analysts groups	82

Note: Index based on weighted ranking of those attending subject meeting.
Source: *Study of Stockbroker Registered Representatives in New England, 1978,* Lowengard & Brotherhood and Marketing Services, Inc., Hartford, Conn.

Get Down to Specifics

As for meeting content, financial analysts do not want broad-sweeping generalities or representation of readily available information. The "absolute worst" get-togethers, one analyst believes, are staged by Roadway Express, which typically has passed out 20-year

Table 12-7
Meeting format favored

Meeting format	Index
Luncheon meeting and presentation	80
Early morning breakfast presentation prior to market opening	79
Late afternoon presentation and reception following market close	74
Dinner and evening presentation	62

Note: Index based on ranking, in order of preference by representatives.
Source: *Study of Stockbroker Registered Representatives in New England, 1978*, Lowengard & Brotherhood and Marketing Services, Inc., Hartford, Conn.

summaries and spent 20 minutes reading them without giving anything away in terms of what it expects in the future and what is happening now. Also wasting his time, he says, are Santa Fe Industries and Seaboard Coastline, which come through every quarter and drone on and on.

Rather than try to cover the waterfront, companies should focus on a specific segment of their operations, a number of analysts advise. And rather than have the vice president of finance play the dominant role, members of the financial community say they would like to see people not as easy to reach, such as certain operating managers. Research among your analysts can determine which operating group they would like to know more about and will make the vice president of finance the program emcee rather than the sole information source.

Answering the Question

Also under fire are the question-and-answer periods that follow the speeches. One analyst recalled unhappily the appearance of one company before an analysts society meeting in which the chairman took up the entire hour and left no time for questions. Even worse, possibly, are the many organizations that are just as unresponsive even though their methods are less obvious. They will talk to, but not answer, the question. The rule of thumb I follow is to allow 5 minutes for questions for each 10 minutes of talking, with two strongly enforced rules. Each speaker, in addition to being rehearsed on typical questions, must answer the questions, and no speech is to last more than 30 to 35 minutes. My experience is that audience interest takes a dramatic nose dive after that length of time regardless of the personality, topic, or special devices.

More enlightening, in the estimation of many analysts, are small gatherings where the company doesn't feel compelled to make everyone happy and can concentrate on the requirements of a select few. In response to this view, I set up alternate monthly breakfast and luncheon meetings for our financial officer. Attendance, by design, was limited to six to eight analysts, and the meetings were usually attended by one additional corporate officer.

In our company, we have an open-door policy for meeting financial analysts. (Surprisingly, not all companies do.) Any analyst can call or meet company representatives at will. Many analysts like the policy and take advantage of it. Many analysts have also been appreciative of return calls when major new announcements generate 40 to 45 calls in one day and not all of them can be answered immediately.

THE ANNUAL MEETING

Nine of the 10 directors sat around the mahogany board table. Eight minutes later, the annual meeting was concluded. There were no questions from the floor because there was no audience—other than the corporate secretary. Thus went the annual meeting of the Square D Company in Detroit in 1958.

Modest to Obscene

Thousands of meetings held by companies in the ensuing years have ranged from the sheer modesty of the Square D meeting to lavish, almost obscene affairs. Regardless of the approach, the annual meeting has been able to generate a yearly storm of controversy. Is it a legally required anachronism, or is it a public relations opportunity?

First, let us examine some annual meeting gems.

At an annual meeting in Boston, W. R. Grace & Co. provided shareholders with a free lunch and plant tour followed by a tour of historic sites in Lexington and Concord. At another meeting in Los Angeles, the company again wooed shareholders with a free lunch, this time a Mexican style meal prepared by a newly acquired restaurant subsidiary.

Wometco Enterprises, Miami, each year treats shareholders to a first-run movie and draws an audience of some 800, or about 10 percent of the company's shareholders. The movie is shown just prior to its public release. The meeting is held in a company-owned twin theater. After the formal meeting, at about 11 A.M., shareholders are escorted through the lobby, where they can pick up complimentary popcorn and soda, into an adjoining theater where the movie is shown. A representative says that the company has always stressed a personal relationship with shareholders and that offering a free movie reinforces that relationship.

Norton Simon, Inc., gives each shareholder a package of products, preferably new products. Cost to the company: about $10 per package, with a higher retail value. Masco Corporation, manufacturer of faucets and other home products, hands out shower heads or other nominal gifts. Alexander & Baldwin, Honolulu, held its 1978 annual meeting at a company resort. Arctic Enterprises, Minnesota-based manufacturer of snowmobiles and thermal clothing, sometimes stages product demonstrations or "fashion shows." Multimedia, Inc., Greenville, South Carolina, played a videotape introducing a recently acquired television station at its annual meeting and carried the meeting on TV monitors around the room.

Some companies use the annual meeting to strengthen their employee communications. Western Union Corporation broadcasts its meeting to employees at 50 locations throughout the United States via the company's microwave and satellite transmission facilities.

In most of the above examples, the company has some special product or service that naturally lends itself to enlivening the annual meeting. But even companies not in that advantageous position are finding ways to improve the meeting or broaden its impact.

Atlantic City Electric Company invites a high school teacher and student from each company service area to the meeting and gives them a blue-ribbon tour of company facilities as part of its economic education effort. At the meeting itself, all motions are made by shareholders. The company contacts shareholders in advance and has found them to be very coooperative. Rainier Bancorporation, Seattle, invited local financial writers to interview senior management, videotaped the session, and then played an edited, 20-minute version at its annual meeting. After the meeting, shareholders were invited on an advance tour of the company's nearly completed new headquarters building.

3M Company, whose meeting draws some 3,000 shareholders, uses a large video screen behind the head table. Donald H. Frenette, director of investor relations, says this "not only allows all stockholders to see what is happening, but gives the meeting an impact it would not otherwise have." A few companies, including Warner Communications and Manufacturers Hanover Corporation, have eliminated all executive speeches in favor of a more informal meeting with added time for questions and answers.

Borg-Warner Corporation is one of a small but growing number of companies that hold regional shareholder information meetings in addition to the annual meeting itself. General Electric holds two separate meetings: the legal one in the spring for formal business, and a follow-up information meeting in the fall.

Armco Steel held its first regional information meeting in Butler,

Pennsylvania. Charles B. Wheat, an Armco spokesman, says the meeting, which drew about 500 shareholders, included a slide show, presentations by four senior officers (including the chairman and president), and a question-and-answer period. Company directors also attended, using the occasion to hold their regular directors meeting before the information meeting. Butler was chosen because of heavy local shareownership and two nearby Armco plants. Many of the attenders were employee shareholders; the meeting began at 4 P.M., just after the day work shift ended. Attendance actually exceeded that of the annual meeting, which is held each year at company headquarters in Middletown, Ohio, and draws about 400 holders.

American Telephone & Telegraph prepares a film of its annual meeting for showing to other audiences, including operating company employees and the parent company's "mini meetings" (regional shareholder information meetings). The film typically covers preparations for the annual meeting, the chairman's address, a sampling of shareholder questions and answers, and the big postmeeting press conference that AT&T holds each year.

Some companies, while not necessarily glamorizing the annual meeting itself, do go out of their way to encourage shareholders to attend. Mid-America Industries, Fort Smith, Arkansas, sends all local shareholders a personal invitation from the chairman (about 10 percent of local shareholders show up). Ametek, Inc., which holds its annual meeting in Wilmington, Delaware, sends personal letters to all holders of 100 shares or more in convenient zip code areas near the meeting site.

Why an Annual Meeting?

Companies that play up the annual meeting generally cite various reasons for doing so:

1. The annual meeting is the most effective medium (indeed, the only one) for giving a large group of individual shareholders face-to-face contact with senior management.
2. A well-run, imaginative annual meeting reflects positively on a company's openness and investor relations style and helps fulfill the company's obligation to be responsive to its owners.
3. The annual meeting can provide a convenient platform for a major corporate announcement, such as an announcement of quarterly earnings, a policy statement on economic or regulatory affairs, or a new product announcement.

Companies which do not play up the annual meeting point out that it follows so closely on the heels of the annual report that some executives don't have enough energy left to go all out on it.

Typically, annual meetings in many corporations run like this: The meeting itself, usually attended by some 200 shareholders, lasts about an hour, after which shareholders receive a small packet of gift products and go their way. Then the board of directors convenes to elect a chairman for the coming year, while visiting analysts meet with corporate officers and divisional vice presidents. The shareholders and management subsequently join for lunch, which is followed by a plant tour.

Reasons against an Annual Meeting

A great deal of tentative interest in improving the annual meeting as a communications tool appears to exist among corporations of all sizes. But this feeling is by no means unanimous.

Surveys I have read disclose strong undercurrents both for and against the annual meeting. Typically, when corporations are asked how important the annual meeting is to their overall investor relations program, 20 percent say "very important"; 50 percent, "fairly important"; 30 percent, "not important/purely a legal obligation."

Many smaller companies, in fact, feel that even when shareholders do show up, the annual meeting tends to be short and dull. Larger companies worry that annual meetings have degenerated into little more than battlegrounds for attacks by shareholder activists. A prominent CEO advised that the best approach is to keep the meeting to two minutes, while an investor relations executive suggested that companies hold their annual meetings in Central America.

William Black, founder and chairman of Chock Full O' Nuts Corporation, traditionally has not even bothered to show up for his company's annual meeting. One proxy explained that Mr. Black "believes he can spend his time more effectively by attending to the management of the company's business affairs." One investor relations director says the company's annual meeting is purposely tucked away each year in an obscure Midwestern town where the only person to show up is the corporate secretary. Neither the chief executive officer nor any of the company's other directors attend, let alone any outside shareholders.

One of the great risks of a full-blown, well-attended meeting is that dozens of things can go wrong. Being in charge of the annual meeting is a terrific pressure spot, and even with the most fastidious planning, goofs sometimes occur.

The classic example dates back to 1961, when AT&T (which is noted for the extreme detail of its advance planning, including a 65-point checklist that specifies every major step from early November through the meeting date in late April) attracted more than 21,000 shareholders to its annual meeting in Chicago with the promise of a free box lunch. The problem: Only 11,000 box lunches had been ordered. A mad scramble ensued as AT&T executives raced around the city searching for more food.

The Style of the CEO

Aside from company size and shareholder mix, a key factor in deciding whether to go all out with the annual meeting tends to be the style of the company chief executive officer. It is the CEO, after all, who puts himself on the line at the annual meeting in terms of having to keep the affair under control and being vulnerable to potential shareholder abuse.

W. R. Grace & Co. is noted for annual meetings that are among the most imaginative in American industry. Grace provides an interesting case study of the detailed planning and the logistical considerations that go into a successful annual meeting. Grace has been rotating its annual meeting site from city to city and back to its headquarters city of New York every third year, actively encouraging shareholders to attend. By far the biggest and most ambitious of these galas was its 1976 meeting, held in Boston both to celebrate the bicentennial and to highlight Grace's rapid rise as a chemicals company. A record 1,600 shareholders attended, of 56,000 holders of record. In addition to the meeting itself, the events included a tent luncheon, complete with roving "soldiers" dressed in Revolutionary War uniforms; a tour of the company's local chemicals unit; and a tour of local historic landmarks. The program lasted nearly six hours, with shareholders and guests transported from site to site by a caravan of buses.

To encourage attendance, Grace mentions the upcoming annual meeting prominently in each annual report and then carries a full-page article on the meeting in its interim report for the first quarter. Although the company uses bulk mailing for most of its quarterlies, it isolates the identities of those shareholders who live near the site of the annual meeting and mails their quarterlies first class to make sure the report (with its feature article on the annual meeting) reaches them in advance of the meeting. In addition, Grace encloses an RSVP postcard with the proxy statement to get a fix on anticipated attendance. And, in the case of the Boston meeting, ads in local newspapers were used. The cost of the meeting—including the hall, luncheon, and transportation—came to between $10 and $15 per person.

Circus or Governance?

As much as a week beforehand, Chairman John deButts of American Telephone & Telegraph holes up at his weekend retreat in Fairfield, Connecticut, to prepare for the ordeal. He takes with him folders full of detailed briefing reports that his division managers have been working on for months.

Chairman Paul Lyet of Sperry Rand, a fact book carefully indexed for quick reference at his fingertips, prepares himself ahead of time by inviting a group of associates to pepper him with their prickliest, nastiest questions.

At Chase Manhattan, a task force of public relations men works for weeks to prepare "appropriate" replies to what shapes up as the toughest public grilling Chairman David Rockefeller ever faces.

So it is that the corporate high and mighty, with butterflies dancing in their stomachs, gird themselves for their annual brush with shareholder democracy—such as it is. Beneath their calm exteriors, most board chairmen are nervous as hell about going before their shareholders, says a veteran investor relations man, and you'd be surprised how much psychosomatic illness there is as meeting time approaches. Such pressure has been a phenomenon in the recent history of annual meetings. When the Vietnam War escalated in the late 1960s, activists of every kind found the annual meeting a handy forum for airing their views.

This is not at all the purpose for which annual meetings were originally intended. Lewis D. Gilbert likes to claim he rescued annual meetings from their "innocuous desuetude" of the 30s and 40s, when they were little more than sparsely attended legal rituals for the election of directors. At first, Gilbert was regarded as a gadfly. In later years, he became the respected champion of annual meetings and corporate governance.

The early period was followed by the circus era, when annual meetings featured free lunches and product giveaways—and drew throngs of lighthearted shareholders. Typically, those interested enough in the proceedings to stay to the end found that early departing shareholders had walked off with the box lunches and free samples.

In the early days, too, corporations were not generally regarded as having social obligations and were not obliged to answer to the outside public. As times changed, the old annual meeting changed too. In the early and mid-1970s, social advocates were in high moral dudgeon about things like illegal political activities, trade boycotts, and bribery by U.S. companies in foreign countries. Today, there are lawyers with briefcases rather than hippies with love beads.

Instead of noisy abuse, today's breed of advocates flood companies with resolutions for consideration at their annual meetings. At first blush, these resolutions would appear to be exercises in futility. Management consistently opposes them, and a majority of shareholders are inclined to follow suit.

But winning the vote is not the main point the advocates are after. There is the publicity. The press covers annual meetings. Ordinary corporate news does not grab headlines nearly as often as allegations called to the attention of management in an open meeting.

The early headline grabbers on consumerism, the environment, and energy have taken back seats to the bottom line. All of the current emphasis on the economic facts of corporate life does not mean that the broad social issues which led to so much spirited confrontation in the 1970s have simply disappeared, or been finally solved. Most of those issues are still alive, and so are most of the groups that led the fight to put them on annual meeting agendas. But hard pressed for funds like everyone else, these protest groups have become more selective about their corporate targets. Indeed, several of the groups appear to have abandoned the fight altogether.

The list of hard economic issues relating to the bottom line includes:

Executive compensation	Accounts receivable
Retirement benefits	Foreign investments
Loans to officers and key	Competitive practices
employees	Product safety
Reduced option prices	Hiring and promoting policies
Directors' qualifications	Discrimination against minorities
Pension costs and liabilities	Energy conservation
Foreign exchange transactions	Pollution control.
Reserves for bad debts	Political contributions
Inventory accounting	

The success of an annual meeting in gaining its objectives depends to a great extent on the way the chairman carries out his responsibilities and exercises his options. One reason the chairman holds the key is that there are no formalized procedural rules which he must follow. Another reason is that few companies have detailed bylaws covering the conduct of the annual meeting. Further, the rules of parliamentary procedure customarily followed at other types of meetings cannot be binding at shareholders' meetings and are generally not well adapted to such meetings.

The annual meeting is largely guided by the chairman. It rests with him to preserve order and to see that the meeting is properly conducted and that all entitled to take part are treated with fairness and good faith. In *The Annual Shareholders' Meeting*, (Corporate Practice Series Portfolio, no. 12 Bureau of National Affairs), Frank Hutson provides an especially lucid and helpful section on the conduct of the annual meeting. Five samples:

1. Shareholders sometimes question the right of management to prescribe the order of business. If the prepared agenda is seriously challenged, the chairman can ask for a voice vote on whether the meeting wishes to adhere to it. On a matter of this kind, a voice vote (rather than a share vote) is appropriate, because only those present are affected by the order in which business is conducted at the meeting.

2. The chairman may be interrupted early in the meeting by a shareholder who asks about recent bylaw changes or matters not described in the proxy statement. Every effort should be made to limit the nature and extent of questions asked at this time. Concern for the wishes and convenience of the overwhelming majority of the shareholders present dictates that the business of the meeting not be delayed by undue discussion of procedural or subsidiary matters. If there have been no bylaw changes, a simple statement to that effect has been sufficient in the past.

3. If no one moves a shareholder proposal at the appropriate time on the agenda, the chairman may proceed forthwith to the next item on the agenda, for the management is under no obligation to introduce a proposal for a shareholder. On the other hand, if the chairman is so inclined, a vote on such a proposal may be called even though the proposal has not been formally introduced.

4. The chairman may adopt reasonable rules concerning discussion, such as a two-minute limit for shareholder statements generally and a three-minute limit on the initial statement made by a proponent of a shareholder resolution.

5. If the chairman is convinced that a shareholder's conduct is seriously disturbing the meeting, he should first advise the shareholder that he is out of order and warn him against continuing his disorderly conduct. If the shareholder persists, the chairman should then request that he sit down. If the shareholder refuses, the chairman should ask him to leave the room. If this has no effect, the chairman may either direct the attendants to conduct the shareholder from the room or he may take a voice vote on the question of ejecting the shareholder and then order him ejected based on such a vote. Submitting the question to a vote should serve to protect the chairman against the charge of arbitrary action and might be helpful if he or the company were sued. On the other hand, the chairman might prefer to handle the matter more simply, without a vote.

Hutson's *Annual Shareholders' Meeting* is an excellent guide for the chairman and the corporate secretary. It is part of the Corporate Practice Series and, as such, may not be available separately. Any inquiries should be addressed to the Bureau of National Affairs, Inc., Washington, D.C. 20037.

Annual Meeting Costs

Following are representative annual meeting costs for the 143 companies that responded with a specific dollar figure to a survey conducted by Corpcom Services, Inc. Also listed are the major cost components.

Company rank	Meeting costs	Sales volume, shareholders, major cost components
Top 10 spenders		
1	$350,000	Approximate annual sales volume: $14 billion. Number of shareholders: 235,000. Hotel expenses, decorations and displays, and transportation.
2	200,000+	Approximate annual sales volume: $3 billion. Number of shareholders: 330,000. Facility rental, mailing of annual meeting materials to stockholders, meeting setup, and other arrangements.
3	200,000	Approximate annual sales volume: $10 billion. Number of shareholders: 200,000. Security, closed-circuit TV, interminable preparation.
4	150,000	Approximate annual sales volume: $480 million. Number of shareholders: 63,000. Travel, hotel, meals, proxy material, and annual report.
5	100,000	Approximate annual sales volume: $30 billion+. Number of shareholders: 688,000. On-site costs, transportation, and local expenses, except mailing and tabulation.
6	90,000	Approximate annual sales volume: $3.5 billion. Number of shareholders: 123,000. Rentals, displays, audiovisual materials, closed-circuit television coverage, luncheon, etc.
7	65,000	Approximate annual revenue: $70 million. Number of shareholders: 42,000.
8	65,000	Approximate annual sales volume: $2.1 billion. Number of shareholders: 47,000. Communications, travel, hotel.
9	64,500	Approximate annual sales volume: $309 million. Number of shareholders: 29,000. Proxy statements, cards, reminder cards, envelopes, train fare New York–Wilmington for 12 people, tallying votes.
10	60,000	Approximate annual sales volume: $225 million. Number of shareholders: 45,000. Meeting legal requirements, $43,000; print and mail report of meeting, $10,000; rental of equipment, $1,000; displays and photos, $3,300; refreshments and luncheon, $700; miscellaneous, $2,000.

Company rank	Meeting costs	Sales volume, shareholders, major cost components
Median group		
71	4,000	Approximate annual sales volume: $304 million. Number of shareholders: 6,500. Audiovisuals, products, room rental.
72	4,000	Approximate annual sales volume: $254 million. Number of shareholders: 3,300. Coffee and cookies, chair rental, sound system rental, slides.
73	4,000	Approximate annual sales volume: $2.4 billion. Number of shareholders: 8,700. Displays and/or giveaways.
74	4,000	Approximate annual sales volume: $450 million. Number of shareholders: 27,000. Computer runs of shareholders—$3,000.
75	4,000	Approximate annual sales volume: $650 million. Number of shareholders: 30,000. Slide presentation is major expense; balance (food, security, etc.) is minor.
Bottom 10		
134	250	Approximate annual sales volume: $50 million. Number of shareholders: 3,600. Rent, coffee.
135	250	Approximate annual sales volume: $630 million. Number of shareholders: 13,900.
136	250	Approximate annual sales volume: $525 million. Number of shareholders: 25,000. Cost given covers room, coffee and rolls, public address, signs, etc.; time of personnel not included.
137	200	Approximate annual sales volume: $40 million. Number of shareholders: 1,500. Coffee and doughnuts, meeting notice, proxy mailing and handling.
138	200	Approximate annual sales volume: $275 million. Number of shareholders: 9,000. Cost of shareholder gift.
139	200	Approximate annual sales volume: $130 million. Number of shareholders: 1,300.
140	100	Approximate annual sales volume: $600 million. Number of shareholders: 20,000.
141	100	Approximate annual sales volume: $11 million. Number of shareholders: 2,400. Chair rental and miscellaneous costs.

Company rank	Meeting costs	Sales volume, shareholders, major cost components
142	80–100	Approximate annual sales volume: $8 million. Number of shareholders: 1,600. Meeting room, refreshments.
143	50	Approximate annual sales volume: $200 million. Number of shareholders: 32,000. Cookies, punch, coffee.

Source: "Annual Meeting Profile," *Public Relations Journal*, May 1978, pp. 32–33. Copyright 1978, Public Relations Society of America.

Annual Meeting Tips

Besides the need for good planning and attention to detail—which almost everybody ever associated with an annual meeting seems to agree are crucial—other tips include:

1. Keep the proceedings as simple and straightforward as possible.
2. Try to avoid long, dull speeches, especially on information known to shareholders.
3. While the CEO dominates the meeting, try to involve senior corporate executives, particularly in the answering of questions.
4. Give each shareholder a printed agenda.
5. Ask security analysts and members of the press to hold their questions until after large, active shareholder meetings. We have always made executives available at informal postmeeting conferences.

Still, shareholders have many complaints about the usefulness of the annual meeting. Some are trivial, such as the charge that there isn't enough time for each shareholder to question management. But others cause considerable anger. Perhaps the most notable is the timing of most annual meetings—usually a weekday morning or afternoon. With so many more people working now, shareholders cannot easily attend such sessions.

Shareholders also gripe about the location of the annual meeting and are increasingly demanding that companies hold more than one meeting and at more than one locale. In addition, shareholders are disgruntled because many of the companies that do hold several meetings with shareholders often use these meetings only to show off new products and allow few or no question-and-answer periods to explore other company matters.

To answer the question as to whether annual meetings are worth the sweat and dollars, *Forbes* noted:

It would be tempting to agree with Fuqua Industries Chairman J. B. Fuqua, who has argued that annual meetings are a wasted effort because only a small percentage of stockholders show up to vote at a meeting where all the decisions have been made in advance. Many companies still show their contempt for annual meetings by holding them in out-of-the-way places like Flemington, N. J., and Portland, Maine, and by scheduling them on the same day. Over 100 Big Board companies, for example, will meet this April 27. But they miss a point. The fact is that businessmen need more, not less, exposure to the outside public. Too often they are sheltered in their paneled offices and their comfortable suburban homes from the fact that—rightly or wrongly—a large part of the general public feels strongly about certain issues. At an annual meeting it is not easy to ignore these public attitudes.

Annual meetings are not, of course, the whole answer. But they can be a useful device in a democracy—a once-a-year event when the corporate mighty must come down out of their skyscrapers and expose themselves to attacks by ordinary mortals. The annual meetings are thus therapy of a sort—costly, sometimes painful therapy—but useful all the same.[1]

---

[1] "Annual Meeting Time," *Forbes*, April 15, 1976, p. 42. Copyright © 1976, Forbes, Inc.

CHAPTER THIRTEEN

On the Offense in Troubled Times

THE BEST MERGER DEFENSE

The old expression "The best defense is a good offense" is very applicable to management in the emergency of the "raid." The history of tender offers since 1960 used to suggest that these raids had only one chance in three of success *if*:

1. The company being raided had taken adequate long-range preventive measures.
2. The company being raided had a detailed battle plan which it implemented quickly and decisively as soon as a tender offer was made.

In recent years, the ratio has changed and quirks have developed in the entire system. The first quirk is that more companies, even those in the billion-dollar class, have been offering themselves up for marriage, for a variety of reasons. The second is that many times when an unwanted suitor makes an offer, two or three other suitors join in the race. As a result, the "victim" is sold to the highest bidder. The advice in this chapter is for the company that believes in itself and wants to remain independent.

There was considerable creative financing connected with tender offers in the 1960s, including such things as warrants and new classes of convertible stocks. Cash tender offers are the rule today. Such offers have quadrupled in number since 1960, and it is not uncommon for the tender offers to be 20 percent or more above the market price. The almost certain profit that cash tender offers bring, regardless of their outcome, should ensure a continued increase in their number.

The historical record shows that companies can reduce their attractiveness as takeover candidates by taking a number of specific preventive measures. And after a tender offer has been made, a number of very effective maneuvers can be used to defeat the offer or to render it so costly as to force its withdrawal.

These measures and maneuvers are similar in nature to general public relations programs that were developed in the 1970s to combat

311

312

unforeseen problems with affirmative action, pollution, product quality, and industrial accidents.

The tender offer defense and battle plan has three parts:

Part I. Yardstick against which to measure, on a continuing basis, corporate vulnerability to tender offers. While this area is primarily the responsibility of the chief financial officer, the communications executive must play a major part.

Part II. Long-range preventive measures to safeguard against tender offers. Here, and the communications executive rather than the CFO is the key planner, but considerable cooperation is required.

Part III. Specific defensive battle plans to combat a tender offer. All troops are called to battle stations.

The steps of this tender offer defense and battle plan are primarily public and investor relations in nature. However, business, legal, financial, political, and other relevant facts and considerations are also involved. Measures ideally suited to one tender offer may be inappropriate and even illegal in another. A legal department must, of course, provide direction on the measures taken. The steps which are clearly not public or investor relations in nature are offered as suggestions for your consideration and should be checked with appropriate resources.

Part I. Yardstick of Attractiveness

An analysis of corporations subjected to tender offers reveals a number of common characteristics. The extent to which these characteristics apply to a company is a measure of its attractiveness as a tender offer candidate. The characteristics that attract corporate suitors are as follows:

1. *Stagnant common stock market price.* This is true particularly if the price is stagnant in relation to that of the general market or the industry segment.
2. *An undervalued stock and a low P/E ratio.* If the stock is undervalued, the raider is almost certain to get its money back even if the attack fails.
3. *Actual or perceived undervalued and/or underutilized assets.* Just what the raider wants.
4. *An earnings downtrend.* This is true particularly if the downtrend is not adequately explained to shareholders and the financial community.
5. *Potential for a sharp earnings improvement.* A turnaround situation that management does not communicate well to shareholders and the financial community.

6. *A recent dividend reduction.* Many companies are afraid to adequately explain the reason, even if the reduction is only for a quarter.

7. *A conservative debt position.* Such a position makes a merged balance sheet better able to absorb indebtedness incurred in the tender offer.

8. *Common stock holdings by executives and employees below 20 percent.* Executives and employees have a high degree of loyalty and are not easily swayed.

9. *Recent abortive merger negotiations.* This situation can prompt a tender offer by the merger rejectee.

10. *A bull market.* Tender offers are less likely in a bear market, when stock prices are on a downtick.

11. *Recent increases in stock trading volume.* Sudden, unexplained daily volume increases, even if they average only 10 percent or so above the daily norm, should trigger a tender offer alert. Large blocks of stock, 5,000 or more shares in one trade, should send storm signals flying.

12. *An executive team that is nearing retirement age.* The offerer may sense management's unwillingness to fight.

13. *A significant amount of the stock held beneficially and in Street name.* Brokers are notoriously on the raider's side because they get a double commission. They are likely to advise their Street-name holders to tender promptly. Beneficial holders, including trusts, favor tenders as the more conservative position.

14. *Large position taken by institutional holders and funds.* Many companies have a target for their stock mix between institutional and individual holders.

There are other telltale signs of tender offer candidacy, but these are the major ones that bear watching. The chief financial officer should be the corporate watchdog on reactions from the financial community on the above points. The communications executive serves as a pair of glasses helping the CFO to focus on the problems and also serves as a sentry from his or her listening post. The degree to which financial community response is known to or shared with the communications executive will have a direct bearing on the ability to establish sound, effective long-range preventive measures.

Part II. Long-Range Preventive Measures

Part I indicates that some of the factors attracting suitors arise from inadequate communications to important corporate audiences. That is why it is imperative to involve the communications executive in the defense against tender offers. Here are suggestions to overcome those factors with communications in the vanguard.

Shareholder relations. Effective shareholder relations assures that shareholders understand the company's long-range prospects and goals. They should know at least the rudiments of the product line, the markets, and, most important, the market potential. A detailed and thorough shareholder survey should be done for a number of reasons:

1. To express the company's interest in shareholders.
2. To provide a benchmark for evaluating the effectiveness of shareholder communications, including the annual report and interim reports.
3. To pinpoint areas in which shareholders lack knowledge.
4. To find any specific bases for shareholder dissatisfaction or concern.
5. To analyze shareholder attitudes toward management.
6. To analyze shareholder attitudes toward dividend policy.

Financial community survey. This survey should ask very specific questions about investment professionals' attitudes toward and understanding of the company's products, markets, goals, and acquisition policies. Personal interviews can be supplemented by an extensive mail survey to get results based on the broadest possible sample. The results of this survey can be used most effectively in planning analyst meetings and designing other communications material.

Initially, at least, both the survey and the interviews should be conducted by trained experts. It will cost more to do them this way than to do them in-house, but the results will be worth it.

Financial analyst meetings. An immediate program of planned meetings with handpicked financial analysts in key financial centers is a vital ingredient to success in preventing a tender offer. It is important that these meetings be held regardless of earnings performance.

If earnings are falling, analyst meetings are very helpful in explaining the reasons for the trend and what is being done to reverse it. If earnings are rising, analysts will need to know why and also to know what conditions will maintain the uptrend or cause it to level off. Either way, effective and believable communications is a powerful tool in slowing runaway tenders. Concentration should be placed on industry splinter groups, advisory services in general, and advisers that serve institutional stockkholders in particular.

Emergency plan to telephone major shareholders. *Plan* is the important word here. The updating of all information on an ongoing basis is a must, since shareholders, managers, and situations change constantly. This should be done annually or sooner if major changes occur on the stock list or in management. The effort will buy two things in the event of a tender offer. The first is a drastic saving of time—time that can never be made up. The second is immediate response. The plan is as follows:

1. Have your transfer agent locate all holders of 1,000 or more shares on a continuing basis. Have their names put in your computer, or arrange to have a direct mail service run them off on 3 by 5 cards. Include telephone numbers and area codes.

2. Set up a management task force team to telephone these shareholders as soon as possible if a tender offer is made. A corporate officer should telephone the company's tender offer position to major institutional holders and advisory services.

3. Prepare a basic statement with details to be filled in as to a specific tender offer. Explain that the company's executives and directors are not tendering and that shareholders have until an offer expires to tender, and urge shareholders not to tender before they have received full information as to the company's position from the company.

Direct mail plan. The telephone plan will give you the edge of immediate response. The direct mail plan will permit immediate dissemination of complete details of the company's position. The steps in this plan are:

1. Have the transfer agent, on an updated basis, keep a set of addressed envelopes under lock and key, ready for stuffing and mailing a message to shareholders.

2. Keep a duplicate set of addressed envelopes under lock and key in the corporate office in case a weekend or holiday mailing is necessary when the transfer agent's office is closed. Designate an employee team to duplicate, stuff, and mail a shareholder mailing from the corporate office.

3. Rough out a draft of a direct mail message that can be used as a guide to a specific message.

4. Develop a media mailing list. Have names, telephone numbers, and addresses of key editors, including business publications, newspapers in plant cities, and radio and TV stations.

Advertising campaign. Advertising lends credence to the telephone and direct mail plans and graphically shows management's seriousness in fighting the tender offer on a broad scale. It also covers shareholders who can't be contacted or don't want to be contacted with the other plans.

1. Develop a media list with schedule deadlines and costs.
2. Design a sample ad, including copy on the major points to be made. Among the points that might be made are:
   a. Question the compatibility of the raider with the company's product line and markets.

  b. Include a statement from the board of directors that the tender offer is grossly inadequate.

  c. If the offer is on a first-come, first-served basis, management can warn shareholders that the raider is trying to stampede them into a hasty decision.

  d. Challenge the terms of the offer. If cash is offered, point out the tax impact. If a stock exchange is offered, question the value of the proffered paper.

  e. If the offer is on a pro rata basis, management can note that there is no point in giving the opposition a free option by tendering prior to the last day of the offer.

  f. Question the source of the funds for the takeover bid.

  g. Challenge the suitor's intent and long-range plans for the company.

  h. Question when payment for shares tendered will in fact be made.

  i. Warn that brokers will urge that tender be made because they will receive a double commission if this is done.

  j. Include an account of appropriate company measures that are being taken against the bid, such as stock split, dividend increase, defensive merger, and legal proceedings against the suitor, along with a reference to the possibility of Justice Department or SEC violation.

Develop an early warning system. The successful execution of the above plans will depend greatly on whether management is given sufficient early warning of an impending offer. Therefore, assign one person to make a daily check stock transfer sheets. This person should look for:

1. Sharp increases in daily trading volume.
2. Buys of 1,000 shares or more.
3. Buys by the same broker over a brief period of time.
4. Abnormal amount of trading in Street name.
5. Changes in institutional holdings.

The same person should check *The Wall Street Journal's* "Abreast of the Market" to spot large blocks traded and should maintain close relations with an investment banker who can help watch the financial community. The corporate secretary, meanwhile, should maintain close relations with your exchange floor specialist so as to give you the name of the broker who is most active in your stock at any given time.

Increase outstanding stock. Smaller companies can be acquired for up to 18.5 percent of outstanding common stock without shareholder, SEC, or NYSE approval. It is possible to dilute a potential raider's position by almost 50 percent with the following steps:

1. Place large blocks of stock in friendly hands.
2. Increase employee holdings. Employee stock purchase plans will not only keep the stock in friendly hands but will also increase employee loyalty.
3. Develop dossiers on potential raiders. To save valuable time, develop a dossier now on firms that might make an offer. Such a dossier will give you insights into the modus operandi of each company.

Proxy solicitation. Since tender offers, unfriendly or otherwise, will involve proxy solicitation, a proxy solicitation firm should be retained in advance.

Begin a systematic search for friendly merger candidates. If all else fails, merger with a company of your choice may be more palatable than a takeover by an unfriendly company. To keep shareholders from tendering their shares, the terms of an equity exchange involving a friendly merger must be at least as attractive as—and preferably better than—that of the unfriendly suitor. And be prepared for the possibility that the raider will either raise the original tender offer price or offer more favorable terms for a merger.

With tender offers surpassing $5 billion, all but a handful of companies are vulnerable to a tender offer. So, begin now to develop dossiers on prospective friendly merger candidates. Hold preliminary discussions with their managements. Set up a merger mechanism for use if either company is threatened by an unwanted offer.

Part III. Tender Offer Battle Plan

Speed and decisiveness are the essence of a successful tender offer battle plan.

The tender offer expires within a specific time frame, usually two weeks. Your opponent will use every device available to influence your shareholders to tender their shares. Every minute wasted by inaction is a gift to the enemy! Thank goodness you have the previously outlined battle plans ready to go.

The very moment a firm notice of a tender offer is received, the battle plan should go into effect. The chairman will orchestrate the plan, utilizing every available resource, including staff, communications, legal counsel, and the corporate secretary.

Here is the outline of a tender offer battle plan.

A. Always heed a meeting request

The offeror's chief executive officer frequently asks for a meeting with the offeree's CEO. It is always advisable to accede to this request.

Such a meeting means an advance warning, since it usually occurs on a weekend or a Friday night. If notified that a tender offer is about to be made, the CEO should contact the communications people immediately so that they can start action over the weekend. He should also call an emergency board meeting to review the plan of action.

B. Reserve space for newspaper advertising

The Wall Street Journal and major metropolitan daily newspapers, such as the *New York Times* and the *Chicago Tribune,* must have *at least* 2 days' notice of insertion. Since the eastern edition of *The Wall Street Journal* is frequently reserved for as long as two weeks in advance, expect at least a five-day delay in getting an ad into that edition. Your agency can utilize this time to finalize the ad and have production work completed for printing.

As noted in Part I, be ready to challenge:

1. The raider's knowledge of your business.
2. The compatibility of your company with the raider's corporate structure.
3. The raider's motives in making the tender offer.
4. The raider's ability to pay for shares tendered.
5. Tax-free aspects of the tender offer. Cash offers are not tax-free.
6. The raider's long-range plans for your company.

Also point out:

1. That a better counteroffer may be forthcoming, one that is tax-free and offers better terms than the cash offer.
2. That if the raider thinks the shares are such a good bargain at the offering price, so should the shareholder. Thus, the shareholder should reject tender offer.
3. Future prospects, such as new products or a boom in the company's major market and improvement of the company's position in that market.
4. Possible Justice Department or SEC violations.
5. That the directors and officers agree that the tender offer is grossly inadequate and that none of them will tender their shares.
6. That if the tender offer is on a pro rata basis, as required for the NYSE-listed companies making a cash tender offer, there is no point in giving the raider a free option by tendering until the last day of the offer. Urge the shareholders to wait. If the tender offer is on a first-come, first-served basis, you can counter by urging shareholders not to be stampeded.
7. Any indefiniteness in the tender offer, such as "outs" in prompt payment for the shares.
8. That brokers get a double commission if the tender offer is acted on, so their blandishments should be ignored.

9. Any defensive measures, such as stock splits, dividend increases, defensive merger, or legal proceedings against the opposition.

C. Start calling major shareholders

Major shareholders must be telephoned to urge them not to tender until they have the full company story. Include holders of 1,000 or more shares and institutional holders.

D. Issue press releases

The public relations department should issue a press release as soon as possible after firm notice has been received of the tender offer and should issue further releases on every change in the company's battle plan strategy and on the company's counters to every change in the raider's strategy. Don't delay; be ready to approve and issue news releases immediately after the raider changes strategy or makes new claims or counterclaims.

E. Do not give your shareholder list to raider

Insist that the raider's legal rights to inspect the shareholder list be established in a court proceeding.

F. Look for weaknesses in tender offer

Watch for such weaknesses as subordinated debentures, which management can point out are really only IOUs not backed up by assets.

G. Know your opponent

From your prepared dossier, you can make a quick study of the opponent's business history, capitalization, management, bylaws and charter, recent registration statements, stock exchange listing applications, indentures, and loan agreements and of any antitrust judgments or consent decrees by which the opponent may be bound. Also identify the opponent's major shareholders, large suppliers, customers, source of capital for the tender offer, banks, and financial advisers. There may be an Achilles' heel that you can exploit.

H. Make your company difficult to acquire

Here are some possible approaches to frustrate the raider's takeover bid:

1. *Raise the dividend.* One third of the companies under attack employ this strategy.

2. *Split the stock.* Ask shareholders to surrender old certificates to you for new ones, instead of sending them additional new shares. This will take certificates out of circulation for a period, so that they cannot be tendered. The raider generally has very little safety factor in a

tender offer, so any increase in outstanding stock could be disastrous to the raider.

3. *Issue stock for cash.* Such stock issuance is not subject to Sections 4(2) and 3(a)(11) of the Securities Act of 1933. For example, encourage management to exercise profitable stock options, particularly if the option plan can be amended to allow acceleration of the exercise privilege.

4. *Purchase stock.* Purchase stock on the open market to reduce the number of shares that can be tendered and possibly drive the price above the tender offer. (Note: Check Rule 10b-5 and Rule 10b-7 under the 1934 Securities Act for the disclosure regulations relating to the method of purchase and the number of shares which may be purchased. It should be explicitly stated that the sole purpose of the bid is to draw shares away from the tender offer and not to manipulate the price of the stock—see Rule 9 under the 1934 Act.)

I. Make your company less attractive

1. *Acquire a competitor of the raider.* Such an acquisition raises the possibility of serious antitrust violations on the raider's part. But make sure the acquisition is airtight. For example, it can contain sanctions that would foil a raider's prior agreement with the Justice Department to sell the acquisition if the tender offer is successful.

2. *Enter into restrictive convenants.* Amend important contracts with major suppliers, customers, and institutional noteholders to provide for some form of renegotiation or acceleration.

3. *Check the raider's indentures.* A restrictive covenant could place restrictions and indentures in violation if the tender offer is successful.

J. Use legal delaying tactics

Use injunctions against the raider's purchase of shares. Check these grounds for an injunction: failure to disclose material facts, such as intention to merge the company with the raider or simultaneous purchase of shares from certain key shareholders at higher prices; alleged conspiracy to violate antitrust laws; and incompleteness of the raider's SEC registration and S-1 prospectus.

K. Consider a counteroffer for raider's stock

A counteroffer by means of a tender offer for the raider's stock could be an effective dampener. Such a ploy could bring the SEC and your stock exchange into the act, with the only possible solution being the mutual withdrawal of bids.

L. Proceed with defensive merger

Proceed with a defensive merger, as noted in Part I.

The danger to a company of offering itself up for marriage is that it does not always get the suitor it wants. Once the trip up the aisle starts, several suitors—not all of the company's choosing—may want to be the groom.

J. W. Van Gorkom, chairman of Trans Union Corporation, solved this problem by getting a definitive agreement with the Marmon Group for $55 per share. The definitive agreement kept suitors unwanted by him at arm's length. But it also kept the price at $55 per share.

Yet, startling odds suggest that a company should have friendly suitors in the wings in the event of an offer from an unfriendly source. Today chances are 85 out of 100 that if a company is the subject of an unsolicited tender offer, it will lose. It may not fall into the hands of the original bidder, but nonetheless it will lose, and if state statutes are removed, the figure is likely to jump to 95 percent. There is nothing illegal or immoral about trying to acquire another company; what it boils down to is simply economic advantage.

A 1978 survey among 177 large industrial companies showed these results:

1. Of those companies that felt vulnerable to a takeover, 45 percent had no formalized defense plans. Of all the companies interviewed, 63 percent had no formalized plan.
2. More than half of the companies, 52 percent, had not made revisions in their corporate statutes to make a takeover more difficult.
3. Three fifths of the companies did not have a list of "white knights" to be approached as a haven in a tender offer attempt.
4. Roughly a third of the companies, 37 percent, had drafted a letter to shareholders asking them to abstain from any action until the board of directors had met.

However, the study did report that companies had intensified their investor relations program to strengthen the loyalty of existing shareholders and to gain additional support for their stock. The reasons the companies gave for feeling vulnerable to takeover attempts were: low P/E ratio, undervalued or hidden assets, book value above market price, high borrowing capacity, and above-average return on net worth.

The odds against a target company successfully fighting an unfriendly takeover are increased by the role of arbitrageurs. Arb houses make their money playing hunches that a merger will go through. On announcement of or on suspicion of an announcement concerning a takeover bid, they will buy as much stock as feasible in the open market with the intent of unloading it as quickly as possible to a willing bidder. This ingenious technique is often referred to as "warehousing."

The problem that arbitrage houses create for target companies is that they represent large amounts of stock held in "unfriendly" hands. The arbitrageur will use any means possible as a shareowner to guarantee that the tender offer takes place. They have no intention of holding the stock longer than necessary, and if an important shareholder vote develops, the target company can rest assured that the arbitrageurs will favor the bidder.

There is serious doubt in some quarters as to the advisability of having a target company's management offer an all-out defense. William Klein II, a senior partner with the New York law firm of Tenger, Greenblatt, Fallon & Kaplan, thinks that the shareholders are poorly served by such defensive maneuvers. An interview with *Fortune*'s Arthur M. Louis went like this:

Q: Doesn't the management have an obligation to its stockholders to automatically oppose any all-cash offer, if only to try to raise the price?

A: Yes, management should always say no in order to try to up the price. My point is not management's talk, which is cheap, but its use of corporate assets, which is expensive. I'm saying—though no court has yet agreed with me—that it is an abuse of discretion and fiduciary duty to hire top lawyers in this field like Marty Lipton or Joe Flom, and a battery of publicists, and to pay $500,000 to investment bankers to fight an all-cash offer. Only the stockholders should do that.

Q: But aren't you really asking management to act like puppets? If they just talk, don't they lose their credibility? The bidder, knowing management won't do anything, sticks by its low price. Don't the stockholders become the losers?

A: No, I'm saying management is the agent for the stockholder, who calls the tune. When the fight is going to cost big money, the stockholders, not management, should take out the ads and do the fighting, if they think it advisable.[1]

Among the reasons for the merger boom are the following: buying a company can be less risky than starting one; the more money a company has, the more tempting it is to buy something with it; the bigger a company grows through acquisitions, the tougher it will be for another company to acquire it; and if a big foreign company wants U.S. operations that will have an impact on its balance sheet, it has to buy a large domestic company.

Among the reasons given for fighting a takeover are independence, "we can do better alone," and "the slump is temporary." One unwritten reason is job security. In some mergers, the swinging door moves

---

[1] Arthur M. Louis, "A Difference of Opinion," *Fortune*, March 12, 1979, pp. 159–60. Copyright © 1979, Time Inc.

so fast and often that the hinges get red-hot. At Trans Union, for example, more than 75 percent of the 180-person corporate staff were fired or quit. And in discussing the takeover of one $1-billion-plus company by another $1-billion-plus company, the winning company's director of human resources said that the entire top staff of the acquired company was fired within 24 hours. But, he added, "They should have known it was coming because they deserved it."

CHAPTER FOURTEEN

How to Organize
Your Communications

Being a good manager, and perceiving yourself as one, is a fundamental step toward doing your job in the most effective and professional manner.
Public Relations Journal

COMMUNICATIONS MANAGEMENT

Becoming a good manager is cloaked in the mystique of climbing the corporate ladder. Financial public relations, now more popularly dubbed investor relations, is subject to the same elusiveness and whims of corporate management as is general public relations.

In the late 1950s, when I applied for the position of public relations manager for a chemical company, I was rejected. The management said that since I was not a graduate chemist, I knew nothing about the product. When I inquired who would teach a chemist public relations, management responded, "That's easy to learn."

Such Neanderthal thinking has not been entirely scrubbed from the minds of corporate management. A new twist is making noncommunicators more popular than ever in communication management positions. Public relations people have succeeded so well in making communications a profession that some managements are no longer willing to entrust this high status to the hands of a communicator. So, engineering companies may want engineers as communicators, banks may want bankers, consumer companies may want to have behavioral scientists respond to consumer activists, and highly regulated companies may want lawyers to serve as their mouthpieces. It is interesting to note, however, that many large law firms, freed from the long-imposed restrictions on advertising, are hiring professional communicators and public relations firms to direct their communications.

These inconsistencies in public relations are small compared with the inconsistencies associated with the growth of investor relations. In this chapter, the troubled history of that growth will be explained first.

324

Then, the chapter will cover the typical investor relations executive, the salary of the investor relations executive, and whether investor relations should utilize in-house or outside counsel. After that, the focus will shift to a very germane topic—how to organize the communications function. The chapter will end with the tantalizing issue of performance measurement.

A Troubled History

Given the management penchant for turning to a market or discipline expert as the panacea for communications, it is not surprising that many corporations turned experts on communications with Wall Street during the yo-yo stock market era of the 1960s and during the mid-1970s, when fluctuations and uncertainty hit the stock market. In response to these developments, management created two new public relations disciplines. The first was financial public relations, where communications-trained individuals were to concentrate on financial audiences. The second was the use of persons not trained in communications frequently financial analysts or treasurers, to communicate to the financial community. Many managements were not concerned about whether their investor relations executive had any knowledge of communications research, word skills, project management, program planning, or results measurement. They wanted someone who "thought like the Street" so they could, in turn, communicate with their brethren on "the Street."

In the go-go stock market era, many managements thought that a professional investor relations effort was the "in" thing for a company that wanted to raise its price-earnings ratio. The job of the investor relations specialist was to point up the company's virtues to institutional portfolio managers, security analysts, and individual shareholders. Staffs and budgets were beefed up substantially into the early 1970s—and then many managements began to have second thoughts.

In more recent years, these second thoughts have turned to downright disenchantment. The euphoria about investor relations has been replaced by doubts at the highest levels of management. There is evidence to back up that judgment. The low level of stock prices has been due largely to the shortcomings of company investor relations programs, according to both investor relations directors and independent observers. The investor relations programs were entrusted to financially oriented people who knew what their brethren in the financial community wanted to hear but had had little or no experience in communications or program planning. Moreover, investor relations departments were partly responsible for the failure to win back the millions of small investors who fled the stock market at the end of the 1960s.

These departments were blamed for not educating the public on the merits of equity investments and thereby failing to attract new shareholders and badly needed capital. Many chief executives saw these failures as a root cause of still other mounting concerns, including persistently low price-earnings ratios and a flood of hostile tender offers. As a result, many corporations have stopped expanding the budgets of their investor relations departments—though no major corporation has actually abolished that function. Other corporations, however, have begun to throw money indiscriminately into desperation efforts, such as crash financial advertising programs and broadsides aimed at financial analysts. The growing impatience of many chief executives is leading them to take steps that are neither selective nor cost effective.

Despite their many shortcomings, the investor relations programs of today are considerably better than those of the 1960s. At first, investor relations programs frequently amounted to little more than letting personnel loose to tout stocks over expensive lunches. In fairness to the financially trained investor relations executive, the entire market was then swamped with major investment shifts and other problems which the best of programs could not have overcome. Now that investors are returning to the stock market—not drawn back by communications, incidentally—many investor relations executives have matured into their roles so that excellent programs may be coming from them. Most large companies and many medium-sized ones have created separate departments under the aegis of a director and have given these departments the task of communicating the corporate story to the investing public. Still, on the whole, far too many investors relations departments are not living up to their promise and are failing to keep the investment community informed in a full, fair, and timely fashion. It is estimated that this holds true for at least one half of the publicly traded companies.

Moreover, the effectiveness of investor relations executives at many companies is hampered by the fact that they must share overlapping responsibilities with public relations departments. Moreover, I have heard many of these executives complain that they frequently do not have the authority from top management to initiate the release of data beyond that mandated by the SEC. Without the backing of the chief executive, they say, investor relations executives are not part of the decision-making process. The job of these executives is simply to put a good face on what has already been decided.

But I see these explanations largely as excuses for investor relations executives and/or their companies letting down on the job. For one thing, many investor relations executives fail to assert themselves in their corporate roles or to grasp the power needed to launch a well-conceived program that exceeds minimum obligations. Also, the quality of many investor relations people is highly questionable. Some come out of the public relations field and/or journalism and are thrust into the job with little training in the specifics of financial analysis. Once in the job, many fail to improve their understanding of the subject, so they often alienate analysts, shareholders, and the financial press with their ignorance of detail.

On the other hand, an accountant or financial analyst with no communications skills may be totally unqualified to handle other analysts and shareholders. If that is the case, it's almost inevitable that the company will suffer from a lack of credibility. I remember one company hiring a former analyst and treasurer without communication experience. One year after he was on the job, he still had trouble explaining the company's relatively simple basic business and figuring out how to set up a luncheon for analysts.

If companies are ever to woo the individual investor and return price-earnings ratios to a level that reflects the true value of their assets, they have no choice but to improve dramatically their investor relations programs, and this will involve finding or training topflight practitioners. The ideal investor relations executive will have well-developed skills in writing, some speaking capability, and an understanding of accounting principles, proxy solicitation, public affairs, marketing, shareholder analysis, and media relations, along with the confidence of top management, so that he or she is a policymaker and not simply a pipeline of stale information.

Investor relations will have to go beyond mundane programs to present a complete, undistorted picture of all significant corporate operations and events. Failing this, there will be more and more regulation. Responsible management will have to provide information that responds to the spirit and the purposes of disclosure requirements.

Typical Investor Relations Manager

In 1978–79, the National Investor Relations Institute (NIRI) made a survey of the investor relations practitioner in 367 major companies.[1] It is interesting that public relations backgrounds were at the low end of the scale of responses, while finance, Wall Street, and accounting backgrounds were at the high end (see Table 14–1).

It is also interesting to note, however, that when the respondents were asked what type of experiences they considered most valuable to prepare someone to do the investor relations job, they gave journalism/public relations a higher rating than Wall Street experience (see Table 14–2).

[1] *A Perspective on Investor Relations . . . a NIRI Survey*, National Investor Relations Institute, July 1979, pp. 1–24.

Table 14–1
What is your background? (check as many as applicable)

	Percent of all companies surveyed	Percent billion dollars and over
Finance	39%	46%
Finance and Wall Street	20	16
Finance and accounting	13	15
Finance, accounting, and Wall Street	6	4
Finance, accounting, and public relations	3	3
Finance and public relations	11	9
Finance, journalism, and public relations	7	6
Other	1	1

Note: Other disciplines mentioned were advertising, employee relations, engineering, corporate planning, and marketing.
Source: *A Perspective on Investor Relations . . . a NIRI Survey*, National Investor Relations Institute, July 1979, p. 9.

Table 14–2
What kind of experience do you consider most valuable to prepare someone to do the investor relations job?

	Percent of all companies surveyed	Percent billion dollars and over
Accounting/finance	43%	50%
Journalism/public relations	22	17
Wall Street experience	19	17
Management	6	8
Marketing/economics	5	3
MBA experience	2	2
Legal experience	1	1
Other*	2	2

* Several other responses appeared: communications training, corporate strategy planning, previous operations responsibility, security analysis experience, and knowledge of specific industries.
Source: *A Perspective on Investor Relations . . . a NIRI Survey*, National Investor Relations Institute, July 1979, p. 10.

However long the argument may rage, neither side or management may ever agree as to which career discipline—public relations or finance—should be responsible for investor relations. But the NIRI survey did provide many other valuable insights into the current state of the art of investor relations (see Tables 14–3 through 14–13).

Table 14–3
Years in investor relations

	Percent of all companies surveyed	Percent billion dollars and over
Less than one year	6%	5%
1–5 years	40	43
6–10 years	33	35
11–15 years	14	12
16–20 years	4	4
Over 20 years	3	2

Source: *A Perspective on Investor Relations . . . a NIRI Survey,* National Investor Relations Institute, July 1979, p. 4.

Table 14–4
Reporting responsibility

	Percent of all companies surveyed	Percent billion dollars and over
Chief financial officer	26%	30%
Chairman	21	15
President	18	9
Director of public relations/ communications	9	12
Treasurer	7	7
Vice president administration	5	
Vice president–secretary	4	
Vice president public relations	4	
Investor relations	1	
Other	5	27

Source: *A Perspective on Investor Relations . . . a NIRI Survey,* National Investor Relations Institute, July 1979, p. 4.

Table 14-5
People supervised

	Percent of all companies surveyed	Percent billion dollars and over
Clerical people	74%	71%
Investor relations assistants	59	58
Investor relations professionals	31	38

Source: *A Perspective on Investor Relations . . . a NIRI Survey,* National Investor Relations Institute, July 1979, p. 5.

Table 14-6
Meetings attended

	Percent of all companies surveyed	Percent billion dollars and over
Operations management meetings only	41%	48%
Operations management and board meetings	6	3
Operations management, board, and top-management planning sessions	23	14
Operations management and top-management planning sessions	30	34

Note: A fraction of a percent attend board meetings and top-management planning sessions or top-management planning sessions only.
Source: *A Perspective on Investor Relations . . . a NIRI Survey,* National Investor Relations Institute, July 1979, p. 5.

Table 14-7
Title

	Percent of all companies surveyed	Percent billion dollars and over
Officer of the company	47%	41%
Director/manager	51	58
Miscellaneous	2	1

Source: *A Perspective on Investor Relations . . . a NIRI Survey,* National Investor Relations Institute, July 1979, p. 6.

Table 14–8
Keeping informed about company operations

	Percent of all companies surveyed	Percent billion dollars and over
Meetings with top management	38%	30%
Meetings with top management and reports	35	42
Reports only	15	18
Meetings with top management and informal discussions with management	4	3
Reports and informal discussions with management	3	3
Informal discussions with management	3	—
Meetings with top management and miscellaneous activities	2	2
Reports and miscellaneous activities	1	2

Source: *A Perspective on Investor Relations . . . a NIRI Survey*, National Investor Relations Institute, July 1979, p. 7.

Table 14–9
Outside counsel

	Percent of all companies surveyed	Percent billion dollars and over
Yes	35%	31%
No	65	69

Source: *A Perspective on Investor Relations . . . a NIRI Survey*, National Investor Relations Institute, July 1979, p. 8.

Table 14–10
Evaluation of outside counsel

	Percent of all companies surveyed	Percent billion dollars and over
An important addition to your staff	97%	97%
Reasonably helpful	2	5
Unimportant to the planning of your program	1	—

Note: Responses include only those with outside counsel.
Source: *A Perspective on Investor Relations . . . a NIRI Survey*, National Investor Relations Institute, July 1979, p. 8.

Table 14-11
Activities and responsibilities

	All companies		Billion-dollar companies	
	Company participates*	Personally responsible†	Company participates	Personally responsible
Analyst contact	351	310	147	134
Analyst mailings	350	320	146	131
Presentations/analyst groups	339	302	149	134
Presentations/broker groups ..	231	206	81	75
Field trips and plant tours ...	207	188	98	91
Speech writing	313	252	141	101
Shareholder relations				
Written/oral correspondence	350	289	146	103
Dividend notices	316	195	133	64
Employee stock purchase plan...................	243	76	118	62
Reinvestment plans	214	113	102	45
Special stockholder events...............	185	140	78	46
Welcome/regret letters	221	147	84	45
Shareholder surveys	177	153	77	60
Publications				
Annual reports	360	284	149	96
Quarterly reports	358	282	149	99
Report/annual meeting	283	204	135	79
Corporate brochure	252	173	114	55
Fact book	195	164	89	70
Management newsletter ...	140	55	70	18
Employee newsletter	260	101	120	27
News releases	346	247	146	74
Broker mailings	204	188	75	62
Other publications	19	16	7	6
Shareholder records				
Shareholder lists	320	107	136	34
Monitor stock transfers	329	216	141	81
Monitor institutional buying	303	218	137	94
Annual meetings				
Preparation of materials/ speeches	344	241	144	91
Arrangements...............	334	188	140	61
Proxy solicit individual	315	87	133	25
Proxy solicit institutional ..	316	92	134	24
Legal documents				
Registration statements	316	46	136	10
Prospectus	317	57	138	18
10-K	330	85	139	28

* Indicates that company participates in activity.
† Indicates that investor relations person is responsible for activity.
Source: *A Perspective on Investor Relations . . . a NIRI Survey,* National Investor Relations Institute, July 1979, p. 12.

Table 14–12
Important activities in getting messages across

	Percent of all companies surveyed	Percent billion dollars and over
To analysts		
Analyst contact	19%	25%
Analyst contact, mailings and presentations to analysts	16	17
Analyst contact and other*	10	14
Publications	9	5
Analyst contact and publishers	9	8
Analyst contact and presentation to analysts	12	10
Analyst contact, mailings and publications	5	2
Presentations to analysts	4	7
Publications	4	3
Other	13	10
To investors		
Publications	45%	45%
Publications and others	13	17
Shareholder relations activities and other	12	14
Analyst contact (institutional only)	10	9
Presentations to broker groups	5	—
Publications and annual meetings ..	4	4
Other	11	12

* Other includes publicity and advertising, most frequently mentioned; government relations information, noted twice.
Source: *A Perspective on Investor Relations . . . a NIRI Survey,* National Investor Relations Institute, July 1979, p. 13.

The Typical Public Relations Manager

For comparison purposes, it is interesting to note that while finance and accounting dominate the backgrounds of investor relations types, public relations communicators have totally different backgrounds and

Table 14–13
Primary reason for financial communications

	Percent of all companies surveyed	Percent billion dollars and over
It helps to obtain a fair market evaluation for the stock	9%	9%
It's the obligation of management to shareholders to communicate	10	11
Both of the above	79	79
It's difficult to measure the impact on the stock price; better than nothing	1	1
Doesn't do much good at all	1	—

Source: *A Perspective on Investor Relations . . . a NIRI Survey*, National Investor Relations Institute, July 1979, p. 14.

other vital statistics, according to *pr reporter* surveys shown in Tables 14–14 through 14–18.

What You Are Worth

While public relations and its investor relations offshoot are relatively new occupations in the corporate world, their values in the perspective of management can be measured on an important scale—

Table 14–14
Previous occupation

Newspaper/wire services	41.0%
Other print media	9.1
Marketing/advertising/sales	9.1
Radio/TV	7.7
Other	33.1

Note: Print media background is declining in importance: half now come from marketing/advertising/sales, broadcasting, and other backgrounds.
Source: *pr reporter*, October 12, 1981, pp. 1–6.
Copyright © 1981, PR Publishing Company, Inc., Exeter, N.H.

Table 14-15
Reporting level

CEO	34.5%
Executive	23.4
Vice president—communications, public affairs, marketing, and advertising	10.8
Other	30.7

Note: Almost 60 percent report to either the CEO or executive/senior vice president.
Source: *pr reporter*, October 12, 1981, pp. 1–6. Copyright © 1981, PR Publishing Company, Inc., Exeter, N.H.

Table 14-16
Age related to salary level

Salary level	20–29	30–34	35–39	40–49	50–59	60+
Less than $20,000	49.0%	11.8%	7.9%	5.5%	5.4%	2.0%
$20–29,000	30.2	39.0	17.5	14.8	9.0	16.0
$30–44,000	17.0	40.9	50.8	40.7	40.1	36.0
$45–54,000	0.0	6.4	15.1	21.4	16.8	24.0
$55,000 and over	3.8	1.9	8.7	17.6	28.7	22.0

Note: As practitioners get older, an increasing percentage (but not all) manage to pull away from the median salary bracket.
Source: *pr reporter*, October 12, 1981, pp. 1–6. Copyright © 1981, PR Publishing Company, Inc., Exeter, N.H.

Table 14-17
Educational level

High school or less	Some college	Bachelor's degree	Master's degree	Ph.D.
1.7%	13.8%	61.1%	25.0%	3.0%

Source: *pr reporter*, October 12, 1981, pp. 1–6. Copyright © 1978, PR Publishing Company, Inc., Exeter, N.H.

salary. Based on various surveys, the corporate communicator appears to be compensated quite well. Generally, the public relations executive fares better in salary than does the investor relations executive, for two reasons. First, investor relations is much newer than public relations. Second, the investor relations executive is responsible for only

Table 14-18
Years in public relations

5 years or less	14.3%
6-9 years	17.0
10-14 years	26.0
15-19 years	11.0
20-29 years	24.0
30 years or over	7.7

Note: About 7 out of 10 practitioners have been in public relations for 10 or more years.
Source: *pr reporter*, October 12, 1981, pp. 1-6. Copyright © 1981, PR Publishing Company, Inc., Exeter, N.H.

one segment of the corporate audience, while the public relations executive is responsible for all corporate audiences. According to the 1979 NIRI survey, investor relations executives receive the compensation shown in Table 14-19.

Table 14-19
Income from job before taxes, including salary and bonus

	Percent of all companies surveyed	Percent billion dollars and over
Less than $15,000	1%	—
$15,000-$19,999	2	1%
$20,000-$29,999	9	5
$30,000-$39,999	24	21
$40,000-$49,999	22	20
$50,000-$59,999	15	17
$60,000-$74,000	12	17
$75,000 and over	15	19

Source: *A Perspective on Investor Relations . . . a NIRI Survey,* National Investor Relations Institute, July 1979, p. 15.

By comparison, *pr reporter* determined the salaries for public relations managers to be those shown in Table 14-20.

A comparison of investor relations and public relations salaries for key jobs in marketing, advertising, and the media can be made from a survey by the *Gallagher Report* (see Table 14-21).

Table 14–20
Comparison of 1981 and 1980 median salaries of top-level public relations/public
affairs practitioners in the United States and Canada, and by type of organization

Type organization	Median salary 1981	1980	1981 Salary range	Median change*
All U.S. organizations	$38,000	$35,000	$16,000–125,000	
All Canadian organizations	38,600	33,000	19,000–200,000	
PR firms	50,000	45,000	16,000–200,000	$5,625
Advertising agencies	38,000	36,500	16,000– 80,000	4,500
Other consulting...............	—	38,000	21,000–100,000	—
Banks........................	35,000	34,000	18,000– 85,000	3,850
Insurance companies	35,000	29,500	11,000–120,000	3,200
Consumer product companies ...	44,700	37,500	26,000–117,000	4,500
Industrials	45,200	36,000	17,000–127,000	4,750
Conglomerates	43,200	42,000	17,000–148,000	4,600
Transportation	—	33,800	8,000– 78,000	—
Utilities......................	41,000	36,500	19,000– 75,000	5,950
Hospitals	30,000	23,650	15,000– 65,000	3,250
Educational	32,800	27,700	14,000– 67,500	2,900
Trade/professional associations ...	38,700	36,000	16,000– 75,000	3,600
Other nonprofits	33,000	30,000	11,000– 72,000	3,000
Government...................	31,000	29,000	15,000– 50,000	2,975

* Calculated on the difference between 1981 and 1980 salaries as reported by *each* respondent.
Note: Median salary and median change are not shown when sample is too small.
Source: *pr reporter*, October 12, 1981, pp. 1–6. Copyright © 1981, PR Publishing Company, Inc., Exeter, N.H.

In a survey of the top 25 corporations in the United States, Larry Marshall, president of Marshall Consultants, Inc., an executive search and management consulting firm, found the results shown in Table 14–22. Marshall reported that

management is viewing its communications function in a new light. Corporations are becoming more responsive to the changing business, political and social environment. They are positioning themselves as proactive, rather than reactive, in their communication of corporate policy.

On the corporate side, salaries for communications executives have escalated dramatically and are on a par with other growing corporate functions. Corporate officers with communications responsibility have compensation packages (base salary, incentive compensation/bonus, profit sharing/pension plan, and, in some cases, other nontaxable benefits such as company-paid auto and life/medical insurance, children's college tuition, expense accounts, housing) often exceeding $100,000, plus other in-

Table 14-21
Average salary

Manufacturing advertisers

Job title	Consumer products marketers	Percent change from 1980	Industrial products marketers	Percent change from 1980
Chairman/president	$130,989	+14.6%	$234,000	+17.0%
Executive vice president	113,750	+25.7	75,000	+ 7.1
General manager	89,400	+14.6	n.a.	—
Vice president/director marketing	65,679	+16.4	45,700	+17.5
Vice president/director sales	81,717	+19.0	50,000	+25.0
Vice president/director advertising	55,000	+15.3	50,344	+11.0
Vice president/director marketing services	58,250	+10.8	48,000	+12.8
Vice president/director public relations	63,000	+13.5	64,800	+11.7
Product manager	44,000	+14.8	39,000	+13.0

Nonmanufacturing advertisers

Job title	Consumer service marketers	Percent change from 1980	Industrial service marketers	Percent change from 1980	Retailers	Percent change from 1980
Chairman/president	$148,714	+ 1.9%	$80,000	+14.3%	$129,167	+10.7%
Executive vice president	n.a.	—	75,000	+ 3.4	n.a.	—
General manager	56,333	+ 7.6	n.a.	—	n.a.	—

Job title						
Vice president/director marketing	62,143	+13.3	73,333	+ 6.3	45,000	+12.5
Vice president/director sales	n.a.	—	40,000	+14.3	n.a.	—
Vice president/director advertising	52,144	+10.7	n.a.	—	50,417	+13.9
Vice president/director marketing services	n.a.	—	35,000	+16.7	n.a.	—
Vice president/director public relations	75,333	+12.0	46,500	+10.7	n.a.	—

Diversified advertisers

Job title	Salary	Percent change from 1980
Chairman/president	$183,600	+ 5.8%
Executive vice president	n.a.	—
General manager	n.a.	—
Vice president/director marketing	74,125	+ 7.6
Vice president/director sales	n.a.	—
Vice president/director advertising	66,750	+11.1
Vice president/director marketing services	92,500	+12.1
Vice president/director public relations	62,250	+16.6

n.a.—Not available. Returns insufficient to provide representative sample.
Source: *The Gallagher Report*, March 22, 1982, Supplement. Copyright 1982, The Gallagher Report, Inc.

340

Table 14-22
What top public relations professionals are earning

Title	Annual compensation package
In the top 25 corporations (over $8 billion in sales):	
Senior vice president	$150,000-$300,000
Vice president public relations/general manager, including: corporate communications director, corporate relations director, public affairs director	80,000- 150,000
Corporate staff services, including directors of government relations, investor relations, press relations, editorial services, consumer affairs, international affairs, community affairs, employee relations, issues management	50,000- 125,000
Division public relations director	50,000- 125,000
In the top 15 counseling firms:	
Principal	100,000- 200,000+
Executive vice president	75,000- 150,000
Senior vice president, including management committee level	75,000- 150,000
Group vice president/manager	50,000- 100,000

Source: Larry Marshall, "The New Breed of PR Executive," *Public Relations Journal*, July 1980, pp. 9-13. Copyright © 1981, Public Relations Society of America.

centives and tax-saving benefits. Across the board, salaries in corporate communications departments have risen an average of 35 percent in the past five years.

Chief executive officers are seeking peer-level thinkers and problem solvers, and this trend will increase. CEOs want to feel confident that their senior communications and public affairs executives are capable of contributing to the management team's decision-making process.[2]

IN-HOUSE VERSUS OUTSIDE COUNSEL

Regardless of the size or the competence of their in-house public relations and investor relations units, most companies make frequent use of outside consultants. To create and establish a department where none now exists; to design a new program relating to a particular corporate public; to provide expertise on a specific issue or problem—

[2] Larry Marshall, "The New Breed of PR Executive," *Public Relations Journal*, July 1980, pp. 9-13. Copyright © 1981, Public Relations Society of America.

these are just a sampling of the reasons corporations hire outside external relations counsel. Companies utilize such firms for dealings with all of their publics and involve these firms in a multitude of programs and projects. The counseling firm can set its own sights regarding the scope of the role it is prepared to perform, and it may involve itself in the narrowest or the broadest aspects of external relations for its clients.

Many companies choose to hire public relations counsel on a project basis. Of the companies that retain outside counsel, the majority utilize the services of more than one such firm at a time. Some retain one principal firm but use others from time to time for special assignments; the rest retain more than one firm on an ongoing basis.

Most often, counsel is brought in by the public relations executive of the company—and only the public relations executive. But, on occasion, the chief executive or someone else in the organization may hire an outside firm. Such occasions usually involve special assignments, such as a new product campaign, a communications training program, or a special program for the financial community.

The counselor would prefer to be brought in by the chief executive. At that level, the counselor would be involved in the broadest management matters. However, the public relations executive sees no appreciable difference in the role the outside firm plays whether the executive or management secures the counsellor.

Outside counsel is not to be discounted as merely a source of assistance for small companies. On the contrary, both large and small companies use outside counselors on a regular basis. "Counsel" is an appropriate name for the public relations, financial relations, or public affairs firm because these firms are called into a corporation for counsel or advice more frequently than for implementation of a program or project. In relation to the media, however, the assistance of the outside firm is sought more often for service than for counsel.

However, outside firms are also relied on heavily for advice regarding investor relations and shareholder relations, as well as advice regarding federal government regulations. One executive says his company retains counsel "as a listening post in Washington." Outside counselors frequently conduct research for the company, to measure the company's image with a particular public or the effectiveness of a particular program. Surveys of institutional investors, for example, are conducted regularly. An excellent resource that the large counseling firms provide is a specialist, or complete department, interfacing with the financial community in New York and frequently in other major cities, such as Chicago. These firms can provide contacts and up-to-date information that are beyond the reach of the average company. The largest counseling firms are shown in Table 14–23.

Table 14–23
50 Largest U.S. public relations operations, independent and ad agency affiliated (for year ended December 31, 1981)

	1981 net fee income	Employees as of October 15, 1981	Percent change from 1980 income
1. Hill and Knowlton*	$46,000,000	1,020	+ 29.8
2. Burson-Marsteller*	41,100,000	945	+ 17.2
3. Carl Byoir & Associates*	18,700,000	454	+ 8.4
4. Ruder Finn & Rotman[1]	15,000,000	390	—
5. Daniel J. Edelman	8,015,145	170	+ 1.8
6. The Rowland Company	7,322,690	121	+ 34.3
7. Manning, Selvage & Lee*	7,070,000	115	+ 17.1
8. Ketchum MacLeod & Grove PR*	6,023,242	115	+ 17.7
9. Doremus & Company*	5,774,282	142	+ 6.6
10. Rogers & Cowan	5,374,000	85	+ 19.6
11. Ogilvy & Mather PR*[2]	5,320,000	90	—
12. Booke Communications Incorporated Group[3]	4,839,467	73	− 6.0
13. Creamer Dickson Basford*	4,518,285	99	+ 23.6
14. Bozell & Jacobs PR*	4,408,000	89	+ 2.5
15. Robert Marston and Associates	4,430,000	61	+ 9.0
16. Fleishman-Hillard	4,185,936	72	+ 41.6
17. Public Relations Board/Financial Relations Board[4]		125	
18. Dudley-Anderson-Yutzy PR	3,284,714	71	+ 19.5
19. Gray and Company[5]		65	
20. Sydney S. Baron & Company	3,241,000	43	+ 5.9
21. Golin/Harris Communications	2,876,820	60	+ 35.0
22. Aaron D. Cushman and Associates	2,548,260	52	+ 21.0
23. Ayer Public Relations Services*		50	
24. Hank Meyer Associates	2,330,918	22	+ 19.0
25. Kanan, Corbin, Schupak & Aronow[6]	2,189,055	33	+ 68.2
26. The Strayton Corporation	2,029,000	30	+ 47.6
27. Gibbs & Soell	1,995,162	40	+ 9.9
28. Henry J. Kaufman & Associates PR*	1,977,000	30	+ 8.7

29. Fraser/Associates	1,946,774	32	+ 54.2
30. Newsome and Company	1,816,872	49	+ 18.6
31. The Rockey Company	1,815,992	41	+ 2.9
32. Geltzer & Company	1,760,550	30	+ 79.0
33. ICPR	1,754,841	36	− 18.0
34. The Hannaford Company[7]	1,752,409	23	+ 91.2
35. Lobsenz-Stevens	1,675,440	32	+ 10.1
36. Anthony M. Franco	1,600,000	41	+ 12.5
37. Gross and Associates/PR	1,518,765	30	+ 9.6
38. Padilla and Speer	1,505,968	26	+ 9.3
39. Public Communications, Inc.	1,465,414	34	+ 24.6
40. Edward Howard & Co.	1,453,747	28	+ 9.5
41. Richard Weiner	1,442,333	39	+ 15.9
42. Porter, LeVay & Rose	1,442,160	19	+ 48.5
43. Zigman-Joseph-Skeen	1,229,000	29	+ 1.3
44. Smith & Harroff	1,212,000	14	+ 8.5
45. Dorf/MJH Public Relations	1,176,433	43	+ 57.9
46. Barking, Herman, Solochek & Paulsen	1,098,263	24	+ 11.3
47. Creswell, Munsell, Fultz & Zirbel*	1,017,884	19	+139.2
48. Sumner Rider & Associates	1,000,275	20	+ 24.7
49. Woody Kepner Associates	1,003,537	25	+ 6.0
50. Paluszek & Leslie Associates	937,856	16	+ 23.0

* Denotes advertising agency subsidiary.

[1] Agency formed January 1, 1982, by merger of Ruder & Finn and Harshe-Rotman & Druck. Substantiation of fees and employees not given.

[2] Founded in late 1980. Acquired Underwood, Jordan Associates in 1981.

[3] Sukon Graphics unit, sold in 1981, not included in 1981 figure. "Booke Communications Incorporated Group" includes Booke and Co., PR firm.

[4] PR Board and Financial Relations Board are separately owned companies that share some facilities and services. They would not provide figures for each company as requested.

[5] Founded March 1, 1981. No financial statement available.

[6] Acquired Scharf, Witchel & Co. in 1981.

[7] Includes $259,328 in fees from Potomac International acquired January 19, 1981.

Source: O'Dwyer's Directory of PR Firms, January 1982. Copyright 1982 by J. R. O'Dwyer Co. Inc., 271 Madison Ave., New York, N.Y. 10016.

The American corporation is becoming increasingly conscious of the face it presents to its various publics: the government, consumers, employees, and shareholders. This image consciousness has spurred a boom in in-house public relations personnel and has given new prestige to the corporate communications department.

Surveys among chief executives of 50 major corporations found that more than 40 believed a communications program could have a positive impact on labor relations, productivity, safety, absenteeism, and quality control. Another survey showed that 72.5 percent of the respondents held more responsibility than they had held over the previous two-year period, that 46 percent used more media, and that 40 percent had larger staffs.

According to Harold Burson of Burson-Marsteller, in-house departments are growing because of management awareness, pressure groups, and media interest. These have contributed to an upgrading in the quality and quantity of public relations. Many communications professionals agree that companies are more open now and are taking an active role in getting information out, so many companies have hired additional communications specialists.

Not everyone connected with public relations associates in-house communications growth with increased candor. Jack O'Dwyer, publisher of *Jack O'Dwyer's Newsletter*, says the increased use of in-house communications and specialists is an attempt by American corporations to build a moat between themselves and the public.

Organizing the Corporate Communications Function

Looking at 368 companies surveyed by the Conference Board in terms of how they have structured their external relations activities, it is evident that the companies fall into one of two broad organizational patterns:

1. There is no single dominant executive below the level of chief executive to whom all external relations functions report.
2. There is one executive—below the level of chief executive—who is responsible for all, or the major segments of, external relations functions.

Analysis of the responses to the Conference Board survey shows a trend toward the second approach: the organization of all external relations under one executive. Of the companies that have this type of structure, more than half indicate that it represents the result of reorganization within recent years. Since not too many years ago the public relations department was a newcomer to the organization picture, the trend seems clear. And even among the companies that do not choose to consolidate external relations structurally, almost all achieve cohesion through some other mechanism.

External relations executives are about evenly split in their preference for one coordinated unit or for separate units. Those in favor of the coordinated approach say that consistency is critical to effective external relations: the company must speak with one voice. Further, they see a commonality among all of the company's publics, and they see each of these publics as part of a whole.

Those executives favoring separate external units stress the special skills required for dealing with different publics. Several note that their organizations are much too large to have one executive handling all external publics. Professional organization planners tend to reach the same conclusions as the practitioners do, though their preferences evolve from a different perspective.

The largest number of respondents have evidently found avenues to coordination that are not strictly structural. In these companies, the executives responsible for one or a few external publics report directly to the chief executive or to a general executive. Other executives in the company are responsible for other segments of external activities, and they also report individually either to the CEO or to a general executive.

This pattern of having a number of executives below the level of chief executive officer, each responsible for one or a few of the company's activities relating to external publics, is quite prevalent among the companies surveyed. This diffuse organizational arrangement occurs in a cross section of industries and in both large and small companies.

In the smaller firms, the chief executives take on the direct responsibility for some of the functions; some other functions may report to the chief executive officer through a staff executive. Most often, in such cases, it is government relations that the chief executive officer feels is most pertinent to his responsibility. He must make the important visits in Washington.

Some of the largest firms—those that are highly diversified in operations and geographically dispersed—find that their need for more specialized knowledge and skills to carry out the various external activities tends to spawn a number of specialized units. A common approach in these companies that have no one overall staff executive coordinator below the level of chief executive is to have one or more units—the public affairs Washington office is typical—report directly to the CEO, while other external activities, possibly public relations or investor relations, report at a low level. Figure 14–1 illustrates such an arrangement in a highly diversified company.

The organization chart shown in Figure 14–2 provides another, more detailed example of this specialized approach to organizing.

346

Figure 14–1
A diversified company with split staff in external relations

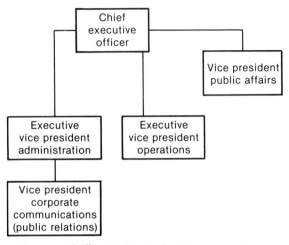

Source: Phyllis S. McGrath, *Managing Corporate External Relations: Changing Perspectives and Responses,* Report no. 679 (New York: Conference Board, 1976), p. 27. Copyright © 1976, The Conference Board, Inc.

Figure 14–2
Partial organization chart showing multiple staff units in external relations

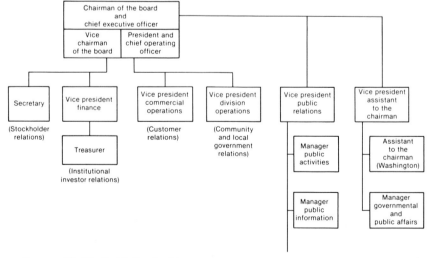

Source: Phyllis S. McGrath, *Managing Corporate External Relations: Changing Perspectives and Responses,* Report no. 679 (New York: Conference Board, 1976), p. 27. Copyright © 1976, The Conference Board, Inc.

Public affairs and government relations report to the vice president/ assistant to the chairman, who reports to the chairman of the board— chief executive officer. Public relations is a separate unit that also reports directly to the chairman. Stockholder relations is handled by the secretary, and institutional investor relations, as part of finance, is handled by the treasurer. Both the secretary and the head of finance report to the vice chairman of the board. Customer services reports to the vice president commercial operations, and community relations and local government relations are handled by the division (regional) managers, who report to the vice president division operations. Both the vice president division operations and the vice president commercial operations report to the president–chief operating officer.

According to the senior officer in charge of public affairs and government relations, this segmented approach is preferable because the "nature of problems and kinds of programs needed to deal with them are too numerous and diverse to expect much benefit from centralizing under one staff executive." In this organization, coordination is achieved for the most part by informal interdepartment consultation, though ad hoc coordinating groups are formed if needed to handle particular problems that arise from time to time.

This line of reasoning is also endorsed by an executive of a consumer products company, who explains that because his company does not view external relations as an "entity," it has not given special organizational consideration to them. Of course, the companies that do not have one executive below the level of chief executive responsible for activities relating to all external publics may combine two or three activities under one of the staff executives in the organization, while the rest are scattered among other units.

While the pattern of more than one external relations executive is still evident, the trend is toward structural unification of external relations functions. Of 303 companies whose external relations executive participated in this survey, 176 reported that one executive was responsible for either all external relations or for the major segments of the external relations function.

An appreciable number of companies follow a middle-ground approach. They have one staff executive who is responsible for several of the company's publics, while the other publics are dealt with by a variety of other executives throughout the corporate structure. Where such an arrangement exists, the most frequent pattern is one in which all of the external publics other than customers and/or investors are grouped under one executive. The constituency most often excluded in such semicoordinated structures is the customer or consumer (see Figure 14–3).

Many public affairs executives distinguish between customer relations and consumer affairs, or between servicing complaints and set-

348

Figure 14-3
Coordinating all but customer relations—a manufacturer

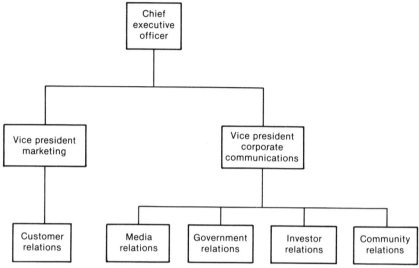

Source: Phyllis S. McGrath, *Managing Corporate External Relations: Changing Perspectives and Responses,* Report no. 679 (New York: Conference Board, 1976), p. 29. Copyright © 1976, The Conference Board, Inc.

ting "consumerism" policy. Where the latter is the activity, they usually feel that it falls within the scope of external relations: "When a company maintains a cohesive attitude toward all of its external communications, that necessarily includes customer 'communication.'"

Second to customers, investors are the public most frequently excluded from the coordinated core group, and most frequently institutional investors rather than individual shareholders. Not only are customers and investors the two publics most frequently excluded from the coordinated reporting structure, but the pattern most often followed is to exclude both. This pattern is illustrated in the organization at General Foods which combines public relations, public affairs, and government relations under the vice president public relations/public affairs, who reports to the vice chairman (see Figure 14-4). Shareholder and institutional investor relations are in the financial organization. Consumer relations and product publicity in women's interest media are under the direction of the vice president consumer affairs. (Public relations handles product publicity in trade and general media.) There is a close working relationship, however, between public relations and the people who handle both consumer affairs and investor relations. The vice president public relations/public affairs sits on committees with the functional heads of the other areas to formulate policy and develop joint programs.

Figure 14-4
Combining public relations, public affairs, and government relations—General Foods Corporation

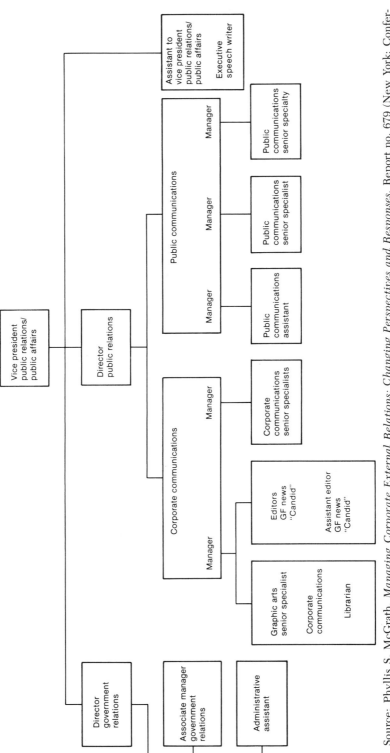

Source: Phyllis S. McGrath, *Managing Corporate External Relations: Changing Perspectives and Responses*, Report no. 679 (New York: Conference Board, 1976), p. 31. Copyright © 1976, The Conference Board, Inc.

At Shell Oil Company, the vice president of public affairs has responsibility for planning and coordinating all corporate communications (see Figure 14–5). His own staff directly handles media relations and a variety of public relations programs. In keeping with the special emphasis oil companies are placing on external relations growing out of the increasing governmental regulation of business, government relations is also part of public affairs. In this company, the vice president is also responsible for consultation on international affairs, an area of growing concern and increasingly active constituencies. Shareholder relations reports to the general counsel, and investor relations reports to the vice president finance. Neither appears on the public affairs chart. This company believes that the importance of coordination and liaison cannot be overstated. Even without structured reporting relations linking all constituency activities, management believes it possible to achieve coordination through the public affairs department.

Some other exclusion patterns include:

1. Coordinating all but government relations (federal, state, and local).
2. Coordinating all but customer relations and community affairs.
3. Coordinating all but stockholders, customers, and community affairs.
4. Coordinating all but community affairs.

Among the companies with a more unified organizational approach to external relations, 41 designated one executive who had responsibility for all of the external relations activities of the company—government relations (federal, state and local), shareholder and institutional investor relations, consumer affairs, and community relations. In many of these companies, this unified external relations structure was the result of recent reorganization.

This trend is clearly evident among all categories of companies. The group of 41 includes manufacturers of industrial and consumer products, insurance companies, extractive resources companies, and utilities. Companies in the group range widely in size—from $330 million to $2.6 billion in net sales.

Allis-Chalmers' chart contains all of the company's external functions (see Figure 14–6). Government affairs, community relations, public relations, and investor communications are coordinated along with other communications units. In addition, the regional vice presidents are in charge of general customer relations and, as the chart indicates, the regional vice presidents report to the staff vice president for communications and public affairs. The company reorganized its external relations group in order to "speak with one voice to the external community."

Figure 14-5
All segments except stockholder and investor relations—Shell Oil Company

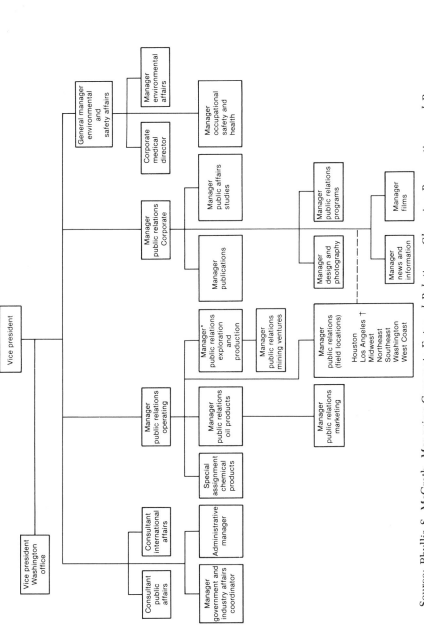

Source: Phyllis S. McGrath, *Managing Corporate External Relations: Changing Perspectives and Responses*, Report no. 679 (New York: Conference Board, 1976), p. 33. Copyright © 1976, The Conference Board, Inc.

Figure 14–6
A coordinated organization—Allis-Chalmers

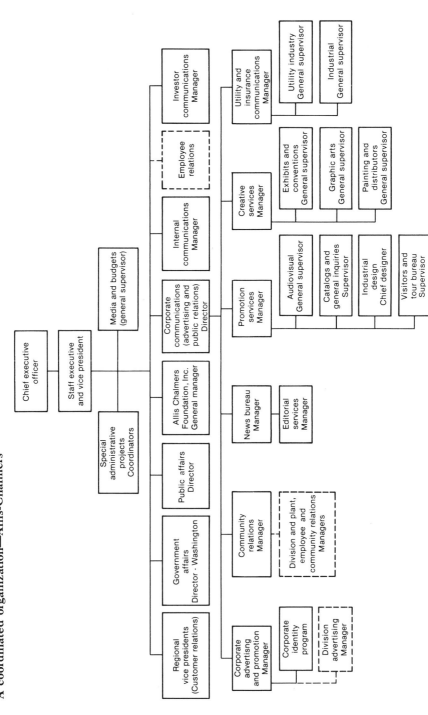

Source: Phyllis S. McGrath, *Managing Corporate External Relations: Changing Perspectives and Responses*, Report no. 679 (New York: Conference Board, 1976) p. 35. Copyright © 1976, The Conference Board, Inc.

The organization chart for Phillips Petroleum illustrates coordination of media relations, state and local government relations, investor relations, education, youth and community relations, and activities involving broader audiences such as consumers (see Figure 14–7). Editorial and graphics personnel provide the support functions for effective maintenance of these relationships. The company's relationship with the federal government constituency is shared responsibility of public affairs and the firm's Washington office, with day-to-day coordination and communication belonging to the latter.

In another variation, the specialized external relations units report to a general executive. A "general executive" is a member of the senior management of the company who has a variety of staff and/or operating units reporting to him; he is not primarily associated with any one specialized activity of the company. Titles typical of such general executives include executive vice president, senior vice president, vice chairman, vice president staff, and vice president administration.

An example of such a corporate organization is depicted in Figure 14–8, the corporate administrative services function at Tenneco. As the chart illustrates, public relations, consumer affairs, community affairs, and government affairs all report to a senior vice president—who is also responsible for a number of other functions, including, in this case, purchasing, office services, and aviation.

At Interlake, Inc., a vice president marketing and public affairs is responsible for all external constituencies—media, government, investors, customers, and community—in addition to his marketing responsibilities (see Figure 14–9). The somewhat unusual arrangement of combining marketing and public relations and public affairs was selected so that one officer could plan and coordinate how the company was "marketed" to the outside world.

Organization structure is not the only means by which a company can arrive at a unified approach to its relations with its publics. Two popular means of coordinating all of the functions are:

1. A committee of all external relations executives.
2. A policy statement for all corporate external relations.

One third of the companies surveyed by the Conference Board have external relations committees, created for the purpose of coordinating all relations with outside publics and providing consistency in communication. Most report regularly, but a few are organized as task force or ad hoc groups to coordinate or determine policy for specific situations. Those that report regularly generally do so to the chief executive officer. The majority of these committees are formal bodies with such names as "public affairs council," "public relations council," or "communications committee."

Figure 14-7
A coordinated approach—Phillips Petroleum

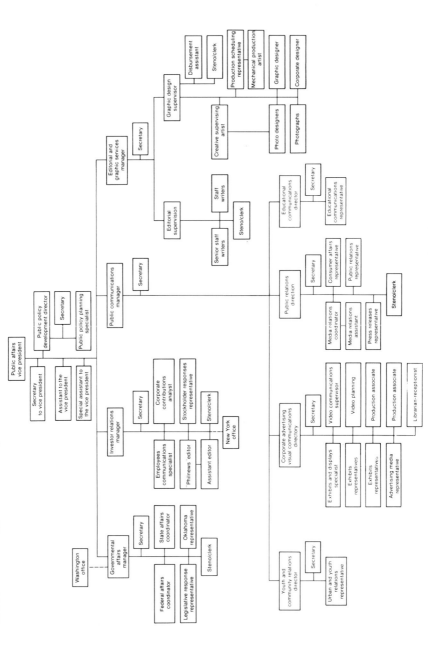

Source: Phyllis S. McGrath, *Managing Corporate External Relations: Changing Perspectives and Responses*, Report no. 679 (New York: Conference Board, 1976) p. 37. Copyright © 1976 The Conference Board, Inc.

Figure 14–8
The general executive as coordinator—Tenneco, Inc.

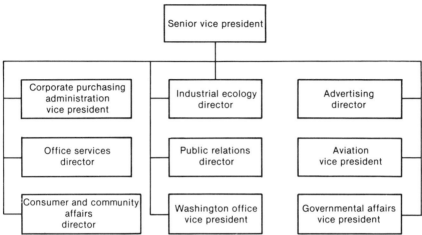

Source: Phyllis S. McGrath, *Managing Corporate External Relations: Changing Perspectives and Responses,* Report no. 679 (New York: Conference Board, 1976), p. 38. Copyright © 1976, The Conference Board, Inc.

Membership on these external relations committees rarely exceeds 10 executives. The members are usually heads of the various external activities throughout the corporation, including those within divisions and subsidiaries. Many companies use the committee approach for coordination among divisions.

The mission and degree of influence of the committees vary from company to company. An oil company reports that its committee on public affairs recommends policies and programs for social responsibility. At another manufacturing company, the communications committee must approve all outgoing corporate communications. Membership on that committee includes public relations, investor relations, employee communications, opinion research, advertising, public communications, and government relations. The committee is chaired by the vice president public affairs. Membership includes all of the company's communications executives and not only those who report directly to the vice president. The communications committee meets once a week. As one example of the extent of the committee's authority, every member of the committee must approve a communication before the investor relations unit issues it to the investment community. Before this committee was established, there was no vehicle for providing consistent information. Now management can be sure that the same information is going to employees and to Wall Street.

Another divisionalized consumer products company has set up a group that meets every two weeks strictly for informational purposes.

Figure 14-9
Combining marketing and external relations—Interlake, Inc.

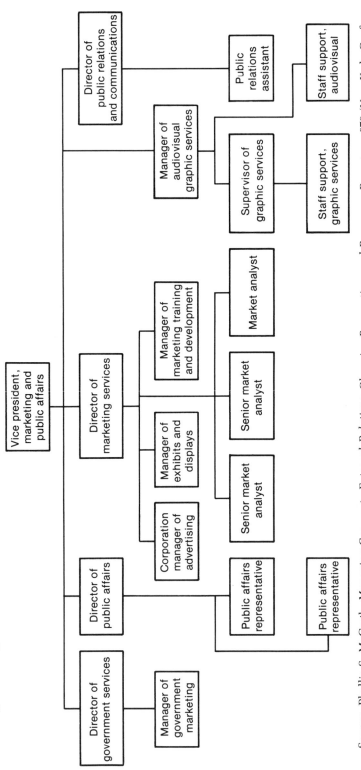

Source: Phyllis S. McGrath, *Managing Corporate External Relations: Changing Perspectives and Responses*, Report no. 679 (New York: Conference Board, 1976), p. 40. Copyright © 1976, The Conference Board, Inc.

The committee is composed of the public relations directors of the company's three divisions, the vice president for corporate communications, and the corporate director of advertising. The chairman is the corporate director of public relations.

Time and time again, corporate executives indicated that the critical factor in achieving effective external relations is the strict observance of corporate policy and the goals the corporation has set for itself in relation to its publics. Through coordination by the external relations staff, adherence to policy and cohesion of action can be achieved throughout the company.

Consistency of action almost assumes a guideline—an enunciated corporate policy. Such policy statements are usually very general, however. To interpret what the corporate policy means in any given situation is the primary function of the person responsible for the company's external relations. Twenty percent of the companies surveyed have one overall policy regarding all external relations.

Most companies have several policies, however, each tailored either to a specific public or to a specific vehicle of communication. Frequently, companies have a policy statement governing the method by which information will be communicated outside the company, how much information will be released and to whom, and what form that information should take. Many organizations also issue corporate statements on the goals of the corporation with regard to particular areas of public affairs—for example, political and civic affairs, corporate contributions, or disclosure.

Of course, external relations activities are not solely the province of corporate headquarters. In divisionalized companies, much of the corporation's external relations activity is carried out at the division level. In all such companies, the organizational questions are: (1) whether to allow the divisions their own external units and (2) how much freedom the divisional units should have, i.e., what relationship should exist between corporate and divisional units.

In some of the divisionalized companies, the divisions have no specialized units at all. The corporate unit provides the service on an "as needed" basis—possibly by lending specialists to the divisions. An insurance company has developed an agency-client approach for dealing with its regional offices. Public relations specialists, who report to the corporate affairs unit, are assigned to various company operations to offer counsel on public relations problems. One person, for example, works with the investment department; several others are assigned to major regional offices.

In a few companies, external relations units are housed at the divisional level but *report* to the corporate head. More often, divisions have their own units principally to handle customers, community, local government, and local or trade media.

358

In the usual pattern, beyond giving advice and assistance, corporate staff monitors and checks divisional activity. Key to the relationship is some understanding of whether a situation is (*a*) of local concern, and thus can be left to the division, or (*b*) of larger concern—affecting the corporation—and thus has to be handled at the corporate level.

Search for the "Optimum"

"One best way to organize a function," "the optimum structure"— these are phrases that organization planners shun. If there is any consensus among top-notch corporate organization planners, it is that there is no "one best way" to organize anything. What way is best depends on a flock of variables. The key is the situation that confronts the company, the weighted or relative emphasis that the company hopes to give a certain effort. Any organization structure usually represents a pragmatic balancing of various trade-offs.

This is clearly the case when it comes to organizing for effective external relations. Analysis of the companies participating in the Conference Board study shows that variations in structure abound. Which is best? Judging from evaluations of a panel of organization planning specialists, the clear answer is: "It all depends." Asked to analyze at least two substantially different ways of structuring external relations activities, they point out strengths and weaknesses in both—in the abstract, of course.

Take Model A (Figure 14–10), a hypothetical construct that might be called a "decentralized" or "fragmented" (depending on one's bias) approach: What are the possible advantages in such a structure?

Figure 14–10
Model A

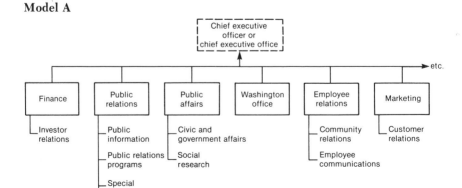

Source: Phyllis S. McGrath, *Managing Corporate External Relations: Changing Perspectives and Responses*, Report no. 679 (New York: Conference Board, 1976), p. 24. Copyright © 1976, The Conference Board, Inc.

The direct involvement of the chief executive in external relations is one of the primary virtues seen in that structure. In such a setup, only the CEO can coordinate all the activities and contribute personal direction to external relations. Furthermore, the fact that there is no intervening layer between the CEO and key functionaries in external relations means shortened lines of communication, which, in turn, contribute to more uncensored feedback and input to the CEO's thinking regarding external involvements.

Another major strength of Model A is that both internal and external activities that are key to total performance in such vital areas as finance and marketing are the job of an individual executive. The structure recognizes that there may well be the need for specialized marketing know-how in dealing with customers, specialized financial know-how in dealing with the financial community. More important, the structure is seen as forcing greater responsiveness to these specialized publics. As summarized by one organization planner: "The responsible officer makes the decisions for dollars and energy and manpower—and is obligated to report in terms of practical achievements."

In citing these possible advantages, the organization planners seemed to be saying, "If forced to say something good about Model A, that's the best I can do." One categorically said "none."

They had far less difficulty in pointing out what they regard as weaknesses—and were more vehement about them. The chief executive's direct involvement in coordinating the effort, for example, is an advantage only if the CEO actually does the job. However, most doubt that he will have, or can have, the time. "The CEO's span of control would be too broad." "It would force delays because he is so busy." "It is inappropriate to expect him to act as coordinator." These are typical expressions of serious doubts about the structure.

Another set of criticisms can be summarized: "It ain't neat." One respondent sees in Model A "fragmented, ambiguous, overlapping responsibilities." Others speculate: "Someone has created jobs to take care of some old war-horses." "Denotes a patchwork approach—with activities added by impulse rather than analysis."

Organization planners evidently view external relations as an area characterized by common problems and common processes. They see in Model A an expensive duplication of effort; they expect conflict among the units not just for the attention of the chief executive but, as one says, "for the eyes, ears, and mouth of the Washington office."

The weakness implicit in Model A that is viewed as most compelling is the difficulty it poses for developing and projecting a uniform or consistent corporate image. Having several spokesmen—who might or might not coordinate their efforts—would present problems in establishing an overall corporate policy and, more important, in interpreting and policing that policy. It "splinters," it "fractionates" the total effort; it "diffuses accountabilility for total corporate image."

360

Figure 14–11
Model B

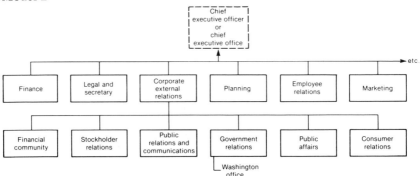

Source: Phyllis S. McGrath, *Managing Corporate External Relations: Changing Perspectives and Responses,* Report no. 679 (New York: Conference Board, 1976), p. 25. Copyright © 1976, The Conference Board, Inc.

Model B (Figure 14–11) is quite the opposite. It hypothesizes a "centralized" or "integrated" structure (again, depending on one's view). Obviously, Model A's weaknesses are its major strengths.

The insertion of one top executive below the level of chief executive to whom all the more specialized external relations departments must report cuts the span of control of the chief executive—with all the improved coordination, attention, and feedback that implies. "It recognizes that coordination is a full-time job." "It allows the CEO to obtain fully developed counsel from one source." "Fixes responsibility on one individual to whom the CEO can look." The possible greater pooling of skills and added developmental opportunities are also mentioned as advantages.

But the advantages cited most frequently and emphatically are succinctly summarized in the comment: "One approach, one viewpoint, one voice, one consistent policy." To some respondents, the major advantage of consistency—plus the more effective monitoring of performance it makes possible—offsets all the disadvantages. But many disadvantages are cited.

It adds a layer to the organization—which can be read as a filter or censor—that removes the chief executive from direct involvement. As one respondent noted, "It builds bureaucracy to combat a bureaucracy." And there is a real question as to whether it is healthy to establish one "Mr. External Relations." Can one person have the competence to harness the varied skills?

Most urgent, to some, is the concern that such a setup may be viewed by operational or line units as relieving them of their external relations job. The fact that Model B sets up a "Mr. Outside" (or "Mr.

Inside") in certain areas of concern—especially finance and marketing—is a related disadvantage. To most of the organization planners, this is the greatest disadvantage. They see finance and marketing losing direct control of external relations with publics critical to their successful performance.

Indeed, in weighing the organizational setups, the responding organization planners seem to offer several guidelines for structuring external relations work:

1. *If* projecting a consistent character to the outside world is crucial, then a structure that coordinates the varied activities serves that purpose best.

2. *If* nurturing special relationships with distinct publics is most critical, then tying external relations to the function most closely linked with the public served takes priority.

3. *If* both consistency and specialized attention are of relatively equal importance, then search for alternatives to Model A or B that give adequate emphasis to both objectives. And there are obviously alternatives—as indicated by actual company practice and in the suggestions of the cooperating organization planners. For example, in reviewing the pros and cons cited, a number of the organization planners make abundantly clear their feeling that relations with the financial community should be a continuing part of the finance function, that relations with customers or consumer groups are integral to the overall marketing function. Few would sacrifice those ties for the sake of consistency. Or, more appropriately, they seem to feel that consistency will not necessarily be sacrificed by maintaining those particular functional ties.

However, when it comes to less readily identifiable publics or constituencies, or to publics where corporate activities overlap, the clear suggestion is that these activities be coordinated by one head. Thus, most would group under one head (title is immaterial) public relations and public affairs (to the extent that they can be distinguished) with government relations and the Washington office.

A few go even further, suggesting that structure be more flexible to permit varying emphases at different times. The need for a focal point to develop, coordinate, and monitor consistency is underscored. But, having set up the focal point, as one planner suggests, allow selected individual central staff units to deal directly with their own constituencies (removing them from the umbrella of the corporate external relations department) on a case-by-case review of the relative importance of the advantages and disadvantages in the particular company at the particular time for the particular function under consideration.

The final caution appended is that flexibility—as detailed above—should not be confused with ambiguity. There is a substantial difference between "It all depends" and "Anything goes."

Status in the Company

Another organizational study was made by Mark J. Appleman, publisher of *The Corporate Shareholder,* to determine how trend-setting companies organize corporate communications to meet today's financial/investor relations needs.[3] Questionnaires were mailed to a sample of 400 large and mid-range companies, with 140 of the replies regarded as sufficiently detailed to warrant analysis. Exactly 100 companies, or 71 percent of the respondents, indicated that their organization for financial communication reflected management's financial/investor relations objectives *primarily.* For 30 companies, or 21 percent, the corporate communications structure reflected management's objectives *secondarily.* The balance of the respondents reported that their communications apparatus was *only incidental* to the company's investor relations aims.

In those companies whose financial communications reflect corporate objectives *primarily,* the appropriate responsibilities are divided mainly between top management and executives with communications titles, such as vice president, director, or manager for public affairs, public relations, investor relations, and corporate communications. A major exception is the preparation of proxy materials, which remains in the hands of corporate secretaries for the most part.

Here is how responsibility for specific activities breaks down among the "primarily" group of 100 companies:

Shareholder communication: communications executives, 40 percent; top management, 37 percent.

Stockholder relations: communications executives, 40 percent; top management, 35 percent; corporate secretary, 13 percent.

Preparation of proxy materials: corporate secretary, 63 percent; financial officer, 10 percent.

Annual meeting: top management, 32 percent; corporate secretary, 28 percent; communications executive, 27 percent.

Financial public relations: communications executive, 53 percent; top management, 25 percent; financial officer, 13 percent.

Contact with investment professionals: communications executive, 40 percent; top management, 30 percent; financial officer, 22 percent.

Corporate financial advertising: communications executive, 52 percent; top management, 19 percent.

Contact with outside consultant: communications executive, 37 percent; top management, 23 percent.

[3] Mark J. Appleman, "New Study Tracks Changing Patterns of Corporate Organization for Communications with Shareholders and Prospective Investors," *Corporate Shareholder,* July 17, 1979, pp. 1–2. Copyright © 1979, Corporate Shareholder, Inc.

Shareholder survey: communications executive, 60 percent; top management, 17 percent; corporate secretary, 15 percent.

For most of these activities, budgetary authority is roughly consistent with functional responsibility. There are exceptions, however. For *shareholder surveys,* top management had budget authority in 17 percent of the companies versus 10 percent functional responsibility, while communications executives had budget authority in 47 percent of the companies versus 60 percent functional responsibility. For *shareholder communication,* communications executives had budgetary authority in 48 percent of the companies studied versus functional responsibility in 40 percent.

In contrast, the key communications responsibilities are divided mainly among financial officers, corporate secretaries, and communications executives, with top management exercising substantially less direct say-so for such activities in the 30 companies, which indicated that the apparatus for financial communication in these companies reflects management's financial/investor relations objectives *secondarily.*

Here is how responsibilities break down among the "secondarily" group of 30 companies:

Shareholder communication: communications executive, 50 percent; corporate secretary, 20 percent.

Stockholder relations: corporate secretary, 40 percent; communications executive, 27 percent.

Proxy materials: corporate secretary, 80 percent; communications executive, 13 percent.

Annual meeting: corporate secretary, 37 percent; communications executive, 23 percent.

Financial public relations: communications executive, 30 percent; financial officer, 23 percent.

Contact with investment professionals: financial officer, 33 percent; communications executive, 23 percent.

Corporate financial advertising: communications executive, 60 percent; financial officer, 27 percent.

Contact with outside consultant: communications executive, 23 percent; financial officer, 20 percent.

Shareholder survey: communications executive, 60 percent; corporate secretary, 20 percent.

Comparison of respondents with "primarily" and "secondarily" orientation toward investor relations turns up broad distinctions:

1. In "primarily" companies, top management tends to exercise more direct responsibility for shareholder communication, annual meet-

ings, shareholder relations, and financial public relations than in "secondarily" companies.

2. In "primarily" companies also, communications executives are likely to be vice presidents or senior vice presidents, while in "secondarily" companies they are likely to carry the title of director or manager.

A BANG FOR THE BUCKS

The question of performance measurement, though urgent, is hardly new. For several years, the *Corporate Shareholder* has been detailing the marketing approach to investor relations, including systematic evaluation of results. Major conferences have explored investor-relations-by-objective, in pursuit of which measurement standards are essential. But in spite of such efforts to provide useful answers, the questions keep simmering at all levels of management.

"How do we know it's cost effective?" is a typical challenge posed by CEOs. "How would results differ if we doubled the investor relations budget or cut it in half?" is a more incisive form of the same challenge. Reams of reports presented to date have not begun to resolve the questions, as demonstrated by the findings of a survey of *Corporate Shareholder* subscribers. Asked to indicate degree of interest in learning more about a number of current topics, a whopping 64 percent of some 150 participating CEOs, financial officers, corporate secretaries, and investor relations and other communications executives gave number one priority to performance measurement of investor relations.

At the same time, however, there are plenty of CEOs and agency people who would prefer not to have a true appraisal of results documented unless success is assured in advance. Hundreds of companies annually spend millions of dollars on investor relations programs which can never be evaluated because the activities are independent of any predetermined corporate objective.

The corporate objective for investor relations is not classified information. It cannot conceivably be used to the company's disadvantage by the SEC or competitors. Companies may differ in size, personality, and financial characteristics, but the ultimate objective of an investor relations program is predictably related to the availability or cost of capital. Any communications program not oriented toward that should not be designated as investor relations. The bottom-line justification for the investor relations budget should be enhancement of the capital picture.

An investor relations executive working for a company without objectives may believe that the important purpose of investor relations is

to educate analysts and portfolio managers to the company's investment merits.

The uselessness of many investor relations programs stems not only
from lack of evaluative objectives but quite often from a babel of
standards. Confusion then merely produces a great deal of activity for
the sake of activity. From among the many yardsticks to measure
performance, which ones apply? The answer is simple. The measurements that matter most are those that can illuminate the path to the
ultimate corporate objective.

Without realistic objectives, clearly defined for all with a need to
know, performance measurement is useless and evaluation of progress
toward the ultimate objective is impossible.

Index